DEVELOPING A PRACTICE IN AMBULATORY SURGERY

Published Volumes

Proportions of the Aesthetic Face
Powell and Humphreys

Facial Reconstruction with Local and Regional Flaps
Becker

Rhinoplasty: Emphasizing the External Approach
Anderson and Ries

Surgery of the Mandible
Bailey and Holt

Lasers in Skin Disease
Wheeland

Dermabrasion and Chemical Peel
McCollough and Langsdon

Free Flap Reconstruction of the Head and Neck
Panje and Moran

Cosmetic Surgery of the Asian Face
McCurdy

Surgery of the Lip
Calhoun and Stiernberg

Principles of Photography in Facial Plastic Surgery
Tardy

The American Academy of Facial Plastic and Reconstructive Surgery

Series Editor: Charles M. Stiernberg, M.D.

DEVELOPING A PRACTICE IN AMBULATORY SURGERY

William H. Beeson, M.D.
Beeson Facial Plastic and
Reconstructive Surgery
Indianapolis, Indiana

Howard A. Tobin, M.D., F.A.C.S.
Facial Plastic and Cosmetic
Surgical Center
Abilene, Texas

1993
Thieme Medical Publishers, Inc. New York
Georg Thieme Verlag Stuttgart • New York

Thieme Medical Publishers, Inc.
381 Park Avenue South
New York, New York 10016

Series sponsored by the educational committee of The American Academy of Facial Plastic and Reconstructive Surgery

DEVELOPING A PRACTICE IN AMBULATORY SURGERY
William H. Beeson
Howard A. Tobin

Library of Congress Cataloging-in-Publication Data

Beeson, William H.
    Developing a practice in ambulatory surgery / William H. Beeson,
Howard A. Tobin.
       p.   cm. — (American Academy of Facial Plastic and Reconstructive Surgery)
    Includes index.
    ISBN 0-86577-412-9. — ISBN 3-13-774901-8
    1. Ambulatory surgery—Practice. 2. Surgery, Plastic—Practice.
I. Tobin, Howard A. II. Title. III. Series: American Academy of
Facial Plastic and Reconstructive Surgery (Series)
    [DNLM: 1. Ambulatory Surgery. 2. Practice Management, Medical—
organization & administration. WO 192 B415d 1993]
RD110.B44   1993
617'.91—dc20
DNLM/DLC
for Library of Congress   93-3095
                                                                           CIP

Important Note: Medicine is an ever-changing science. Research and clinical experience are continually broadening our knowledge, in particular our knowledge of proper treatment and drug therapy. Insofar as this book mentions any dosage or application, readers may rest assured that the authors, editors, and publishers have made every effort to ensure that such references are strictly in accordance with the state of knowledge at the time of production of the book. Nevertheless, every user is requested to carefully examine the manufacturers' leaflets accompanying each drug to check on his own responsibility whether the dosage schedules recommended therein or the contraindications stated by the manufacturers differ from the statements made in the present book. Such examination is particularly important with drugs that are either rarely used or have been newly released on the market, but the user of *all* drugs should rely on the drug manufacturer's information as current at the time of use.

Some of the product names, patents and registered designs referred to in this book are in fact registered trademarks or proprietary names even though specific reference to this fact is not always made in the text. Therefore, the appearance of a name without designation as proprietary is not to be construed as a representation by the publisher that it is in the public domain.

The statements in this book are solely those of the authors and not those of the Educational and Research Foundation.

Copyright © 1993 by Thieme Medical Publishers, Inc., and the Educational and Research Foundation of the American Academy of Facial Plastic and Reconstructive Surgery. This book, including all parts thereof, is legally protected by copyright. Any use, exploitation or commercialization outside the narrow limits set by copyright legislation, without the publisher's consent, is illegal and liable to prosecution. This applies in particular to photostat reproduction, copying, mimeographing or duplication of any kind, translating, preparation of microfilms, and electronic data processing and storage.

5 4 3 2 1

Printed in the United States of America

TMP ISBN 0-86577-412-9
GTV ISBN 3-13-774901-8

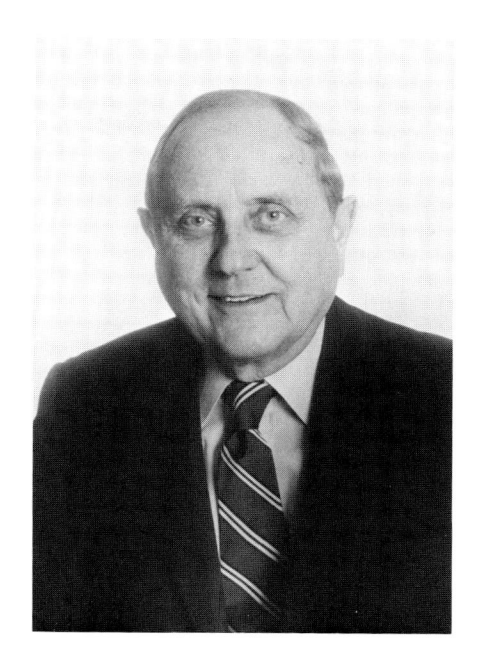

For James E. Davis, M.D., whose *Major Ambulatory Surgery* has inspired and informed us, and whose professional leadership has made such a lasting contribution to physician organizations everywhere.

Contents

	Preface viii
	Acknowledgments ix
	Contributors x
1.	Overview of Ambulatory Surgery 1
2.	Staffing the Office Surgical Center 14
3.	Anesthesia and Outpatient Surgery 51
4.	Equipment and Facilities 58
5.	Marketing 68
	Howard A. Tobin, M.D., F.A.C.S.
6.	Quality Assurance and Risk Management 75
	Howard A. Tobin, M.D., F.A.C.S.
7.	Financing a Practice 99
	Steven J. Beck
8.	Office Computerization 109
	Dot Sellars, C.M.A.-A., C.O.A.P.
9.	Space Planning Your Medical Facility and Negotiating an Office Lease 115
	Russell D. Richardson
10.	Office Surgical Facility—How I Do It 134
	Appendixes, Forms, Protocols, and Guidelines
	Appendix 1. Anesthesia 147
	Appendix 2. Employee Training 160
	Appendix 3. Quality Assurance 163
	Appendix 4. Risk Management 169
	Appendix 5. Handling of Infectious or Hazardous Medical Waste 172
	Appendix 6. Employee Forms 178
	Appendix 7. Patient Care Forms 203
	Appendix 8. Patient Instruction Forms 215
	Appendix 9. Administrative Forms 230
	Appendix 10. Perioperative Patient Care Quality 238
	Appendix 11. Recommended Practices for Laser Safety in the Practice Setting 240
	Appendix 12. Recommended Practices for Operating Room Environmental Sanitization 245
	Appendix 13. Recommended Practices for Selection and Use of Packaging Materials 251
	Appendix 14. Recommended Practices for Sterilization and Disinfection . 255
	Appendix 15. Recommended Practices for Surgical Tissue Banking 269
	Index 274

Preface

Ambulatory surgery in a non-hospital setting has dramatically increased over the past 20 years. Today it is more than simply having a designated treatment room in the office dedicated to surgical procedures; instead it may be one of the tools that can be used by physicians to directly affect access to cost-efficient, quality medical care. Ambulatory surgery is not only clinically better for the physician and staff, but patients often report dramatic preferences in the quality of care received in such a setting. Developing an ambulatory surgical practice is not a project to be taken lightly. The complications of bureaucracy and regulation, in combination with financing, construction standards, personnel issues and partnerships, can seem overwhelming.

Thomas Jefferson once said, "he who receives an idea from me, receives instruction himself without lessening mine; as he who lights his taper at mine, receives light without darkening me. That ideas should freely spread from one to another over the globe, for the moral and mutual instruction of man, and improvement of his condition, seems to have been peculiarly and benevolently designed by nature, when she made them, like fire, expansible over all space, without lessening the density in any point, and like the air in which we breathe, move, and have our physical being, incapable of confinement or exclusive appropriation."

In the spirit of Jefferson, medicine builds upon the shared experience and expertise of others. This book is no exception. It is the fruits of the labors of a number of individuals. It is hoped that this publication will serve as a reference and as a catalyst to spur physicians involved in ambulatory care on to greater heights and to facilitate development of ambulatory surgical practices by other physicians. While this book does have a topical orientation to facial plastic surgery, the concepts are applicable to physicians of any specialty.

Quality, access, and cost are the focus of significant attention by both the general public and organized medicine. All three principles must be part of the driving philosophies in all practices. Ambulatory surgery is helping us to achieve those goals.

William H. Beeson, M.D.
Howard A. Tobin, M.D., F.A.C.S.

Acknowledgments

Developing a Practice in Ambulatory Surgery required the combined talents and efforts of a large number of individuals. We are indebted to the American Academy of Facial Plastic and Reconstructive Surgery for their technical support and encouragement regarding the production of this book. Mr. Steve Duffy, Executive Vice President, and Mr. Tom Rhodes, legal counsel, were invaluable in their assistance. We are grateful to the many editors, and transcriptionists, who assisted with this project and to Carrie Van Dyke and Pam Blow, R.N., for their production assistance.

We are also appreciative of the Association of Operating Room Nurses (AORN) for their excellent protocols which are reproduced in this publication, and to Bent Ericksen, Ph.D., for his valuable contribution to the personnel section of this manuscript. Special thanks also go to Chris Damon, Executive Director of the Accreditation Association for Ambulatory Health Care (AAAHC) for his invaluable assistance with the development of this publication.

Our sincere thanks go to Jim Costello and Chris Goldsbury of Thieme Medical Publishers, Inc., for their support, understanding, encouragement and guidance of this book through to completion. Dealing with individuals of such high caliber made the production of this book a pleasure.

We extend our sincere gratitude and appreciation to our office staffs and families for their endless help and encouragement. Without their continued assistance and support this project would never have evolved beyond an idea.

Our sincere thanks and gratitude go to the following individuals for their contributions to this monograph:

> Steven J. Beck
> Jim Gilmore, M.D.
> Robert Lehman, J.D., M.B.A.
> Devinder Mangat, M.D.
> E. Squier Neal
> Louie Patseavouras, M.D.
> Russell D. Richardson
> Dot Sellars, CMA-A, COAP
> Ronald Strahan, M.D.

We are all well aware of the time and effort they put into preparing their chapters and their dedication to medical education.

William H. Beeson, M.D.
Howard A. Tobin, M.D., F.A.C.S.

Contributors

William H. Beeson, M.D.
Beeson Facial Plastic & Reconstructive Surgery,
 Indianapolis, Indiana
Assistant Clinical Professor, Indiana University School
 of Medicine
President, Indiana State Medical Association
Secretary, American Academy of Facial Plastic &
 Reconstructive Surgery
Treasurer, American Academy of Cosmetic Surgery

Howard A. Tobin, M.D., F.A.C.S.
Director, Facial Plastic & Cosmetic Surgical Center
Abilene, Texas

Steven J. Beck
Senior Vice President
Huntington National Bank of Indiana
Indianapolis, Indiana

Bent Ericksen
Practice Personnel Systems
Lake Forest, California

Jim E. Gilmore, M.D., F.A.C.S., F.I.C.S.
Associate Clinical Professor, Dept. of Otolaryngology
University of Texas Southwestern Medical School at
 Dallas
Jim E. Gilmore, M.D. Associated
Dallas, Texas

Devinder Mangat, M.D., F.A.C.S.
Associate Clinical Professor, Facial Plastic Surgery
Dept. of Otolaryngology, Head & Neck Surgery
University of Cincinnati, Cincinnati, Ohio
Mangat Facial Surgery Center
Cincinnati, Ohio

E. Squier Neal, J.D.
White and Raub
Indianapolis, Indiana

Louie L. Patseavouras, M.D., F.A.C.S.
Private Practice–Facial Plastic Surgery
Greensboro, North Carolina

Russell D. Richardson
Eaton & Lauth
Carmel, Indiana

Dot Sellars, C.M.A.-A., C.O.A.P.
Richmond, Virginia

Ronald Strahan, M.D.
A Medical Corporation
Los Angeles, California

1 Overview of Ambulatory Surgery

INTRODUCTION TO OFFICE SURGERY

Ambulatory surgery is on the rise. In 1982, 24 million surgeries were performed in the United States. The President of the American Medical Association at that time estimated that 8 million surgeries (one third) could have been performed on an outpatient basis. That figure has continued to increase dramatically. Three years later in October 1985, it was stated in *Ambulatory Care* that 60% of all surgeries could be performed on an ambulatory basis.

Office surgery has long been popular in the plastic-surgical realm. *Plastic and Reconstructive Surgery* in 1976 stated that 75% of plastic surgeons in the states of California and Florida performed procedures in their offices.

There are numerous reasons for the dramatic increase in office surgery. Several of those are improved anesthesia, improved surgical techniques, and increased desire to contain medical costs and the realization that postoperative infections might well be decreased in an ambulatory versus a hospital setting. Improved anesthesia has resulted in significantly less postoperative nausea and vomiting. This enables patients to return home for their convalescence much earlier than with prior anesthetic techniques. Pharmacologic advances have resulted in much improved *anoesia* during the recovery period.

Improved surgical techniques have resulted in a reduction of intraoperative time. In addition, advances have lessened the degree of tissue trauma, thus facilitating a recovery and reducing postoperative ecchymosis and pain. Improved hemostatic techniques have decreased the need for postoperative transfusions. The list could go on and on.

The desire to contain medical costs has been paramount in fostering the increase in office-based surgery. At a time when the average annual rate of health care expenditures in the United States was over 12.6% of the gross national product, the Health Care Financing Administration studies showed free-standing facility charges were approximately 16% less than hospital outpatient charges.

Some studies have shown a reduced infection rate for surgery performed on an outpatient basis. The Division of Epidemiology and Preventive Medicine at the University of Texas Southwestern Medical School has reported that 1 of 20 patients acquires an infection during hospitalization. Approximately 1% of these individuals die each year. In 1982 the American Medical Association reported in the publication "Establishing a Free Standing Ambulatory Surgery Center" that there is a decreased risk of nosocomial infection associated with office surgery.

HISTORY OF AMBULATORY SURGERY

It is important to review briefly the history of outpatient surgery and the obstacles that have been overcome, in order to place the future course for ambulatory surgery in a better perspective. According to Dr. James Davis, author of *Major Ambulatory Surgeries*, the first ambulatory unit in the United States was established at Butterworth Hospital in Grand Rapids, Michigan. Subsequent to this event, Dr. Wally Reed and Dr. John Ford established the first free-standing surgery center in Phoenix, Arizona, in 1970 with the opening of their surgicenter. Dr. Joe Belshe of St. Cloud, Minnesota, is frequently credited with establishing the second such facility in the United States.

In 1972, Davis and Detner published a study in the *Annals of Surgery* that documented that the quality of care in ambulatory surgery was satisfactory and comparable to inpatient care. In addition, they noted that it was approximately 25% cheaper.

In June 1971 the American Medical Association House of Delegates endorsed the concept of ambulatory surgery. However, not all facets of organized medicine held this same point of view. In 1972 the regents of the American College of Surgeons expressed a preference for hospital-affiliated or hospital-based ambulatory programs. This was based on the feeling that nonhospital-based programs had a potential for decreased quality of care.

Again in 1981, the American Medical Association House of Delegates recognized the increasing quality of free-standing surgery centers and passed a resolution that advocated such care. That same year, the American College of Surgeons revised its earlier position and endorsed ambulatory surgery in hospital outpatient and in free-standing centers when "appropriate quality assurance measures are enforced."

Quality of care is of paramount importance to both physicians and patients. It is important to address the issue of quality care factually, whether that care is rendered as an inpatient or outpatient, in the hospital or in an office or in a freestanding surgical center.

The Orkand study is often recognized as the best structured, best implemented, and most authoritative study assessing the quality of care in ambulatory surgery. That study showed that quality of care in ambulatory surgical units was no less than that obtained by hospital inpatients. In 1974 the then Department of Health, Education, and Welfare awarded the Orkand Corporation of Silver Spring, Maryland, a 3-year contract to study costs, quality, and the effect on the American health care delivery system of surgery performed in various settings. The study studied 900 patients in seven facilities in Phoenix, Arizona. Care in four different settings was assessed: (1) traditional hospital inpatients, (2) traditional hospital outpatients, (3) hospital ambulatory surgical centers, (4) surgical care rendered in freestanding centers.

The findings are impressive. Independent free-standing units cost approximately 42.5 to 61.4% less than care rendered in an inpatient setting. Independent free-standing units costs approximately 14.3 to 44.9% less than similar care rendered in hospital ambulatory units. Most important, however, was the fact that overall quality of care rendered in free-standing units was noted to be *at least* as good as care rendered in the three other settings. Understandably, such an extensive and expensive study as the Orkand project has not been repeated.

PROS AND CONS OF OFFICE SURGERY

There are many pros and cons to performing surgery in an office-based unit. Some legal authorities feel that there is a yet to be tested standard of care for procedures performed in such a setting. Traditionally, the community standard required that one perform surgery and render care equal to hospital standards, regardless of the location where such care was rendered. Today, many believe that as more and more surgery is done in an office surgical setting, a new standard may be evolving. This standard would be set specifically for ambulatory surgical patients in a free-standing or office surgical center. Some legal authorities believe that the standards of such care regarding preoperative and postoperative instructions, postoperative monitoring, and follow-up care might actually be higher than that rendered in an inpatient setting. These opinions further emphasize the importance of establishing a thorough and effective risk-management program in the office surgical center.

WHAT DOES OFFICE SURGERY REQUIRE?

Performing surgery in your office requires that you will establish protocols and operating procedures that are similar to those utilized in a hospital setting and that are designed to maximize patient safety. A primary tenet is close observation of the patient in the immediate postoperative period. This dictates that vital signs be appropriately monitored and that recovery be provided in an area that affords the patient both privacy and convenience while making emergency resuscitation equipment, readily available, should that be necessary.

Many believe that better patient education is required when surgery is performed in an office setting. Normally, the nurse on the hospital floor would be responsible for reviewing postoperative instructions with the patient prior to discharge. When surgery is performed on an outpatient basis, the physician and the physician's staff provide this instruction. Obviously, the patient cannot care for himself immediately following surgery. For this reason, one must be sure that a responsible adult is both staying with the patient and is also cognizant of the postoperative instructions. Such a person must be able to deal effectively with the normal postoperative sequelae that the floor nurse would ordinarily be responsible for. The dressing changes, the nausea and vomiting, the minor discomfort that may be associated with surgical procedures must all be considered as potential items for the patient's caretaker to deal with.

Consistent with a friend, family member, or ancillary medical person caring for the patient following discharge from the office surgical area is the necessity for the physician and his staff to be readily available to answer questions or to deal with emergency situations in the unlikely event that they should arise. It is vital that adequate backup systems be employed in order that events such as a dead paging beeper battery does not preclude the patient or the patient's caretaker from obtaining a quick medical response to questions. Many physicians find that giving the patient not only the office answering service number, but also their home telephone number sufficiently deals with this problem. Other physicians find that it is advantageous to have their nursing staff also carry pagers in order that they may serve as backup if the solo practitioner is unable to be reached.

Documentation has always been of medicolegal importance. It is extremely critical in the outpatient setting. Oftentimes the degree of documentation that is required is something that the physician who has operated in the hosptial setting takes for granted. It is customary for the hospital record to be all encompassing and for nurses to record data, a responsibility that now becomes that of the physician and his office staff when surgery is performed in the office surgical area. Inpatients have their vital signs, symptoms, and condition frequently documented on the patient record by the attending nurse. On an outpatient basis, a telephone call that the patient is having some nausea or has a decreased oral intake of fluids might well be important at a later time. It is extremely important that such information obtained from telephone calls be recorded on the patient's chart in a very timely manner. Physicians performing surgery on an ambulatory basis must have a system by which such phone calls and patient contacts can be recorded appropriately in the patient's medical record.

Documentation has taken on a new dimension. In 1987, Medicare standards dictated that outpatient Medicare surgical services be reviewed. This has resulted in increased documentation standards for Medicare patients. It appears that new requirements as to what are appropriate histories and physicals, appropriate discharge summaries, and other documentation regarding ambulatory patients will continue to be established. It will be extremely important for physicians performing surgery in the office surgical area to be aware of what new standards the Federal Government requires in regard to Medicare patients. Such standards may well become the community standard and would affect the documentation practices for the surgeon performing facial plastic surgery.

QUALITY OF CARE

Quality of care has always been of primary importance to physicians. With today's health care market being so competitive, health care consumers are looking for the best value for their health care dollars. National corporations and various business coalitions throughout the country are monitoring the quality of care their employees receive. At the present time, numerous organizations are attempting to establish means by which employers can direct their employees to various health delivery entities in order to obtain a better value for their health insurance premiums. With many large corporations being self-insured, this issue becomes an important cost factor in the overall corporation budget.

Tom Peters, noted author of *In Search of Excellence*, points out in his new best-seller *Thriving in Chaos* that when quality increases, cost often decreases approximately 40%. If an operation is performed once and the patient is able to return home following surgery and to work after a very short convalescence, it is a better dollar value than a less expensive surgery performed twice.

The American Medical Association recognized the importance of dealing with quality of care and formed a special division within its organization to deal specifically with quality of care issues.

For a variety of reasons, many physicians believe that quality of care should actually increase when surgery is performed in the office surgical unit. There is increased supervision in the office surgical unit. The physician is constantly available to monitor all stages of the patient's care, including preoperative sedation, postoperative recovery, and discharge, which is not the case in the hospital setting. The physician is readily available to handle any complications that arise during the patient's treatment. The physician is also available to supervise all employees directly. This direct supervision and direct accountability should help to increase the quality of care delivered.

There is increased specialization when surgery is performed in the office surgical area versus the hospital setting. The physician's staff is familiar with the routine being performed and have the specialized equipment and expertise necessary to carry out efficiently and effectively the treatment of the patient. In the hospital setting it is common to have operating room nurses who are not familiar with the procedure being performed or scheduling conflicts result in equipment being unavailable.

Office surgery provides for increased productivity and time efficiency. The surgeon is free to perform other tasks while waiting for the patient to be prepared for surgery or moved to recovery. There is no problem with accessibility of the operating room because of emergency procedures or complications with another surgeon's procedure, resulting in the need to delay your surgery.

Many surgeons find that there is a significant reduction in wasted resources with surgery performed in the office surgical area versus the hospital setting. When employees are directly accountable for resources and supplies and when these are under the scrutiny of the physician and his supervisory staff, waste dramatically decreases.

Many believe that office-based surgery is more cost effective and perhaps provides better quality of care than surgery performed in the hospital setting. However, there is increased responsibility that the physician assumes when office surgery is undertaken. Risks can increase dramatically if the surgeon does not prudently execute those responsibilities. Office surgery requires a change in philosophy and a change in standard operating procedures. Economic factors have been the initial catalyst for change. However, the choice for surgery being performed on an inpatient or an outpatient basis is no longer available. Factors such as diagnosis related groups (DRGs), third party reimbursement, and other restrictions dictate that surgeons perform surgery in the most cost-effective surroundings and that there be no sacrifice in the quality of care they render.

CERTIFICATION AND ACCREDITATION—IS IT ALL WORTH IT?

One of the first legal problems faced by surgeons desiring to open an office surgical unit is whether or not to obtain a certificate of need or state licensure. Certificate of need and licensure laws vary from state to state. It is important for the physician to check with his State Board of Health or other health care regulatory agency regarding these issues. Oftentimes, consultation with legal counsel is also advisable.

In most states, a physician's office exemption exists. However, one must check closely with the aforenoted regulatory agencies. In some states if your office practice is primarily surgical, your office could be defined as an ambulatory surgical center that is operating without a license and that would be subject to state regulation.

There are several steps that can be taken to lessen the possibility of regulation. The first is to limit the use of your operating room facility to yourself and members of your organization. Physicians who allow their "colleague down the hall" to utilize their facilities are opening themselves to state regulation. The second is to refrain from identifying your facility as anything but your office to the general public. Finally, it is imperative that each individual check the law to determine if there is a risk of legal action for operating an ambulatory surgery center without a state license.

Authorities point out that you could be an ambulatory surgical facility for reasons of Medicare reimbursement and still maintain a physician's office exemption for reasons of state licensure. To be Medicare certified, you must comply with state licensure standards. However, this does not necessarily mean that you have to have a state license. One needs to check with legal counsel regarding this issue.

REASONS FOR CERTIFICATION

There are many reasons to obtain certification:

1. "Mobil Five Star rating"—there is a certain satisfaction that is derived from knowing that an outside group has placed its "stamp of approval" on your operation. The service industry has long recognized the promotional value that can be obtained from such recognition in the fact that it serves to attest that an organization has established and continues to meet specific standards in important areas.
2. Specialty society requirements—some specialty societies require that their members establish a mechanism for peer review and quality assurance in order to maintain membership in their organizations. The American College of Surgeons has such a position for its members who perform surgery primarily in an office surgical setting.
3. Liability—with the ever-increasing litigious climate, it may well be advantageous to have certification should an untoward event occur in your office surgical facility. Many legal authorities feel that certification would help to establish that you have met or exceeded the local community standards for quality of care in such a facility.
4. Reimbursement considerations—many third-party carriers will reimburse an office surgical unit for the facility fee or supply charge only if the facility is certified or accredited by specific organizations. While this activity is not uniform among various carriers or areas of the country, it is an important consideration and one that should be investigated on an individual basis.

TYPES OF CERTIFICATION/ACCREDITATION

Basically, there are two levels of certification or accreditation for office surgical or freestanding surgery centers. (See Addendum at the end of this chapter.) The first level is Accreditation Association for Ambulatory Health Care (AAAHC) or Joint Commission on Accreditation of Healthcare Organizations (JCAHO). Both organizations are nonprofit and nongovernmental and provide independent review and accreditation for ambulatory surgical and office surgical facilities. AAAHC site reviews are performed by physicians and administrators who volunteer their time and who themselves are members of accredited facilities. The JCAHO, on the other hand, utilizes employees of their organization to perform such site surveys. Both organizations place an emphasis on procedures and protocols that assure that a high level of quality of care is being delivered in surveyed facilities. Accreditation by AAAHC or JCAHO may be granted for 1 to 3 years.

The second level of accreditation or certification is state licensure or Medicare certification. In some areas, a Certificate of Need may be required in order to obtain Medicare certification or state licensure. The cost of obtaining "second level" certification is extremely significant. There are increased administrative costs in applying for such certification. There is considerable paperwork that must be completed. Assistance from paid consultants is often required to complete the various forms and applications. In addition, there are strict physical plant requirements that may be extremely expensive. Many physicians have found that the structural cost for a facility that would meet state licensure or Medicare requirements may be twice that for a facility that would be approved by AAAHC or JCAHO. It is advisable to contact your state health care planning agency or board of health regarding specific physical plant requirements and regulations for freestanding surgical centers. Assistance from an architect experienced in building such medical facilities is imperative.

LIABILITY ISSUES IN OFFICE SURGERY

Some hold the belief that office surgery has increased liability. This is based on two premises. The first is that facilities in an office may be inadequate when compared with surgical facilities in a hospital setting. It is believed by these individuals that equipment insufficiency may actually increase the risks involved in a surgical procedure and thus increase the doctor's liability. The second premise is that the hospital is liable for acts of its employees that result in injury to a patient. In the office surgical setting, liability is increased because of the loss of this agency relationship between ancillary health care personnel and the employer. The second premise emphasizes the importance of hiring well-qualifed nursing personnel to assist in the office surgical facility and emphasizes the importance of establishing continuing education for such individuals.

The technical aspects of executing a surgical procedure will be the same regardless of where that procedure is performed—in an office or in a hospital. Thus, the mechanical aspects will be scrutinized closely in any legal proceeding. The emphasis will be placed on evaluating the patient immediately before surgery, monitoring during surgery, and monitoring during the postoperative recovery phase. Many individuals feel that under such close scrutiny, the office surgical center may actually fare much better than a hospital setting. This is because the physician in his office might well be immediately available to correct a problem, which would not be the case had the procedure been performed in a hospital setting. In addition, the office surgical nurse customarily performs multiple functions in contrast to the hospital, where nursing personnel work only in preoperative preparation, surgery, recovery and other areas. Personnel in the office are acquainted with the patient through all phases of care. Thus, there is a decreased possibility of error due to lack of knowledge about the patient or a communication error pertaining to a specific patient. This is certainly not the case in the hospital setting where one nurse may prepare the patient for the operation and another nurse in a separate area may be responsible for caring for the patient during the surgical procedure. In addition, many nursing personnel may rotate through the operating suite during the specific procedure. Oftentimes, these individuals have no prior knowledge as to the specific case and might have, in fact, very little experience with the procedure being performed.

The fact is, if one has a problem in an office surgical facility, he must be able to demonstrate clearly a capability to deal with this emergency just as if it had occurred in a hospital facility. This standard of care issue is primary in any legal proceeding. Many individuals feel that accreditation or certification by a nationally recognized organization or governmental entity markedly strengthens the case for the office surgical facility.

CERTIFICATION IMPROVES QUALITY OF CARE

Without doubt, the best reason for seeking accreditation or certification is to improve the quality of patient care. Certification requires establishment of well thought out protocols and procedures for each stage of patient care and requires documentation and monitoring of such. It is doubtful that the physician in an office surgical setting would develop the fire and disaster protocols, the routine medical equipment checks, the complex quality assurance studies, conduct the medical in-service training sessions, or establish the complex peer review mechanisms that are required for accreditation. Although some diligent physicians might establish such protocols, it is doubtful that even they would maintain them on a regular basis if it was not required for certification.

A study conducted by the General Motors Corporation showed that if a task was not monitored or supervised, its "life expectancy" or longevity was only 7 weeks. This appears to be true in corporate America and is undoubtedly true in the office surgical facility. Thus, accreditation requires the physician to set standards and to monitor those standards. It is the old song that "what gets measured gets done."

An ancillary reason for obtaining accreditation or certification is the positive public relations effect it has in the community and the positive marketing effect that can result. In a competitive medical environment it is important to distinguish oneself from the competition. Accreditation of an office surgical facility is certainly a positive distinction.

CHAPTER 1 ADDENDUM

Accreditation Standards

> The following standards are <u>extracted</u> from the 1987-88 edition of the Accreditation Handbook for Ambulatory Health Care, and are provided for the general reference of participants at the American Academy of Cosmetic Surgery Office Surgery / Risk Management course. Those who are considering accreditation should obtain the complete handbook by sending $25. to the **Accreditation Association for Ambulatory Health Care; 9933 Lawler Ave; Skokie, Ill 60077-3702.** Request *the 1977-88 Accreditation Handbook for Ambulatory Health Care.*

Governance - An accreditable organization has a governing body that sets policy and is responsible for the organization. Such an organization has the following characteristics.

A. The organization is a legally constituted entity in the state(s) in which it is located and provides service. The organization is constituted by at least one of the following: 1. charter 2. articles of incorporation 3. partnership agreement 4. franchise agreement 5. legislative or executive act

B. The governing body addresses and is fully responsible, either directly or by appropriate professional delegation, for the operation and performance of the organization. Governing body responsibilities include, but are not limited to,
   1. determining the mission, goals, and objectives of the organization
   2. assuring that facilities and personnel are adequate and appropriate to carry out the mission
   3. establishing an organizational structure and specifying functional relationships among the various components of the organization
   4. adopting bylaws or similar rules and regulations for the orderly development and management of the organization
   5. adopting policies and procedures necessary for the orderly conduct of the organization
   6. assuring that the quality of care is evaluated and that identified problems are appropriately addressed
   7. reviewing all legal and ethical matters concerning the organizations and its staff, and, when necessary, responding appropriately
   8. maintaining effective communication throughout the organization
   9. establishing a system of financial management and accountability appropriate to the organization
   10. determining a policy on the rights of patients
   11. approving all major contracts or arrangements affecting the medical care provided under the auspices, including but not limited to, those concerning a. the employment of practitioners b. the provision of radiology services and pathology and medical laboratory services d. the provision of care by other health care organizations, such as hospitals e. the provision of education to students and post graduate trainees
   12. formulating long-range plans in accordance with the mission, goals, and objectives of the organization
   13. operating the organization without limitation because of race, creed, sex, or national origin
   14. assuring that all marketing and advertising concerning the organization do not imply that it provides care or services that it is not capable of providing
   15. developing a policy on risk management appropriate to the organization including, but not limited to, a. periodic review of all litigation involving the organization and its staff and health care practitioners b. periodic review of all incidents reported by staff and patients c. review of all deaths, trauma, or adverse reactions occurring on premises. d. resolution of patient complaints
   16. determining a policy on continued education for personnel.

C. The governing body provides for full disclosure of ownership
   1. The names and addresses of all owners or controlling parties (whether individuals, partnerships, trusts, corporate bodies, or subdivisions of other bodies, such as public agencies or religious, fraternal, other philanthropic organizations) are furnished to the Accreditation Association for Ambulatory Health Care, Inc. (AAAHC).
   2. For corporations, the names and addresses of all officers, directors, and principal stockholders, either beneficial or of record, are available to the public upon request and are furnished to the AAAHC.
   3. Accredited organizations must notify AAAHC within 30 days of any significant change in ownership (such as merger, change in majority interest, consolidation), name change, scope of services, or additional services or locations.

D. The governing body meets at least annually and keeps such minutes or other records as may be necessary for the orderly conduct of the organization.

E. If the governing body elects, appoints, or employs officers and administrators to carry out its directives, the authority, responsibility, and functions of all such positions are defined.

F. When a majority of its members are physicians, the governing body, either directly or by delegation, makes (in a manner consistent with state law and based on evidence of the education, training, experience, and current competence of the physician) the initial appointments, reappointments, and assignment or curtailment of medical privileges. When a majority of the members of the governing body are not physicians, the organization's bylaws or similar rules and regulations specify a procedure for establishing medical review for the purpose of making (in a manner consistent with state law and based on evidence of the education, training, experience, and current competence of the physician) initial appointments, reappointments, and assignment or curtailment of medical privileges.

G. The governing body provides (in a manner consistent with state law and based on evidence of education, training, experience, and current competence) for the initial appointments, reappointments, and assignment or curtailment of privileges and practice for non-physician health care personnel and practitioners.

QUALITY OF CARE PROVIDED An accreditable organization is administered in a manner that assures the provision of high-quality health services and that fulfills the organization's mission, goals, and objectives. Such an organization has the following characteristics.

A. All health care practitioners have the necessary and appropriate training and skills to deliver the services provided by the organization.

B. Health care practitioners practice their professions in an ethical and legal manner.

C. All personnel assisting in the provision of health care services are appropriately trained, qualified, and supervised and are available in sufficient numbers for the care provided.

D. The provision of high-quality health care services is demonstrated by at least the following:
    1. education of, and effective communication with, those served concerning the diagnosis and treatment of their medical conditions, appropriate preventive measures, and use of the health care system.
    2. accessible and available health services.
    3. appropriate and timely diagnosis based on findings of the initial assessment(history and physical examination)
    4. treatment that is consistent with clinical impression or working diagnosis.
    5. appropriate and timely consultation
    6. absence of clinically unnecessary diagnostic or therapeutic procedures
    7. appropriate and timely referrals
    8. patient cooperation
    9. continuity of care
    10. provision for services when the organization's facilities are not open
    11. appropriate, accurate, and complete medical record entries
    12. adequate transfer of information when patients are transferred to and from other health care providers
    13. patient satisfaction

E. When clinically indicated, patients are contacted as quickly as possible for follow up regarding significant problems and /or abnormal laboratory or radiologic findings.

F. When the need arises, patients are transferred from the care of one health care practitioner to another. 1. Adequate specialty consultation services are available by prior arrangement.
2. Referral to a health care practitioner is clearly outlined to the patient and arranged with the accepting health care practitioner prior to transfer.

G. Concern for the costs of care is demonstrated by the following:
    1. the relevance of health care services to the needs of the patients
    2. the absence of duplicative diagnostic procedures
    3. the appropriateness of treatment frequency
    4. the use of the least expensive alternate resources when suitable
    5. the use of ancillary services that are consistent with patients' needs

H. When the need arises, provisions are made for health care practitioners and other staff to communicate with patients in the language primarily used by them.

QUALITY ASSURANCE PROGRAM In striving to improve the quality of care and to promote more effective and efficient utilization of facilities and services, an accreditable organization maintains an active, organized, peer-based, quality assurance program as an integral part of professional and administrative practice. Such an organization has the following characteristics.

A. The professional and administrative staff understands, supports, and participates in the quality assurance program, through an organized mechanism responsible to the governing body.

B. At least two physicians are involved in quality assurance activities in order to provide peer based review. (In solo physician organizations, such as office based surgical practices and independent practice associations, an outside physician is involved in quality assurance activities to provide peer-based review.)

C. The quality assurance program addresses clinical, administrative, and cost-of-care issues does not fulfill this requirement.

D. Quality assurance activities conducted by specific clinical disciplines within the organization (individual medical specialties, nursing, and so forth) are consistent with the characteristics of the organization's overall quality assurance program.

E. The organization provides ongoing monitoring of important aspects of the care provided.

F. Health care practitioners participate in the development and application of the criteria used to evaluate the care they provide.

G. Data related to established criteria are collected in an ongoing manner.

H. Collected data are periodically evaluated to identify unacceptable or unexpected trends or occurrences that influence patient outcomes (results of care).

I. Quality assurance activities have the following characteristics.
  1. Important problems or concerns in the care of patients are identified. Sources of identifiable problems include, but are not limited to,
     a. unacceptable or unexpected results of ongoing monitoring of care, such as complications, hospital transfers, malpractice cases, lack of follow up on abnormal test results, radiology film retakes, prescribing errors for medications, specific diagnoses, and so forth.
     b. the clinical performance and practice patterns of health care practitioners
     c. medical record review for quality of care and completeness of entries
     d. quality controls for and use of diagnostic imaging, pathology, medical laboratory, and pharmaceutical services
     e. other professional and technical services provided
     f. assessment of patient satisfaction
     g. direct observation
     h. staff concerns
     i. accessibility
     j. medical/legal issues
     k. wasteful practices
  2. The frequency, severity, and source of suspected problems or concerns are evaluated. Health care practitioners participate in the evaluation of the problems or concerns identified.
  3. Measures are implemented to resolve important problems or concerns that have been identified. Health care practitioners as well as administrative staff participate in the resolution of the problems or concerns that are identified.
  4. The problems or concerns are re-evaluated to determine objectively whether the corrective measures have achieved and sustained the desired result. If the problem remains, alternate corrective actions are taken as needed to resolve the problem.
  5. Through the organization's designed mechanisms, quality assurance activities are reported, as appropriate, to the proper personnel, the chief executive officer, and the governing body.

J. To permit flexibility and encourage innovation and variation, no particular method of conducting quality assurance activities is specified or required for accreditation. However, exclusive concentration on ongoing monitoring of care, without evidence of resolving problems, does not fulfill this standard.

K. Findings of quality assurance activities are incorporated into the organization's educational activities.

L. Appropriate records of quality assurance activities are maintained.

MEDICAL RECORDS An accreditable organization maintains a medical record system from which information can be retrieved promptly. Medical records are legible, documented accurately in a timely manner, and readily accessible to health care practitioners. Such an organization has the following characteristics.

A. The organization develops and maintains a system for the collection, processing, maintenance, storage, retrieval, and distribution of patient medical records.

B. An individual medical record is established for each person receiving care.

C. All clinical information relevant to a patient is readily available to authorized health care practitioners anytime the organization is open to patients.

D. Except when otherwise required by law, any record that contains clinical, social, financial, or other data on a patient is treated as strictly confidential and is protected from loss, tampering, alteration, destruction, and unauthorized or inadvertent disclosure.

E. There is a person designated in charge of medical records whose responsibilities include, but are not limited to
1. The confidentiality, security, and physical safety of medical records
2. the timely retrieval of individual medical records upon request
3. the unique identification of each patient's medical record
4. the supervision of the collection, processing, maintenance, storage, retrieval, and distribution of medical records
5. the maintenance of a predetermined organized medical record format

F. Policies concerning medical records address, but are not limited to,
1. the retention of active records
2. the retirement of inactive medical records
3. the timely entry of data in medical records
4. the release of information contained in medical records

G. Except when otherwise required by law, the content and format of medical records, including the sequence of information, are uniform.

H. Reports, histories and physicals, progress notes, and other patient information (such as laboratory reports, x-ray readings, operating reports, and consultations) are reviewed and incorporated into the medical record in a timely manner.

I. If a patient's medical record is complex and lengthy, a summary of significant past surgical procedures as well as past and current diagnoses or problems is conspicuously documented in that patient's medical record to facilitate the ongoing provision of rational medical care. The summary is legibly recorded in the same location in all patient charts. The summary does not repeat problems or diagnoses that recur during ongoing treatment. The summary includes, but is not limited to, 1.significant surgical conditions , including major procedures
2. significant medical conditions, including medical diagnoses of conditions for which the patient receives medication or treatment on a repeated or continuing basis
3. conditions that are likely to significantly influence future care. If a patient's medical record is not complex and lengthy, the record should contain appropriate and adequate information to facilitate the ongoing provision of rational medical care.

J. The presence or absence of allergies and untoward reactions to drugs is recorded in a prominent and uniform location in all patient charts on a current basis.

K. Entries in a patient's medical record for each visit include, but are not limited to,
1. date, department (if departmentalized), and provider name and profession (for example, PT, MD, RN, and so forth)
2. chief complaint or purpose of visit
3. clinical findings
4. diagnosis or medical impression
5. studies ordered, such as laboratory or x-ray studies

6. therapies administered
7. disposition, recommendations, and instructions given to the patient
8. signature or initials of practitioner

L. Significant medical advice given to a patient by telephone is entered in the patient's medical record and appropriately signed or initialed.

M. Entries in patient's medical records are legible to the clinical personnel in the organization.

N. Any notation in a patient's medical record indicating diagnostic or therapeutic intervention as part of clinical research is clearly contrasted with entries regarding the provision of non-research related care.

O. When necessary for assuring continuity of care, summaries or records of a patient who was treated elsewhere (such as by another physician, hospital, ambulatory surgical service, nursing home, or consultant) are obtained.

P. When necessary for assuring continuity of care, summaries of the patient's records are transferred to the health care practitioner to whom the patient was referred and, if appropriate, to the organization where future care will be rendered.

7. **Professional Improvement** - An accreditable organization strives to improve the professional competence and skill, as well as the quality of performance, of the health care practitioners and other professional personnel it employs. Such an organization has the following characteristics.

A. The organization provides for convenient access to library services that include materials pertinent to the clinical, educational, administrative, and research services offered by the organization.

B. The organization provides adequate orientation and training to familiarize all personnel with the organization's policies, procedures, and facilities.

C. The organization encourages participation in seminars, workshops, and other educational activities pertinent to its mission, goal, and objectives.

D. When attendance at educational activities is required of professional personnel, the organization accepts evidence of participation in relevant external educational programs.

E. The organization provides a monitoring function to assure the continued maintenance of licensure and/or certification of professional personnel.

8. **Facilities and Environment** - An accreditable organization provides a functionally safe and sanitary environment for its patients, personnel, visitors. Such an organization has the following characteristics.

A. The organization assures that its facilities
1. comply with applicable federal, state, and local building codes and regulations
2. comply with applicable federal, state, and local fire prevention regulations
3. are inspected at least annually by the local or state fire control agency, if this service is available in the community
4. contain fire-fighting equipment to control a limited fire, including appropriately maintained and placed fire extinguishers of the proper type
5. have prominently displayed illuminated signs with emergency power capability at all exits from each floor and hall
6. have alternate lighting, as appropriate to the facility, to provide adequate evaluation of patients and staff in case of an emergency
7. have stairwells protected by fire doors.

B. The organization has the necessary personnel, equipment, and procedures to handle medical emergencies that may arise in connection with services sought or provided. At a minimum the organization provides
1. periodic instruction of all personnel in the proper use of safety, emergency, and fire-extinguishing equipment

2. a comprehensive emergency plan to address internal and external emergencies, including a. a provision for the safe evacuation of patients during an internal emergency, especially patients who have difficulty walking
   b. a provision for the most efficient use of available facilities and services during an external emergency
   c. a requirement for at least four drills a year of the internal emergency plan
3. personnel trained in cardiopulmonary resuscitation and the use of cardiac equipment present in the facility during hours of operation.

C. Smoking is prohibited in such areas as operating rooms, anesthetizing locations, rooms where oxygen and other volatile gases are administered or stored, and other hazardous areas. Smoking is permitted only in designated areas.

D. Hazards that might lead to slipping, falling, electrical shock, burns, poisoning, or other trauma are eliminated.

E. Reception areas, toilets, and telephones are provided in accordance with patient and visitor volume.

F. When appropriate, adequately marked patient and visitor parking is provided.

G. Provisions are made to reasonably accommodate handicapped individuals.

H. All examination rooms, dressing rooms, and reception areas are constructed and maintained in a manner that assures patient privacy during interviews, examinations, treatment, and consultation.

I. Adequate lighting and ventilation are provided in all areas.

J. Facilities are clean and properly maintained.

K. Food, snack services, and refreshments provided to patients meet their clinical needs and are prepared, stored, served, and disposed of in compliance with local health department requirements.

L. Procedures should be available to minimize the sources and transmission of infections, including adequate surveillance techniques.

M. A system exists for the proper identification, management, handling, transport, treatment, and disposition of hazardous materials and wastes whether solid, liquid, or gas.
   1. This system includes, but is not limited to, infectious, radioactive, chemical, and physical hazards.
   2. The system provides for the protection of patients, staff, and the environment.

N. The space allocated for a particular function or service is adequate for the activities performed therein, including space allocated for pathology and medical laboratory services, radiology services, pharmaceutical services, examination and treatment rooms, offices, operating rooms, recovery areas, storage rooms, reception areas, medical records, and other special function areas.

O. Appropriate emergency equipment and supplies are maintained and readily accessible to all areas of each patient care service site.

P. Equipment is properly maintained and periodically tested.

Q. Alternate power adequate for the protection of the life and safety of patients and staff is available. Special attention is given to
   1. operative and recovery areas for surgical services
   2. treatment areas where emergency services are provided.

R. New facilities constructed by accreditable organizations comply with Section 12-6 "New Ambulatory Health Care Centers," Chapter 26, and other sections as may be applicable, of the 1981 edition of the *Life Safety Code* (NFPA 101)*, published by the National Fire Protection Association, Inc., unless otherwise provided for by state law, local code, or appropriate jurisdiction having authority.

S. Existing facilities of accreditable organizations will, over a reasonable period of time, be brought into compliance with Section 13-6 "Existing Ambulatory Health Care Center," Chapter 27, and other sections as may be applicable, of the 1981 edition of the *Life Safety Code* (NFPA 101)*, published by the National Fire Protection Association, Inc., unless otherwise provided for by state law, local code, or appropriate jurisdiction having authority . * *Life Safety Code* and 101 are registered trademarks of the National Fire Protection Association, Inc., Quincy, Massachusetts .

Although revisions have been made, the 1981 edition is the only edition applicable for accreditation purposes.

9. **Anesthesia and Surgical Services** - Anesthesia services and surgical procedures in an accreditable organization are provided and performed in a safe and sanitary environment by qualified health care practitioners who have been granted privileges to perform those procedures by the governing body. Such an organization has the following characteristics.

A. Anesthesia services provided in the facilities owned or operated by the organization are limited to those techniques that are approved by the governing body upon the recommendation of qualified medical personnel.

B. Adequate supervision of anesthesia services provided by the organization is the responsibility of one or more qualified physicians who are approved by the governing body upon the recommendation of qualified medical personnel.

C. Anesthesia is administered by anesthesiologists, other qualified physician or dentist anesthetists, qualified nurse anesthetists, or supervised trainees in an approved educational program.

D. A person qualified to provide anesthesia services is available as long as clinically indicated.

E. Policies and procedures are developed for anesthesia services which include, but are not limited to,
   1. education, training, and supervision of personnel
   2. responsibilities of non-physician anesthetists
   3. responsibilities of supervising physicians
   4. use and degree of supplemented local anesthesia

F. Anesthesia is not administered unless the operating surgeon or anesthesiologist has evaluated the patient immediately prior to surgery to assess the risk of the anesthesia relative to the surgical procedure to be performed.

G. Patients who have received anesthesia are evaluated by the operating surgeon or anesthesiologist after recovery from anesthesia, prior to discharge.

H. Patients who have received anesthesia, except unsupplemented local anesthesia, are discharged in the company of a responsible adult.

I. No patient shall receive general anesthesia unless one or more additional health care practitioners besides the one performing surgery are present or immediately available.

J. All machines in use for general anesthesia shall have not less than one annual testing by technicians with appropriate training and a log of this testing will be maintained.

K. Surgical procedures performed in the facilities owned or operated by the organization are limited to those procedures that are approved by the governing body upon the recommendation of qualified medical personnel.

L. Adequate supervision of surgery conducted in the organization is a responsibility of the governing body, is recommended by an anesthesiologist or another physician, and is provided by appropriate personnel.

M. Surgical procedures are performed only by health care practitioners who
   1. are licensed to perform such procedures within the state in which the organization is located
   2. have been granted privileges to perform those procedures by the governing body of the organization, upon the recommendation of qualified medical personnel and after medical review of the practitioner's documented education, training, experience, and current competence.

N. Surgical procedures to be performed in an office surgical practice are reviewed periodically as part of the peer review portion of the organization's quality assurance program.

O. An appropriate and current history, physical examination, and pertinent preoperative diagnostic studies are incorporated into the patient's medical record prior to surgery.

P. The necessity or appropriateness of the proposed surgery, as well as any available alternative treatment techniques have been discussed with the patient prior to scheduling for surgery.

Q. Registered nurse(s) and other personnel assisting in the provision of surgical services are appropriately trained and supervised and are available in sufficient numbers for the surgical and emergency care provided.

R. Each operating room is designed and equipped so that the types of surgery conducted can be performed in a manner that protects the lives and assures the physical safety of all persons in the area. At least one operating room is available for surgery.
   1. Only nonflammable agents are present in an operating room, and the room is constructed and equipped in compliance with standards established by the National Fire Protection Association (NFPA 56G, Standard for Inhalation Anaesthetics in Ambulatory Care Facilities, 1980)and with applicable state and local fire codes.

S. An anesthesiologist or another physician qualified in resuscitative techniques is present or immediately available until all patients operated on that day have been discharged.

T. With the exception of those tissues exempted by the governing body after medical review, tissues removed during surgery are examined by the pathologist, whose signed report of the examination is made a part of patient's medical record.

U. The findings and techniques of an operation are accurately and completely written or dictated immediately after the procedure by the health care practitioner who performed the operation. This description is immediately available for patient care and becomes a part of the patient's medical record.

V. A safe environment for treating surgical patients, including adequate safeguards to protect the patient from cross-infection, is assured through the provision of adequate space, equipment, and personnel.
   1. Provisions have been made for the isolation or immediate transfer of patients with communicable disease.
   2. All persons entering operating rooms are properly attired.
   3. Acceptable aseptic techniques are used by all persons in the surgical areas.
   4. Only authorized persons are allowed in the surgical area.
   5. Suitable equipment for rapid and routine sterilization is available to assure that operating room materials are sterile.
   6. Sterilized materials are packaged and labeled in a consistent manner to maintain sterility and identify sterility dates.
   7. Environmental controls are implemented to assure a safe and sanitary environment.
   8. Suitable equipment is provided for the regular cleaning of all interior surfaces.
   9. Operating rooms are appropriately cleaned before each operation.

W. When hospitalization is indicated or to evaluate, stabilize, and transfer when emergencies or unplanned outcomes occur, the organization either has a written transfer agreement for transferring patients to a nearby hospital when hospitalization is indicated or permits elective surgery only by practitioners who have admitting and similar surgical privileges at a nearby hospital.

X. Procedures have been developed for obtaining blood and blood products on a timely basis.

Y. Emergency power adequate for the type of surgery performed is available in operative and recovery areas.

Z. Periodic calibration and/or preventive maintenance of equipment is provided.

AA. The informed consent of the patient or, if applicable, of the patient's representative is obtained before an operation is performed.

BB. A procedure has been established for the observation and care of the patient during the preoperative preparation and postoperative recovery period.

CC. Protocols have been established for instructing patients in selfcare after surgery, including written instructions to be given to patients who receive regional and general anesthesia.

2 Staffing the Office Surgical Center

Personnel are probably the most vital component to the successful office surgical center. The number of personnel required to staff an ambulatory surgical center and the qualifications of these individuals may vary widely. A variety of factors will influence personnel needs. These include the nature of the practice, the physical structure of the facility, the capabilities of the particular employees, and the personal preferences of the surgeon or surgeons. For these reasons, it is difficult to standardize the personnel needs for such facilities. However, the typical facility requires three general classifications of employees: medical, clerical, and custodial.

The primary responsibility of medical personnel is to assist the surgeon in the delivery of quality patient care. Individual state licensing requirements as well as accrediting association guidelines may dictate that individuals have certain qualifications or certifications in order to perform a particular task or to function in a particular capacity. For this reason, it is imperative for each physician to consult with regulatory and certification agencies within his or her state in order to assure compliance with legislative mandates. Medical personnel used in an office surgical facility may include Registered Nurses, Licensed Practical Nurses, Physician Assistants, and Surgical Technicians. Although many surgeons elect to "train" individuals of varying backgrounds to assist them in providing patient care, it is important to recognize that there is an increasing trend nationally for utilization of Registered Nurses for such functions. Many hospitals are utilizing Registered Nurses to perform functions that were previously performed by Surgical Technicians or Licensed Practical Nurses. In order to be consistent with the "practice standard" in your community, it is important to keep abreast of such practices at hospitals in your locale.

If devastating cardiopulmonary complications are to be avoided, observation and monitoring of patients for recognition of the earliest signs and symptoms of difficulty must be second nature to the ambulatory surgery staff. It is imperative that center staff be able to provide appropriate emergency care if each situations should arise. For this reason, many facilities require all medical personnel to be trained in basic cardiac life support. In addition, many facilities are now requiring their medical personnel also to be certified in advanced cardiac life support.

The qualifications and character of office and clerical personnel are extremely important to the success of an office surgical center. Medical terminology is obviously of benefit for clerical staff. However, it is not mandatory. State of the art computer software packages for word processing can easily be adapted to enable secretarial staff of varying backgrounds to function efficiently and effectively in the medical office. The specific qualifications for clerical personnel may vary widely between facilities, but all need to possess a pleasing personality and the ability to get along with people. Clerical personnel make the initial contact with prospective patients and are often the primary liaison between patients and physicians. Their importance in this capacity cannot be overemphasized.

In a smaller facility clerical personnel may be asked to function in a multitude of capacities. However, clerical personnel should not give medical information to patients without first consulting directly with the physician on the subject in question. The importance of this cannot be overstressed.

The custodial staff are indispensable for the maintenance of an office surgical facility. The qualifications of custodial personnel must be considered carefully. Previous custodial work, training, and experience are necessary. In order to maintain a medical facility properly, cleaning procedures and protocols must be established. Proper cleaning of such a facility varies significantly from routine commercial office custodial care. Newly employed custodial staff must be instructed in surgical facility cleaning procedures and be made aware of the great importance of maintaining proper environmental control, especially in the operating room.

In addition to specific qualifications for individuals filling specific job categories within the office surgical facility, it is extremely important that employees possess common personal attributes. A mature person who is attuned to the fears and anxieties of surgical patients is vital. A stable personal life reduces the potential for distractions from work responsibilities. In addition, the ability to interact with other personnel amicably is essential in order for the center to function appropriately.

Most hospital staff ratios are approximately three staff members (exclusive of physicians) per patient. The ratio of staff member per patient is often able to be significantly reduced in the ambulatory surgery center. This is due to the fact that patients are usually healthy, treatment is nondiagnostic, and personnel in office surgical centers are usually selected for their initiative and energy in execution of their duties. For this reason, a ratio of one staff member per patient is frequently found in ambulatory and office surgical facilities. However, it must be stressed that the number of personnel must be adequate to ensure that patients receive quality medical care and are adequately supervised until they are released from the facility. One scrub nurse and one circulating nurse are needed for each surgical procedure. A separate recovery room nurse is also necessary. In a small facility with one operating room and a single recovery area, a circulating nurse may be able to function as a circulating-recovery room nurse. However, each facility should closely scrutinize its personnel needs to be sure that it is not understaffed and it is able to provide patients with the same standard of care that would have been rendered had the procedure been performed in the hospital setting.

Litigation involving personnel is one of the most frequent problems noted in business today. Courts have made significant monetary awards to individuals who have been wrongly discharged. In addition, sexual harassment suits filed against employers are increasingly common. As "proprietor" of a medical facility, you are subject to the same risks in the area of personnel management as any other business. For this reason, it is imperative that certain policies and procedures be developed in order to protect the organization from legal liability as well as to ensure efficient and effective management of the facility.

ORGANIZATIONAL DECISIONS

The quality of the medical staff is extremely important. The number of staff your organization will need is related directly to the quality of individuals you are willing to hire. Some surgeons believe they can reduce overhead by hiring individuals with less training and experience. Far too often, they find that not only do such staff members lack the skills to act interchangeably, but they often require you to spend more time in supervision. If temporary help is needed to assist in carrying out office functions, operating costs can significantly escalate.

CHAIN OF COMMAND

With only a few employees, it is easy for individuals to report directly to you. This allows you to maintain close personal control of the daily operations without spending an inordinate amount of time on supervision. However, as a practice grows, serious consideration needs to be given to establishing a formal chain of command. This will enable some individuals to report directly to an office manager or supervisory person and relieve you of routine decisions and management responsibilities. This is extremely important in order to maintain office efficiency and productivity.

It is extremely important, however, for the physician never to relinquish command completely. Employees work better when they receive personal words of encouragement and direction from their boss. Also, direct contact keeps you in touch with staff sufficiently to resolve minor employee problems before they materialize into significant conflicts.

Some physicians choose to hire an office manager. There are various management consulting firms that can be utilized for this purpose. If an office manager is hired, it is important for the physician to review the manager's qualifications closely. It is also important for the physician to work with the office manager to establish a chain of command that will allow the office manager to function efficiently and to perform his or her job in the most appropriate manner. Far too often, a practice matures to the point where an office manager is needed. However, long-term employees who have become accustomed to reporting directly to the physician refuse to accept the new organizational structure and thus defeat the primary advantages of having an office manager, that is, relieving the physician of routine decision-making and supervisory functions. This is an important issue to consider and to address directly with all employees whenever an office reorganization is undertaken. Many facilities find that an excellent way to avoid confusion about the chain of command is to create a formal organizational chart that shows precisely who reports to whom.

JOB DESCRIPTIONS

Job descriptions are essential to recruiting and interviewing qualified personnel. They should reflect your feelings concerning performance responsibilities, job qualifications, terms of employment (full or part time, permanent or temporary) and method and frequency of evaluation. It is also vital that the job description be explicit as to whom an individual reports. This allows a new employee to recognize from the beginning of their employment how they fit into the overall office structure.

Two other elements are useful in a job description. First, always conclude the performance responsibilities with the statement that the job holder will "perform other tasks as needed." That gives the job supervisor latitude to ask the employee to help out when another person is busy without hearing the "not my job" refrain.

Second, provide signature lines at the end of the document. When both the physician and the employee have signed, you have a document that shows mutual agreement about the job (Fig. 2-1).

You therefore have a safeguard when evaluating or terminating the employee based on criteria in the job description. Only a few job descriptions are needed in a medical office: nurse, office manager, secretary, receptionist, and bookkeeper. (Note that, in some states, creation of signed, written job descriptions may create a contract. Legal advice may be indicated if you use such descriptions.)

SAMPLE JOB DESCRIPTION

TITLE: Medical office receptionist
QUALIFICATIONS:
1. High school diploma
2. Typing skills (60 wpm)
3. One-year's experience in medical office
4. Such alternatives to the above qualifications as the surgeon may find appropriate and acceptable.

REPORTS TO: Surgeon

SUPERVISES: [Not applicable]

JOB GOAL: To assure that all office inquiries are properly channeled, and that all visitors—especially patients—receive a courteous welcome

PERFORMANCE RESPONSIBILITIES:
1. Prepares to greet each day's patients by pulling their charts, looking at their photographs so that patients can be identified and called by name.
2. Cheerfully acknowledges patients by name upon arrival.
3. Answers all patient inquiries in a courteous and helpful manner.
4. Explains any lengthy delays in the surgeon's schedule, and offers to re-schedule if patients desire.
5. Notes receipt of any patient gifts in patient files, placing files on surgeon's desk each evening so he can write personal thank-you notes.
6. Handles all incoming calls, recording each in telephone log.
7. Assists all other visitors with their inquiries.
8. Performs such other tasks as may be assigned.

TERMS OF EMPLOYMENT: Permanent, full-time position; salary to be established by surgeon.

EVALUATION: Performance of this job will be evaluated over an initial 3-month probationary period, then again after six months, and at regular annual intervals thereafter.

Approved by: _____ Date: _____

Reviewed and agreed to by: _____ Date: _____

SOURCE: Beeson Facial Plastic and Reconstructive Surgery, Indianapolis, Indiana

---

Figure 2-1.

POLICIES AND PROCEDURES MANUAL

"He governs best who governs least" is a philosophy adopted by many physicians. While this may sound appropriate in theory, in practice it frequently leads to discontent and misunderstandings among office staff. This is especially true when the office staff grows.

Many studies have shown that individuals work best when they know exactly what is expected of them. Statements about what is expected by the legal owner of the business are called policies. Policies are viewed as broad statements that usually start with a word about why a particular goal is worthy and conclude with what the goal is. An example of such would be "The———Facial Plastic Surgery Center believes that smoking is dangerous to the health of staff and patients, and damaging to their skin; therefore smoking will not be permitted on office premises."

Written policies have various uses. In an interview situation, a professional-looking policy manual shows potential employees that you have thought out issues important to them. A new employee can read such a manual as an orientation to office goals. Current employees can read the manual to clarify procedures.

For yourself, a well thought out, up-to-date policy manual can help you treat employees fairly and equally. This is of significant importance in protecting yourself from potential litigation.

The key word to all policies is "reasonableness." For instance, you should not expect employees to work beyond established office hours unless you are prepared to pay overtime (this is true even if the employee volunteers for extra hours). If you allow one employee 3 months off with pay for a medical problem, then the same option must be available to all other employees, including pregnant employees. This is especially important since the Courts now view pregnancy as a medical disability. If one employee is merely reprimanded for tardiness, another may not be fired for the same violation.

Violations of standard of reasonableness can leave the physician open to suit under State or Federal legislation outlawing employment discrimination. A well-structured policy and procedure manual that has been reviewed by your attorney will help to ensure that you maintain a reasonable and consistent attitude when dealing with employee problems. (Note that, in some states, a manual may give the employee contract rights that would not otherwise arise. In those states a manual would be contraindicated. Obtain legal advice if you plan to adopt such a manual.)

Every employee should get a copy of the office policy manual. Some surgeons ask new employees to sign their copy, signifying their having read and understood the manual.

When developing personnel policies, certain topics should be considered and reduced to writing. These include office goals and philosophy, codes of ethics, employee rights, salary and fringe benefit packages, sick leaves and holidays, evaluations, professional development, and disciplinary actions.

Office Goals and Philosophy

Let staff know that patient care is your top priority and that the highest possible quality of care is your goal. State explicitly that all other office policies derive from this commitment—including office personnel policies—which means that you recognize the ultimate fairness of providing good pay and working conditions in return for good performance and shared commitment.

Code of Ethics

Because the legal system often holds physicians responsible for an employee's breach of conduct, such a policy has a second purpose: By demonstrating your active pursuit of the highest possible conduct by all office personnel, it places the responsibility for personnel conduct more squarely on employees. Specific rules should be spelled out: Staff will honor patient confidentiality, will not abuse drugs or alcohol, will not deliberately falsify office documents, and so on. Here is the place to require compliance with basic office rules—no excessive tardiness, observance of office hours, observance of a professional appearance in personal grooming and dress.

Employee Rights

Employees have rights as well as responsibilities and these too should be spelled out in the policy manual and reviewed by your attorney to ensure their accuracy and completeness. The legal system will not protect an employer whose arbitrary or capricious behavior or simple ignorance of relevant law results in the violation of an employee's rights.

Another provision of your policy on employee rights should cover an employee's right to voice complaints, air grievances, and appeal decisions that affect his working conditions. A sensible mechanism for voicing complaints can defuse otherwise explosive personnel problems. Key policy elements are:

1. If the complaint involves another employee, require the grieving employee first to talk out the problem directly with the other employee.
2. If they cannot resolve the situation between them, then require the employee to talk to his immediate supervisor.
3. If the situation is not resolved there, the employee may continue to appeal on up the chain of command until the buck stops in your office.

Salary and Fringe Benefit Package

It is almost impossible to compete successfully for top job candidates without a competitive salary and fringe benefit package.

Even if, without such a policy, you do manage to attract a highly competent individual, be prepared to lose them. High turnover, low productivity, unhappiness, and even enbezzlement are not unknown in offices that do not spell out how top performance of assigned duties will be rewarded and that bonuses might be earned for work above and beyond the call.

To learn your area's salary range for various medical office staff positions, contact the local medical society, the chamber of commerce, and local hospitals. Ask for the starting-, mid-, and high-point for each position.

Some simple rules for setting up a salary/fringe benefit package were shared by business consultant Roger L. Rusley in *Medical Economics* (June 11, 1984):

1. Set a minimum and maximum for each position. Tie these to each job description. Indicate that, if the job grows, so will the salary range—this gives employees incentive to take on new responsibilities.
2. Establish how an employee can move from minimum to maximum pay. Include a time frame. If the probationary period concludes with a satisfactory performance rating, for instance, note that the salary will increase by so much. A good rating after another 6 months might merit a second increase, with successive raises possible for each satisfactory annual performance rating.
3. Conduct performance or salary reviews regularly. Within 30 days of the date when an employee becomes eligible for a raise, you should conduct an official performance evaluation. Your policy might suggest that poor results would warrant probation for 30 days, followed by either award of the raise or termination. Says Rusley, "People on probation seldom overcome their problems, so you're probably just postponing the job of dismissal."
4. Spell out fringe benefits. Life, health, and disability insurance; medical and dental reimbursements; retirement plans—various combinations of these and other benefits frequently amount to as much as 25% of an employee's stated salary. Let employees see the full scope of your benefit package; competing employers will. "But keep bonuses unstructured," advises Rusley. "The regular $100 bonus every quarter soon becomes an expected salary supplement."
5. Give separate cost-of-living increases. On some date other than the day you award merit increases, take a look at your salary range for each job. Compare it to the annual inflation rate. Adjust the entire range upward accordingly, raising employee salaries to the new level. Employees should understand that cost-of-living increases may come automatically, but merit increases will not; they are tied to performance.
6. Start sharp new employees above the minimum. Says Rusley, "If you think they're worth it and they ask for it, give it." You may just have hired a receptionist who will grow into the job of office manager. "But don't hire at the maximum," warns Rusley, who believes that any new person needs time to catch onto your way of doing things.

Leaves and Holidays

How many days of paid sick leave will you grant (10 or 12 per year is standard)? Will any restrictions apply (you might restrict eligibility to employees who have worked with you at least 6 months).

Employees will expect a certain number of paid vacation days per year. You might increase the number granted with each additional year of employment, up to a certain maximum. Since the rationale behind vacation days is to give employees a needed respite from job duties, it is a good policy to require that vacation days be used in the year they are earned. This policy is fiscally responsible, too, because it means that you pay employees for days at the same rate at which they are earned.

A day or two of personal or emergency leave is also common practice. You might state that pay for such days will be awarded at your discretion and that each request is handled on an individual basis.

Leave for jury duty is something you must grant. Most employers state that they will pay the employee the difference (if any) between his daily rate and whatever per diem the government pays.

Evaluations

Evaluations of employee performance are both a management prerogative and a management necessity. And yet, evaluations must be employee-oriented. There is no payoff to secret, behind-closed-doors appraisals of performance that deny an employee an opportunity to hear charges against them.

The goal of evaluations, after all, is to enhance not punish performance. This requires a rather open, even-handed evaluation policy that states objective criteria against which performance will be measured and at what (regular) intervals evaluations will occur.

Evaluations may be as formal or informal as you like, although safeguards should be built into any procedure. You may choose to submit an employee to a period of official "observation," ask him to complete a self-evaluation that you then discuss together, rely on peer and/or patient appraisals, or any combination of these methods. Whichever you do, the procedure (to be legal) must include only job-related criteria and be based on direct observation of performance (not hearsay). It should include a means of appeal. Also, it should note that any deficiencies found will result in a plan of assistance to help the employee improve, and that good reports will result in either a bonus or raise (depending on your salary policy).

Professional Development

Many physicians require regular professional development activities. The rationale: Patient care improves as the staff improves. Most employees, you will find, appreciate the opportunity to upgrade their skills.

In-service training can be very informal (one facial plastic surgeon requires his nurses to read two professional magazines each month). More formal training opportunities might include: developing a library of videotapes on procedures you perform and conducting regular staff seminars with these visual aids, or paying registration fees for staff to attend training programs conducted by their professional associations. For a very promising staff member, you might want to offer tuition reimbursement for job-related courses at area institutions.

The importance of in-service training and continuing medical education cannot be overemphasized in the office surgical center. In the hospital, weekly in-service training sessions are routine. They enable staff to keep abreast of newer techniques and to obtain a more in-depth understanding as to the various principles behind certain practices or procedures.

It could be argued that nursing staff in the office setting obtain similar information on a daily basis by virtue of their increased personal exposure to the physician and by virtue of the fact that they function constantly under the doctor's direct supervision—much the same as would a medical student or resident on rotation. However, well-organized, formal sessions that address specific needs of the nursing staff are vital if the quality of patient care is to increase continually. Such educational programs are an integral part of the Accreditation Association for Ambulatory Health Care or the Joint Commission on Accreditation of Healthcare Organizations.

Considering the devastating consequences of acute cardiopulmonary problems that can be associated with surgery, it is imperative that the entire nursing staff be proficient in dealing with the various emergencies that can arise. In-service training sessions dealing with problems such as cardiac arrest, acute drug reactions, and hyperthermia are examples of how in-service training sessions can both serve to improve patient safety and be an integral component of overall facility risk-management.

Disciplinary Action

If a doctor sees an employee violate established office policy and fails to do anything about it, he gives tacit approval to the inappropriate conduct. This happens far too often in medical offices, largely because discipline is one of the most disagreeable of all management jobs.

Yet consider the effect on patient service if your nurse of 20 years gradually develops a serious drinking problem; or your promising young receptionist starts a family and requests increasing amounts of time off to handle childcare problems. In both cases, it's clear, job performance is affected critically.

Most employee problems creep up like this slowly, visible only after small offenses are repeated so often that they finally become critical. Either that, or they are evident before the initial probationary period concludes.

Three types of disciplinary actions are possible, and your policy should spell them out: a new or extended probationary period, suspension, or dismissal. State and federal regulations concerning termination and antidiscrimination laws can be very complex. You may wish to consult with an attorney specializing in employment law to be sure your actions are legal.

Dismissal obviously is easiest during the initial probationary period—no notice is required. If you cannot summon the courage to dismiss at that time, no doubt you will be even less able to do so in the years to come. If you have any doubts, extend the probationary period rather than offer the job with reservations.

Dismissal is much harder, legally and personally, the longer an employee has been with you. In some states you must afford your employee his due process rights under the law—that is, his right to hear complaints against him and to give his side of the story. And you must be able to provide proof of misconduct (Fig. 2-2).

The main task is to be able to back your decision with good personnel records. Written evaluations of performance, warning notes, letters showing your plans to assist the employee overcome deficiencies—all belong in the employee's file.

Personnel Records

Beyond documentation for disciplinary action, complete and up-to-date personnel records contain a wealth of management information. You need it all; to meet payroll requirements, file tax returns, administer your fringe benefit program, verify employment to credit agencies, control leaves and absences, and evaluate, promote, and transfer employees.

IF YOU MUST TERMINATE EMPLOYMENT

Should you give an employee two weeks' notice, or ask her to leave immediately now that the decision is made, the job is over?

Neither choice is right for every instance.

If a vital function will go unstaffed, you may want to ask the employee to continue—unless the reason for termination was behavior that grossly affected the health or safety of patients and staff. Or perhaps your partner is not in total agreement with your wish to terminate an employee you simply do not like. A compromise: Preserve your partnership, but give the employee time to find another job.

If no extenuating circumstances exist for giving notice, immediate termination is best. It is best to do it in your office, at the end of the day, at the end of the week, with only you and the employee present. (The presence of another employee in the outer offices is advisable for your personal security.) Have ready the employee's personnel folder, all reasons for termination carefully documented. Also have a check made out for a sum that includes wages due to that hour, compensation for any unused vacation time, and any severance pay offered in lieu of notice. If appropriate, have a letter of reference ready, too.

Be honest and helpful, stating your case without interruption. This will help you retain command of the situation and impart a sense of finality to it. Do not conclude before having asked for the return of office keys or other property.

Some physicians ask employees to sign a form stating that they understand the reasons for their termination. This goes into their permanent file.

Another tip: Depending on the reason for termination, you may want to change locks and any security codes for office alarm systems.

Figure 2-2.

Some medical offices separate their records into operating files (current employees) and permanent files (those who are no longer with you). Operating files sometimes are further divided into those of applicants, those of assigned employees, and those for payroll purposes of assigned employees.

Employee records should be accessible, but confidential. Employees have a right in some states to review their contents whenever they ask. You should review contents of all files at least annually, or whenever an employee leaves. Permanent files can be stored out of the main business office, and the rule of thumb is, if a file is not referred to for 5 years, discard it.

Nepotism

Hiring friends or relatives is almost always a disaster. Partners feel they have no control over the "special" employee and staff cannot appreciate the inevitable special exemptions from duty or special privileges. You may find that you have hired someone you cannot fire. Best to set the no-relative-as-employee policy early in your medical career.

RECRUITING AND INTERVIEWING

Screening job candidates is a difficult and time-consuming task. For this reason, many physicians choose to turn over the job to an employment agency, which will want a job description from you, and a considerable sum of money.

For what often amounts to thousands of dollars (usually a percentage of the annual salary you offer the applicant), agencies will weed out all but those individuals who fit the description you provide.

Local medical societies, in some areas, also provide this service. Others catalog resumes of would-be medical office staffers and local physicians are welcome to browse.

If you want to find and screen your own employees, try looking first at technical training schools in the area. These institutions, which provide special training for paramedics, secretaries, and others, are eager to place their graduates—many of whom make up in energy and ambition what they may lack in experience.

Another source of excellent help are your colleagues and friends. Word of mouth spreads amazingly fast among the medical community, and the extensive network almost always produces results.

Some physicians wish to remain more anonymous in their search for candidates. For them, a discreet notice can be placed in the newspaper (asking that inquiries be sent to an anonymous box office number) or on a bulletin board notice located in an area where likely candidates might see it.

Whether a candidate comes to you prescreened by an agency or unscreened from the newspaper, it is still up to you to ask the questions that tell you whether this person is the right person.

There are two things to keep in mind as you interview. The first is that questions helpful to a personnel manager in a large industrial plant may not be entirely helpful to you, and the second is that the law does not allow you to ask many questions that, on the surface, sound perfectly innocent.

You undoubtedly will share any personnel manager's keen interest in a candidate's appearance, intelligence, skills, honesty, reliability, education, and so on. Yet, as head of a small office, you must go deeper and look for a personality that is compatible with you and other employees.

"In a large industrial plant, incompatibility might not create a problem (because an employee can be transferred), but in a small office, it is crucial," says industrial psychologist Robert M. Hecht. His case files show that "personality conflicts" account for 80% of the failures to select the right person for the right job.

To get at key personality traits, you cannot merely rehash what's on an application, says Hecht in *Medical Economics* (September 13, 1982). His suggestions:

- Ask which previous boss the applicant liked the best, and why. If she cannot stand "bossy types," she probably will not get along with your no-nonsense office manager.
- Ask how the applicant handles it when she opposes a decision made by her current boss.
- Ask why the applicant thinks he or she will succeed at this job. The person probably does not have a good understanding of the job if she responds, "Oh, it sounds interesting" or "It's glamorous to work in a doctor's office" or "There's no overtime, is there?"
- Ask what might cause the applicant to fail at the job. If she admits to getting queasy at the sight of blood, or thinks it might be depressing to be around patients all day, she is not the person for you. Nor is she, perhaps, if she cannot bring herself to ask patients about delinquent bills.
- Ask how the person would like you to assist her if she gets the job. You will be looking for the perfect answer, that the person expects to learn, ask questions, proceed under supervision, then ultimately wean herself and work independently. What you want to listen for is any sign that the person will be too independent or remain dependent forever.

Listening is the key to a successful interview. Too many interviewers do all the talking. Instead, take time to put the applicant at ease and ask some "netural-friendly" questions to establish rapport. Talk enough to make sure the potential employee gets a good understanding of the job, but then ask questions that let the applicant tell you about himself.

There are some questions you may not ask. There are specific laws and regulations that restrict the questions you may ask either in interviews or on job application forms. Although it is fine to ask anything related to the ability to perform the job, questions that even hint at discrimination in hiring practices must be avoided.

You may ask, for instance, a woman's full name but not her maiden name, unless she worked under her maiden name and you must know it to check her work record. Likewise, you may ask an applicant's current mailing address and length of time there, but you may not ask where the person lived previously. Ask about convictions only, not arrests. Ask a person's age or birthdate only if it relates to the job (a requisite of bonding, for instance). Ask about impairments that would interfere with the job, but stay away from questions about pregnancy, contraceptives, family planning, disability, past treatment for particular diseases. Ask about ability to work overtime, but not whether any religious beliefs affect availability. Ask about language skills if job related, but do not inquire about ancestry, national origin, mother's native tongue.

You may ask whom to contact in case of an emergency. Checking references is absolutely permissible, as is inquiring into past work experience and special skills. Do not ask, however, for a spouse's name or place of employment, childcare arrangements, height or weight, race or creed.

When the interview is over, tell each applicant that there are a few more people you plan to talk with, and that you will contact her in a week or so. This gives you time not only to talk to other applicants, but also to check references and prepare for a second interview with the top three candidates. In a second interview, facets of an applicant's personality often surface that remained hidden or unnoticed at the first.

ORIENTATION

Orientation is whatever happens to employees that first day or week on the job. Done well, it will start them off smoothly. Done poorly, it can turn them off forever.

A good approach requires an uninterrupted period of time, during which the employee is introduced to other staff members as well as to office protocol. Give her enough information to get her through the first day with minimal confusion, and if she is new to the community, be sure to tell her about banks, restaurants, and other area features.

Gradual immersion in the complexities of the job works better than the drill sergeant approach. Let someone experienced explain and demonstrate how insurance forms are filled out, for instance; then let the new employee perform the tasks under supervision; leave her with written instructions for future reference but check in and monitor her work so no bad habits settle in early.

Several orientation steps are especially important in a medical office—teaching empathy for patients, warning of medical and legal pitfalls, and stressing the importance of patient confidentiality.

Also teach independence. Your time is valuable. Set guidelines about when you should be interrupted and when not. These, together with the office policy manual, should give you the framework you need to put together a solid staff.

CHAPTER 2 ADDENDUM: STAFFING AN OFFICE SURGICAL FACILITY

THE HIRING PROCESS

This section on the hiring process is reprinted with permission from *Practice Personnel System* published by Practice Personnel Systems, 21476-H Lake Forest Drive, El Toro, California 92630. The editors wish to thank Dr. Bent Ericksen for this important contribution. The editors have found Dr. Ericksen's publication, *Practice Personnel System*, to be excellent and highly recommend it to physicians and office managers.

HOW TO ATTRACT QUALITY STAFF

No management function is more critical than the ability to hire qualified and competent people.

The Small Business Administration states that one of the reasons so many businesses fail is because of poorly selected employees.

Most doctors agree that their success depends on their ability to surround themselves with a skilled and dedicated staff.

One doctor who had experienced a number of staff changes in a short time put the above statement in perspective when he said "unless I can hire good staff, I'm not going to make it".

Going through a staff change can be a time of severe stress for everyone in the practice. There is the fear of hiring a stranger, and the important questions of, how well will she fit in? How well will she relate to the patients? Will she have the necessary skills to do the job? Can she handle my "special situation" here in the office? How long will she stay with me? How long will it take to find the new staff member? What will it cost in terms of time, advertising and lost production? Will we need to get a temporary to fill in? etc. etc.

If it takes a prolonged time to find a replacement, or the practice has to go through several new hires before finding the right person, the damage to morale and production can be severe.

And to complicate matters, it is becoming increasingly difficult to find and hire staff at any level of experience. And once hired, staff don't stay long. The average staff member will stay in one office for an average of 21 months and then go to work for another office or leave the profession entirely. The cost of each staff member turnover is between $10,000 - $12,000, although in many cases it can be much higher.

Dr. Phil Whitener told his audience at a seminar nine years ago, "times have changed and we better change with it". Most doctors are doing an excellent job in keeping their clinical skills updated to meet the needs of their patients, while not aware that their staff has needs, and that those needs have changed and are not being met.

HOW TO ATTRACT QUALITY STAFF (cont'd)

The noted author, lecturer and management consultant Peter Drucker writes that "employees are a companies greatest resource". Can we afford to continue to neglect the needs of the doctor's greatest resource, the staff?, and what are those needs anyway?

Recent surveys show that the attitude of employees have changed. They are more interested in the quality of work life than the quantity of work output. And they interpret quality of work life to mean "a place where they can be recognized as an individual - where they can have the opportunity to develop a sense of self-worth and self-fulfillment".

Let's take a look at another study. John Cotton, assistant professor of organizational behavior at Purdue's Krannert School of Management says that most studies show a weak correlation between job satisfaction and productivity. What they find is a correlation the other way, "the more productive a worker is, the happier he is on the job."

In the author's survey, here is what the staff said would contribute to their productiveness and sense of satisfaction on the job. We call it working within a "Success-directed Climate".

PERFORMANCE FACTORS

THOSE QUALITIES THAT RELATE TO AN INDIVIDUAL'S ABILITY AND MOTIVATION NECESSARY TO FUNCTION EFFECTIVELY WITHIN A SPECIFIC POSITION.

ANALYTICAL ABILITY: Able to evaluate and categorize pertinent information needed for the planning and performance of duties.

ATTENTION TO DETAILS: Aware of the details and attends to them. Good memory.

DECISIVENESS: Can make a decision and come to a final conclusion.

MANUAL DEXTERITY: A talent for using tools or instruments.

MENTAL ALERTNESS: Comprehension. Anticipates unusual occurrences and is prepared to act immediately. Understands directions quickly.

ORGANIZATIONAL ABILITY: Able to take a concept and put it into operation. Can organize materials, activities and time.

RESOURCEFULNESS: Ability to devise new methods in an imaginative and practical way.

RESPONSIBILITY: Carries through with duties and commitments.

SELF CONFIDENCE: Convinced of one's personal ability to achieve goals.

SELF DIRECTION: Perceives what needs to be done and proceeds with a minimum of supervision.

PERSONAL DISPOSITION FACTORS

PERSONAL DISPOSITION FACTORS ARE THOSE QUALITIES WHICH DETERMINE AN INDIVIDUAL'S COMPATIBILITY AND EFFECTIVENESS IN DEALING WITH OTHERS.

ABILITY TO HANDLE CRITICISM: Can accept critique without feeling personally rejected.

ADAPTABILITY: Maintains flexibility to accommodate the needs of the doctor as well as those of the patients.

ATTITUDE: Desire to do the job as well as possible. Responds to instructions with interest and concern.

CREDIBILITY: Sincerity in dealing with patients. Trustworthiness as an employee.

ENTHUSIASM: The energetic, dynamic quality that inspires others.

FRIENDLINESS: Realistic empathy and concern for others.

OBJECTIVITY: Separates facts from feelings. Able to remain poised and level-headed.

PERSUASIVENESS: That extra energy that gives importance to a message.

STABILITY: Will maintain a friendly and cooperative attitude, even while working under pressure. Will not be negatively influenced by the moods and reactions of others.

VERBAL SKILLS: Communicates effectively with staff and patients.

That's a lot to ask for. It's easy to understand the feelings of helplessness a doctor experiences when faced with the challenge of having to hire a new staff member. With the many requirements imposed by state and federal laws and regulations, a good hiring process must include steps to minimize the risk of litigation later. Charges of discrimination, wrongful discharge, emotional stress, etc., are common, and the cost to the employer in terms of anxiety, lost time/lost production, legal fees, and damages rewarded the former employee, can have devastating economic consequences for the small professional employer.

Through many years of trial and error, we have developed a hiring technology that works - a systematic technique that takes much of the guesswork out of hiring. We call it.

SIX STEPS TO SUCCESSFUL HIRING.

STEP 1. **DEFINE JOB RESPONSIBILITIES.**

Write a detailed job description. Use the job description located in the JOB DESCRIPTION section. Here are the key elements to consider:

* **TITLE:** title of position.

* **STATUS:** exempt or non-exempt. (The term "exempt" means from the requirements to be paid overtime. Non-exempt staff members must be paid overtime.)

* **RESPONSIBILITY:** a statement of the major purpose and function of the position.

* **SUPERVISION:** who assigns, reviews and approves the work.

* **DUTIES:** describe the specific tasks in order of importance. State frequency i.e., daily, weekly, etc.

* **AUTHORITY:** what authority (the right to command, influence or judge) is vested in the position. Make clear what decisions the person is responsible for making, and what decisions are reserved for management — for example: "can spend up to $125.00 for supplies without prior approval").

* **ADDITIONAL INFORMATION:** list any other information that would be of help in understanding the responsibilities of the job.

SIX STEPS TO SUCCESSFUL HIRING (cont'd)

STEP 2.   **ATTRACT APPLICANTS.**

In his book THE ART OF NEGOTIATING Herbert Cohen writes: "if you want to deal effectively with people you have to approach them based on **their** needs."

Staff has told us what their needs are.

a. If it doesn't presently exist, it's now time to create that Success-Directed Climate.

b. Decide what you have to offer. How much are you willing to pay? What is the salary scale - entry level and top? The date of the next increase? and how much?

c. Do you have an incentive program? What is the ending date of the present program? Will you extend the date or start another program - or do you know yet?

CAUTION: If you hire a new staff member and have told her that the practice has an incentive or bonus program, without also saying that this program may be discontinued at any time, you are leaving her with a false impression that is sure to cause problems later.

d. What benefits do you provide? Healthcare, vacations, holidays, sick-leave/well pay, etc.?

e. Consider what you are willing to commit to regarding training. How and where will the training take place? Who will do the training? (on the job, management consultant, seminars, etc.). How much will the training cost? Is that expense planned for in the budget?

f. How much skill and experience do you require the new person to have in each of the areas covered by the job description. In what areas of expertise are you willing to compromise? (refer to JOB DESCRIPTIONS and THE EMPLOYMENT INTERVIEW EVALUATION FORMS).

SIX STEPS TO SUCCESSFUL HIRING (cont'd)

WHERE TO FIND APPLICANTS

Sources:

- Friends and acquaintances of your present staff.
- Suppliers.
- Vendors.
- Employment agencies.
- Professional Associations.
- State Employment Development Department.
- Patients.
- Advertisement in one or more newspapers through an effectively written classified ad.

HOW TO WRITE AN EFFECTIVE AD

The following are guidelines to assist you in composing employment advertisements for filling positions in your practice.

When writing the ad use the 100-year-old AIDA PRINCIPLE for effective advertising, generate: **Attention, Interest, Desire, Action.**

Do not abbreviate words in the ad.

TITLE OF POSITION:

What you want to draw is an executive secretary type of personality with the skills to handle the variety of important front office responsibilities.

Use as descriptive a title for the position as possible. Say "Appointment secretary", "Financial Secretary", "Front Office Secretary" or "Dental secretary" as the title best applies to the position you are trying to fill.

SIX STEPS TO SUCCESSFUL HIRING (cont'd)

Do not call the position "Receptionist", since that is a misnomer for the front office position in most healthcare offices. (A receptionist is a person who directs people and phone calls and handles matters that do not require the skills and responsibilities inherent with the front office position. The quality person you are looking for will not respond to an ad calling for a receptionist).

DIRECT ANSWER ADVERTISEMENTS GET THE BEST RESULTS:

- Use both day and evening telephone number for an immediate response.

- Requirements to answer to a P. O. Box gets very little response. (Unless you are looking for a partner, associate or a manager/administrator for a large practice).

USE WORDS THAT DESCRIBE THE JOB IN AN APPEALING WAY:

Words like: Meaningful, Responsible, Quality, Challenging, Rewarding, Special, Caring, Pleasant, Friendly, Great doctor to work for, etc.

Do not use words like: 5 day week, group practice, busy office, fast-paced, downtown (unless parking is free).

CAUTION: To avoid legal problems later, <u>do not</u> either verbally or in writing, <u>anywhere</u> during the hiring process use words like: Career opportunity, long term employment, permanent employment, or any words that might imply other than an "At Will" employment relationship.

<u>State absolute requirements only:</u>

For Example:

- Typing.
- Insurance Processing.
- X-ray license.
- RDA Licence.
- Expanded duties.
- Bookkeeper.
- Computer experience.

SIX STEPS TO SUCCESSFUL HIRING (cont'd)

Mention benefits that will draw applicants:

- Medical insurance.

- Four-day work week (or number of hours if less than 40).

- Bonus or Incentive Plan. (Be careful here. Refer to Step 2c above.)

- A specific high salary that you are willing to pay a quality person with top qualifications - <u>follow that amount with "if qualified"</u>. Make the figure realistic and attainable. Since no one is going to do as well the first few months on the job as they are required to after six to twelve months, you can start the person out with less than the stated amount. And yes, this is both ethical and legal, and if the salary is at the high end of what competition is paying for a like job, you are more likely to draw quality applicants.

- Will train (if that's the case).

Mention the qualities that portray an attractive office image.

- Modern

- Quality oriented

- Growing

- Desirable area

- Team oriented

- Warm, caring, friendly

EXAMPLES OF EFFECTIVE ADVERTISEMENT FOR STAFF

R D A

Cheerful, warm, enthusiastic and very special are the words that best describe our dental team and office environment. We seek your superior chairside expertise and caring personality to help provide quality care for our fine patients. Excellent benefits. $ _____ if qualified. Ph. # _____ . Location _____ .

DENTAL SECRETARY

We seek a very special person to join our enthusiastic, warm and very dedicated dental team. Must be experienced in all facets of front office duties. If you are that person, you will love this pleasant and professional work environment. $ _____ if qualified. Phone # _____ . Location _____ .

SIX STEPS TO SUCCESSFUL HIRING (cont'd)

DENTAL SECRETARY

We are looking for an outgoing, efficient people person to complement our great team of dental professionals. Beautiful modern office and a pleasant quality oriented work environment. $ _____ if qualified. Phone # _____. Location _____.

STEP 3. EVALUATE APPLICANTS.

    A. WHEN APPLICANTS CALL IN RESPONSE TO THE AD.

    The primary goal is to briefly qualify the applicant and to sustain or increase an interest in the position.

        1. Ask questions regarding caller's work experience. (If you have decided that you <u>must</u> have an RDA with ortho experience and the applicant has never worked in a orthodontic office, there is no point in going any further).

        2. Briefly answer questions about the job. Answer questions about salary with "the salary will be determined during an interview with the doctor and will depend on your qualifications. The doctor does believe in paying an excellent salary for the right person" (or words to that effect).

        3. Encourage applicant to come in to fill out an application. If this is not possible, offer to mail one.

        4. Give the name and address of the practice.

    B. WHEN APPLICANTS ARRIVE IN THE OFFICE.

    The purpose here is to get as much information about an applicant as possible in order for the employer to decide whether to interview or not to interview. Interviewing as many applicants as possible does not ensure that the best person is picked for the job. (A survey reported in ROBERT HALF ON HIRING states that when several people were interviewed the person interviewed last would get the job 55.8% of the time).

    It is important to maintain good public relations throughout the screening and interviewing process. Look upon every applicant as a potential patient and treat them with the same courtesy and respect.

SIX STEPS TO SUCCESSFUL HIRING (cont'd)

1. A good screening process starts at the first personal contact with the applicant. Use the PRE-INTERVIEW REACTION FORM to start the information gathering process. The purpose of the form is to record your impression of the person's voice, appearance, mannerism, attitude or anything of an unusual or informative nature.

2. Give each applicant an APPLICATION FOR OFFICE EMPLOYMENT FORM* to complete.

    * The PPS APPLICATION FOR MEDICAL AND DENTAL OFFICE EMPLOYMENT FORMS have been specially designed for the medical and dental professions and comply with all federal and state legislative requirements. The information provides the doctor with the necessary information about an applicant with which to decide to interview or not to interview. This three page form may be ordered directly from our office. (please specify your preference - the dental, chiropractic or medical form?)

3. Review the application form after it has been completed and is being returned. Make sure all the questions have been answered and the applicant has signed and dated the form.

4. Answer any questions and inform the applicant that "Doctor (name) will review all the applications and the applicants he feels are qualified will be called within the next few days to set up an interview."

STEP 4. THE EMPLOYMENT INTERVIEW

An employment interview may be conducted with job applicants _if_ the information received on the employment application, test results or other sources indicate the applicant meets the specific requirements of the job. The purpose of the interview is to confirm and build upon the information you already have.

CAUTION: Be careful to adhere to all Equal Opportunity Employment Laws and Regulations. Don't ask questions you cannot legally ask. (Refer to LEGAL PRE-EMPLOYMENT INQUIRY GUIDE.)

SIX STEPS TO SUCCESSFUL HIRING (cont'd)

Although you may not be able to ask the following questions directly, here are **the real questions** you want to have been answered when you are through with the interview: How smart are you? How skilled are you? Do you work hard? Can you work and share authority and decisions with others? Do you have a reasonably satisfying personal life that will not interfere with work? Do you like yourself? Can we enjoy working together? Do you take care of yourself? How do you behave when you are angry, scared or frustrated? Are you honest? How dependable and loyal a person are you? How long will you stay? What do you want from this job? What do you want from me?

Here is what usually happens during an interview - and the reasons most interviews are ineffective:

* The employer does most of the talking.

* A decision is made during the first few minutes based on first impressions.

* Non-job related negatives are given more weight than job-related positives. (Children, divorced, clothing, wealthy, too heavy, too old.)

* Time is spent on irrelevant topics - what is relevant is neglected.

To interview effectively, and to get all the information you need within the proper and **legal boundaries**, is both a skill and an art. Here are some practical steps to take:

A. **The Preparation**

1. Know the information you must gain from the interview. Study the items needed to assist you. They are: The Employment Application Form, The Employment Interview Evaluation Form and related forms, and Useful Questions for Interviewers. For questions you cannot legally ask, refer to: Legal Pre-Employment Inquiry Guide.

2. Review all the information you have available about the applicant from the Pre-Interview Reaction Form, the Application form, resume, letters of recommendation, other sources, etc. Also consider that studies have proven that applicants provide false information about 67% of the time.

3. Highlight the areas you need to discuss during the interview and write down any additional information you need to receive from the applicant.

SIX STEPS TO SUCCESSFUL HIRING (cont'd)

4. Set up a convenient time for the interview so you won't feel rushed.

5. Hold the interview in a place where you can have privacy.

6. Do not allow interruptions from phone calls or other staff members while the interview is taking place.

B. **The Process**

1. As an interviewer, your primary job is to ask questions, to listen and observe the response. A good rule of thumb is that the applicant should do about 75% of the talking.

2. The first thing to do is to create a relaxed, stress-free atmosphere where both you and the applicant can feel relaxed. Make every effort to put the applicant at ease, be friendly and courteous. Be seated in such a way that you don't have any large object, such as a desk, between yourself and the applicant. Your objective is to create an environment that invites trust and straightforward communication.

   It's common for the interviewer to be a little nervous. You tend to remember the stress everyone is going through in the office, and the importance of making the right hiring decision. Just start talking. In fact, during the first part of the interview is where the personnel professionals do most of their share of talking. Talking releases nervous energy, and people tend to relax at the sound of their own voice. Small talk like: "Did you have any problems finding the office?" "What do you think of this rather lengthy application form?" "It gave me some excellent information about your background and brought you here - and I sure appreciate you taking the time.

   You are doing fine and now that you are both feeling relaxed, just continue talking.

3. Give pertinent information about the practice: patients, general business philosophy, work schedule, benefits, working conditions and environment, etc., and describe the various job responsibilities very clearly. Then move on to the actual interview.

SIX STEPS TO SUCCESSFUL HIRING (cont'd)

4. Ask questions and <u>listen with a purpose</u>: Are your questions being answered? <u>Listen for meaning</u>: What is she really telling me? And listen without interrupting or correcting the speaker. Do not use stress interview techniques (like asking applicants to demonstrate how they would collect a bill from a patient.) Ask open ended questions, that require more than a "yes" or "no" response. Open ended questions begin with a "what", "how", and "why." Be careful to ask "why" or "how come" questions in a nurturing or factual, rather than a judgmental tone of voice.

   Let the applicant talk. You can nod your head at appropriate points, make neutral statements like "I understand," "uh-huh" and compliment the applicant where fitting. Don't interrupt unless the applicant strays off the subject and you need an answer. Avoid disagreeing. An interview is an opportunity for you to get information, not to make a point.

   Pausing is a powerful tool for getting another person to talk. When you ask a question (and ask only one question at time,) give the applicant time to answer it. If necessary, use the pause to create the psychological pressure to respond. Frequently the applicant will add more to an answer if the interviewer doesn't immediately go on to another question.

   Make summary statements of facts. After you have gathered information, for instance, about what the applicant liked best and least on the last job, you can summarize the contents of that information and then pause. The chances are that the applicant will add more to what you have stated.

   You might make a statement that reflects back what you have perceived. This is sometimes referred to as "active listening."

   If the applicant has told you about something unpleasant you might say something like, "I understand you were feeling upset about that." This is likely to invite further comment.

5. Check out the information you have received from the application form, resume and other sources. Ask questions about job record and gaps of time between employment. Clear up discrepancies wherever you find them. Ask about prior pay and present wage requirements, etc.

6. Ask about each job the applicant has held, specific duties, job responsibilities. Ask what specific contributions the applicant made to the success of that prior employer's practice.

7. The length of the interview will depend upon the type of job you are trying to fill or how the applicant is responding to your questions. It can be as short as a few minutes or take one or even two hours.

SIX STEPS TO SUCCESSFUL HIRING (cont'd)

8. A final decision depends on a careful consideration of the skills and personality factors of the candidate. In evaluating prospective staff members, it is essential to appraise the "whole person". Job applicants bring with them their life script (hopefully it is: I am OK, you are OK), diverse experiences, family environment, their unique circumstances and possible problems. All of this, and much more, will affect their performance on the job.

9. The purpose of the interview is to share information. In order for the employer to get the necessary data about an applicant on which to base a sound hiring decision, it's important that the conversation be as frank and forthright as possible. The interviewer will know that a question is probing a sensitive area when the applicant responds in one of the following ways:

   - A sudden change of pace in talking or in the rate of reply.

   - An attempt to change the subject or to laugh it off.

   - Sudden nervousness, blushing, stammering, fidgeting.

   - Not answering the question.

   - Insists on giving more information before answering.

   - Repeats the question either loud or to self.

   - Asks another question back.

   - "I don't remember".

   - Defends, rationalizes or justifies.

   - "What did you say, I didn't hear you".

   - Being vague, inaudible, or apologetic.

   - Silence.

   - "I would rather not talk about it".

   - Gives more than one answer.

   - When the question "How do you feel about .....?", is followed by these words: "that, she/he, they, if, how, it, my, you, or whenever", your question is not being answered.

   Take into consideration that an applicant is likely to be nervous and therefore not interview to best advantage. If you suspect this to be true and are interested, you may want to schedule a second interview.

SIX STEPS TO SUCCESSFUL HIRING (cont'd)

10. At the point you decide that the individual does not meet your requirements, it's time to discontinue the interview. Do not leave anyone hopeful of a job she will never get. A short statement such as the following is in order:

    "You have some good qualifications, they do not, however, meet the job requirements. I appreciate your time and interest - it's been a pleasure to talk to you. Good luck in your job hunting". (No further explanation is necessary)

    If you say "no" clearly at the time of the interview, you will not waste time later with needless phone calls or letters.

11. **If you like the applicant at this point, ask these questions:**

    * As you probably know, every employer is now legally required to inspect certain documents to verify employment eligibility status. Should you be hired will you be able to show us the documents that will verify that you are legally authorized to work in this country? (Refer to section THE NEW FEDERAL IMMIGRATION LAW.)

    * What additional information can you give me that I should know about you at this point?

    * What else would you like to know about the job? The practice? The staff? anything else?

    * We have a Staff Policy Manual that spells out several commitments the doctor and staff has made to each other, and we are all obligated to live by these commitments. Do you think that making such a commitment will be a problem for you?

    * Can vacations be arranged around the office schedule?

    * When would you be available for employment?

    * May I contact your present and prior employers? Is there anything I should know before talking to them? What do you expect your references to tell me? Why?

    * End the interview with a clear understanding of the applicants continued interest.

    * Give a date by which the applicant will be notified.

SIX STEPS TO SUCCESSFUL HIRING (cont'd)

C. The Post-Interview Evaluation

1. Immediately after the interview:

    a. Write your comments and finalize your evaluation using the EMPLOYMENT INTERVIEW EVALUATION FORM.

    b. Review the notes you have made. What does the factual information you have received add up to?

    c. Relax and concentrate on how you feel about the applicant. Mentally, see her on the job, responding to you, the staff and the patients. Is the total feeling good or bad?

STEP 5. CHECKING REFERENCES

MOST DIFFICULTIES AFTER HIRING RESULT FROM AN EMPLOYER NOT CHECKING REFERENCES.

"The single most important indicator of how an employee will perform in the future appears to be how he or she has performed in the past. Employees with a history of success tends to continue their successful performance. The others, despite their best intentions, rarely are able to turn over a new leaf." Arthur A. Witkin, Chief psychologist, Personnel Sciences Center, New York, NY.

Each applicant is expected to furnish information concerning their work history. Although business references are of more value, personal references are also important. For personal references, request business or professional people who are not related to the applicant.

The person who has conducted the employment interview should also carry out the reference checks. If possible speak to two persons the applicant has worked for on each job; the immediate supervisor and that person's superior. Be cautious about any extreme comments you hear, good or bad, unless they are verified from other sources.

SIX STEPS TO SUCCESSFUL HIRING (cont'd)

Many former employers fear being sued for defamation of character and will only, as a matter of policy, furnish information concerning a former employee's dates of employment, position held and final wage rate. However, it is worth noting that no employer is legally prohibited from furnishing, upon special request from an authorized source, a truthful statement concerning a person's work performance, the reason for a former employee's discharge or voluntary termination.

Questions to ask a former employer when checking references:

1. Was he/she punctual and conscientious in carrying out work assignments?

2. What was applicant's beginning and ending date of employment?

3. What was applicant's salary at termination?

4. Why did he/she leave employment?

5. How was applicant's punctuality and attendance history?

6. Would you rehire the applicant?

7. What were the applicant's major job responsibilities?

8. How would you rate the applicant's quality of work?

9. How would you rate the applicant's quantity of work?

10. How would you characterize the relationship between the applicant and other employees?

12. What were the applicant's principal strengths? Outstanding successes? Significant failures?

13. How would you compare the applicant's performance with the performance of others with similar responsibilities?

14. Were you satisfied with the applicant's management skills? (If applicable.)

15. How would you describe the applicant's success in training, developing and motivating subordinates? (If applicable.)

16. What other information do you have that would help to develop a more complete picture of the applicant?

SIX STEPS TO SUCCESSFUL HIRING (cont'd)

STEP 6. **THE DECISION**

Make a decision as quickly as possible - good people don't stay unemployed for long. If you need to interview one or two of the candidates a second time, do so right away.

CAUTION: Involving your staff in the decision making process is usually not a good idea. (There are some exceptions which we will discuss later). Here is why:

- Staff are not skilled interviewers, nor have they been privy to all pertinent information about the applicant. Therefore, they can only give an opinion based on feelings and not on facts.

- If you are not very satisfied with the performance of your present staff and are trying to hire someone with superior skills, your present staff is likely to recommend someone that is not going to show them off. The superior person will be rejected. If you take their advice what have you gained?

- If you hire someone they did not recommend, they will soon prove that **your** selection was wrong.

Involve the staff in the decision making process only if: 1) you are very happy with the quality of your present staff, 2) you have two equally qualified applicants, and 3) you are willing to hire the person they recommend.

Evaluate each applicant against the other applicants you have interviewed. Review all the following sources of information. However, none of these items should be relied upon solely, or given disproportionate weight.

. The Pre-Interview Reaction Form.

. The Employment Application Form.

. License Verification (If applicable).

. Copies of certificate of training.

. Resume.

. Your notes on the Employment Interview Information Form.

. References from prior employers.

. Bonding Verification. (if applicable)

. Test results to ascertain skill and potential job performance. (if applicable.)

SIX STEPS TO SUCCESSFUL HIRING (cont'd)

Document your reasons for hiring or not hiring each of the applicants. This documentation will assist you if charged with discrimination. Save those records for a period of 24 months. However, should you receive information that a charge of discrimination has been filed, or might be filed, all relevant records and files must be retained until the complaint has been fully and finally resolved.

Make your decision, call the applicant right away and make the job offer. (In today's job market you can expect to have to negotiate, before getting that final yes. I suggest you lay the groundwork during the interview as to approximate wages, benefits, etc. that you might be willing to offer, to avoid any surprises at this point.)

Mail the CONFIRMATION OF EMPLOYMENT letter to the new staff member.

CAUTION: There will be times when you decide to make the job offer prior to having checked references. If that's the case, make the offer pending upon receiving a satisfactory response from the references. However, if you later withdraw the offer, be prepared to have to prove in court that you had a valid reason to change your mind, (the applicant may claim to have lost out on another job opportunity.) It just isn't worth the potential trouble; check references first, then make the offer.

After your offer has been accepted, call the other applicants you interviewed and inform them of your decision.

Answer the applicants who call to inquire why they didn't get the job with, "We have hired the person who best matched our job requirements". You are not obligated to give more information.

The Personnel File

Create a Personnel File for the new staff member. Place the records and forms you have used to make your hiring decision in that file. (Refer to The Personnel File section in THE DOCTORS ADMINISTRATIVE CONTROL MANUAL OR THE PERSONNEL FILE KIT.)

USEFUL QUESTIONS FOR INTERVIEWERS

Below are listed some useful questions grouped into various subject areas.

Work Experience:

1. What do you think are your strongest qualities, skills or abilities?

2. How long did you work at - - - ?

3. What did you find most attractive about the job?

4. What did you find the least attractive about the job?

5. What specific skills did you learn - - - ?

6. How did you get along with your supervisor(s)?

7. How did you get along with your co-workers?

8. Were you ever disciplined? Why?

9. Were you ever praised or recognized for your work? Why?

10. How did you feel about your progress at - - - ?

11. Describe the best boss you ever had? The worst one?

12. If you could make one suggestion to your last employer, what would it be?

13. Do you feel you were treated fairly at - - - ?

14. Would you rate your work as excellent, good, fair or poor?

15. Do you have any special abilities or talents that were never recognized by - - - ?

16. Please describe in detail the kind of work you did in your last job.

17. Why did you specifically leave each of your former jobs? If currently employed, also ask: Why do you want to leave your present job?

18. Describe the type of criticism most frequently made of your work by former employers.

USEFUL QUESTIONS FOR INTERVIEWERS cont'd

Leisure Activities and Interests.

1. What are your leisure activities that you feel will make you a better employee?
2. What led you to these activities?
3. Have you ever had any part time work of special interest to you? What?
4. What talents or interests do you have?
5. What extracurricular activities are you involved in?

Attendance and Punctuality

1. How many days of work have you missed the last 2 years? For what reasons?
2. How many times were you late or left early in the last two years?
3. What do you think constitutes having a good attendance record?
4. What illnesses or accidents have caused you to miss work?
5. What do you consider a legitimate reason for missing work?

Education and Training

1. What was your major course of study?
2. Why did you select that?
3. What courses did you prefer? Why?
4. What courses did you dislike? Why?
5. What school did you attend? Why?
6. Who was your favorite teacher? Why?
7. What training have you had that would help you in this position?
8. Do you anticipate obtaining further training or education? In what areas?

USEFUL QUESTIONS FOR INTERVIEWERS cont'd

Motivation

1. What led you to apply for work here?
2. What are your reasons for working generally?
3. What do you know about us?
4. Why do you think this would be a good place to work?
5. What have you done that you are proud of?
6. What part of your education did you pay for?
7. What are your short-term career goals?
8. What are your long-term career goals?
9. What would you want to avoid in future jobs?
10. In your past jobs, has anyone tried to hold you back or keep you from getting ahead?
11. What does "success" mean to you?
12. What do you consider to be the most important quality for being successful?

Persuasive Skills

1. What sales work have you done?
2. What kind of training in sales do you have?
3. What school activities involved persuasion?
4. What do you do to convince others to agree with you?

Social Skills

1. How do you get along with others?
2. What do other people think of you?
3. Have you ever been selected as a leader or representative of a group?
4. What are your best social skills?
5. Do you prefer group or one-to-one situations? Why?

USEFUL QUESTIONS FOR INTERVIEWERS cont'd

Comunication Skills

1. What speech or communication courses have you taken?

2. What speeches have you given in the past?

3. What is important in communicating with others?

4. What kinds of written communication have you composed? Describe them.

5. What further information would you like to add about your qualifications? Yourself?

LEGAL PRE-EMPLOYMENT INQUIRY GUIDE

Subject

	Permissible	Inquiries to Avoid
1. Name	"Have you worked for this company under a different name?" "Is any additional information relative to change of name, use of an assumed name or nickname necessary to enable a check on your work and educational record? If yes, please explain."	Inquiries about name which would indicate applicant's lineage, ancestry, national origin, or descent. Inquiry into previous name of applicant where it has been changed by court order or otherwise. Inquiries about preferred courtesy title: Miss, Mrs, Ms.
2. Marital and Family Status	Whether applicant can meet specified work schedules or has activities, commitments or responsibilities that may hinder the meeting of work attendance requirements. Inquiries as to the duration of stay on job or anticipated absences which are made to males and females alike.	Any inquiry indicating whether an applicant is married, single, divorced, or engaged, etc. Number and age of children, information on childcare arrangements. Any questions concerning pregnancy. Any such questions which result in limitation of job opportunities.
3. Age	Requiring proof of age in the form of a work permit or a certificate of age -- if a minor. Requiring proof of age by birth certificate after being hired. Inquiry as to whether or not the applicant meets the minimum age requirements as set by law and requirement that upon hire proof of age must be submitted in the form of a birth certificate or other forms of proof of age. Inquiry as to whether or not an applicant is younger than the employer's regular retirement age.	Requirement that applicant state age of birth. Requirement that applicant produce proof of age in the form of birth certificate or baptismal record. The Age Discrimination in Employment Act of 1967 forbids discrimination against persons between the ages of 40 and 70.
4. Handicaps	For employers subject to the provisions of the Rehabilitation Act of 1973, applicants may be "invited" to indicate how and to what extent they are handicapped. The employer must indicate to applicants that: (1) compliance with the invitation is voluntary; (2) the information is being sought only to remedy discrimination or provide opportunities for the handicapped; (3) the information will be kept con-	An employer must be prepared to prove that any requirements for the job are a "business necessity" and needed for the safe performance of the job. Except in cases where undue hardship can be proven, employers must make "reasonable accommodations" for the physical and mental limitations of an employee or applicant. "Reasonable accommodation" includes alteration of duties, alteration of

LEGAL PRE-EMPLOYMENT INQUIRY GUIDE

	Permissible	**Inquiries to Avoid**
	fidential; and, (4) refusing to provide the information will not result in adverse treatment. All applicants can be asked if they are able to carry out all necessary job assignments and perform them in a safe manner.	work schedule, alteration of physical setting, and provision of aids. (The Rehabilitation Act of 1973 forbids employers from asking job applicants general questions about whether they are handicapped or asking them about the nature and severity of their handicaps.)
5. Sex	Inquiry or restriction of employment is permissible only where a <u>Bona Fide Occupational Qualification</u> exists. (This BFOQ exception is interpreted very narrowly by the courts and EEOC.) The burden of proof rests on the employer to prove that all members of the affected class are incapable of performing the job. Sex of the applicant may be requested (preferably not on the employment application) for affirmative action purposes but may not be used as an employment criterion.	Sex of applicant. Any other inquiry which would indicate sex. Sex is not a BFOQ because a job involves physical labor (such as heavy lifting) beyond the capacity of some women nor can employment be restricted just because the job is traditionally labeled "men's work" or "women's work". Applicant's sex cannot be used as a factor for determining whether or not an applicant will be satisfied in a particular job. Questions about an applicant's height or weight, unless demonstrably necessary as requirements for the job.
6. Race or Color	General distinguishing physical characteristics such as scars, etc., to be used for identification purposes. Race may be requested (preferably not on the employment application) for affirmative action purposes but may not be used as an employment criterion.	Applicant's race. Color of applicants skin, eyes, hair, etc., or other questions directly or indirectly indicating race or color.
7. Address or Duration of Residence	Applicant's address. Inquiry into length of stay at current and previous address. "How long a resident of this state or city?"	Specific inquiry into foreign address which would indicate a national origin. Names and relationship of persons with whom applicant resides. Whether applicant owns or rents home.
8. Birthplace	"Can you, after employment, submit a birth certificate or other proof of U.S citizenship?"	Birthplace of applicant. Birthplace of applicant's spouse, parents or other relatives. Requirements that applicant submit birth certificate before employment. Any other inquiry into national origin.

LEGAL PRE-EMPLOYMENT INQUIRY GUIDE

		Permissible	Inquiries to Avoid
9.	Religion	An applicant may be advised concerning normal hours and days of work required by the job to avoid possible conflict with religious or other personal conviction. However, except in cases where undue hardship can be proven, employers and unions must make "reasonable accommodation" for religious practices of an employee or prospective employee. "Reasonable accommodation" may include voluntary substitutes, flexible scheduling, lateral transfer, change of job assignments, or the use of an alternative to payment of union dues.	Applicant's religious denomination or affiliation, church, parish, pastor, or religious holidays observed. Any inquiry to indicate or identify religious denomination or customs. Applicants may not be told that any particular religious groups are required to work on their religious holidays.
10.	Military Record	Type of education and experience in service as it relates to a particular job.	Type of discharge.
11.	Photograph	May be required for identification after hiring.	Requirement that applicant affix a photograph to his application. Request that applicant, at his option, submit a photograph. Requirement of photograph after interview, but before hiring.
12.	Citizenship	"Are you a citizen of the US?" "Do you intend to remain permanently in the US?" "If not a citizen, are you prevented from becoming lawfully employed because of visa or immigration status?" Statement that, if hired, employee must submit proof of citizenship or employment eligibility (Form I-9).	"Of what country are you a citizen?" Whether applicant or his parents or spouse are naturalized US citizens. Date when applicant or parents or spouse acquired US citizenship. Requirement that applicant produce naturalization papers prior to hiring.
13.	Ancestry or National Origin	Languages applicant reads, speaks or writes fluently. (If another language is necessary to perform job.)	Inquiries into applicant's ancestry, national origin, descent, birthplace, or native language. National origin of applicant's parents or spouse.

LEGAL PRE-EMPLOYMENT INQUIRY GUIDE

		Permissible	Inquiries to Avoid
14.	Education	Applicant's academic, vocational, or professional education; school attended. Inquiry into language skills, such as reading, speaking, and writing foreign languages.	Any inquiry asking specifically the nationality, racial, or religious affiliation of a school. Inquiry as to how foreign language ability was acquired.
15.	Experience	Applicant's work experience, including names and addresses of previous employers, dates of employment, reasons for leaving, salary history. Other countries visited.	
16.	Conviction, Arrest, and Court Record	Inquiry into actual convictions which relate reasonably to fitness to perform a particular job. (A conviction is a court ruling where the party is found guilty as charged. An arrest is merely the apprehending or detaining of the person to answer the alleged crime.)	Any inquiry relating to arrests. Any inquiry into or request for a person's arrest, court, or conviction record if not substantially related to functions and responsibilities of the particular job in question.
17.	Relatives	Names of applicant's relatives already employed by this company. Names and address of parents or guardian (if applicant is a minor.)	Name or address of any relative of an adult applicant.
18.	Notice in Case of an Emergency	Names and address of persons to be notified in case of accident or emergency.	Name and address of _relatives_ to be notified in case of an accident or emergency.
19.	Organizations	Inquiry into any organizations which an applicant is a member of providing the name or character of the organizations does not reveal the race, religion, color, or ancestry of the membership. "List all professional organizations to which you belong. What offices do you hold?"	"List all organizations, clubs, societies, and lodges to which you belong." The names of organizations to which the applicant belongs which would indicate through character or name the race, religion, color, or ancestry of the membership.
20.	References	"By whom were you referred for a position here?" Names of persons willing to provide professional and/or character references for applicant.	Requiring the submission of a religious reference. Requesting reference from applicant's pastor.
21.	Credit Rating	None.	Any questions concerning credit rating, charge accounts, etc. Ownership of car.

3 Anesthesia and Outpatient Surgery

Cosmetic facial surgery can be performed using either general or local anesthesia. Popularity of local anesthesia is increasing significantly. Some physicians prefer local anesthesia, feeling that there is significantly less bruising than when general anesthetics are used. This, however, has not been definitively substantiated. An advantage of local anesthetics is that they can be safely administered on an outpatient basis at substantially less cost to the patient than general anesthesia. These are two points that may account for the increase in popularity of local anesthetics in cosmetic facial surgery.

Many surgeons, however, utilize general anesthesia. Oftentimes general anesthesia may be supplemented with the infiltration of a local anesthetic with a vasoconstrictor as the primary technique. This has the advantage of allowing the anesthetist complete control of the patient, while still providing the surgeon the advantage of hemostasis obtained through the use of a vasoconstrictor.

The use of local infiltration anesthesia with vasoconstrictors instead of vasoconstrictor alone gives three additional advantages. First, the local anesthetic allows for the use of lower level of general anesthesia. In addition, the local anesthetics allows for analgesia in the early postoperative phase. Finally, lidocaine provides some degree of arrhythmia protection. Cardiac arrhythmias can be produced with utilization of epinephrine alone.

Many patients prefer the "luxury" of being completely asleep during facial plastic surgery. The main argument that has been levied against the use of general anesthesia has been the fact that there is more bleeding. Many surgeons take exception to this point.

There are two general anesthetic options available to the facial plastic surgeon: a potent inhalation agent, and narcotic technique utilized in combination with a tranquilizer.

Isoflurane (Forane) is a commonly utilized inhalant used in combination with nitrous oxide and, of course, oxygen. Forane is the newest of the halogenated inhalation agents. Induction and emergence is prompt and, although there is frequently a decrease in blood pressure, cardiac output remains stable. This is due to the fact that the lowered blood pressure is a result of vasodilation.

Many facial plastic surgeons avoid halothane (Fluothane) because of its sensitization of the myocardial conduction system to the actions of epinephrine. Isoflurane appears more stable in this respect. There has been no indication of liver toxicity following the use of isoflurane, but its two main disadvantages are an unpleasant odor and the fact that it is a more potent respiratory depressant than halothane.

A narcotic-tranquilizer technique is frequently employed in general anesthesia. This is used in combination with endotracheal inhalation. These drugs are frequently used in conjunction with muscle relaxants and nitrous oxide. Innovar is a combination of a narcotic (fentanyl citrate) and tranquilizer (droperidol). Innovar is frequently used as a combination drug or the component drugs themselves may be used in various combinations.

Regardless of which type of anesthetic agents are employed, patient selection is the most important factor when dealing with anesthesia in an outpatient setting.

Most procedures performed on an outpatient basis should be confined to patients in anesthesia class I or II. All patients should have appropriate laboratory and physical examinations prior to undergoing any elective cosmetic surgical procedure.

PREOPERATIVE CONSIDERATIONS

The following items should be considered prior to surgery:

1. Signed consent form.
2. Appropriate laboratory tests (some physicians favor a very thorough laboratory evaluation, which could include Chem-12, urinalysis, complete blood count, prothrombin time (PT), and partial thromboplastin time (PTT). Other physicians favor a more limited laboratory profile for preoperative evaluation. A few years ago it was common to have extensive blood testing and routine radiographs of the chest for every patient undergoing surgical procedures. This "cookbook" method of workup proved to be extremely cost-ineffective. For this reason, many third party reimbursement plans have significantly limited the scope of preoperative laboratory profile for which they will compensate. These companies point to articles in the medical literature that indicate that the initial history performed by the physician followed up with an appropriate physical examination will markedly reduce the number of laboratory tests needed.

3. Physical examination (including vital signs). It is well known that the most important aspect of preoperative evaluation is patient history. It is recommended that patients be given a patient information sheet to complete in order to obtain a more adequate and thorough patient history. Such a patient information sheet asks, in summary form, for history related to any general illness. It also inquires as to previous operations, medications, and allergic reactions. Such a patient information sheet may help the surgeon to evaluate thoroughly areas in which a patient may be reluctant to converse. Such areas may have to do with previous venereal infections, genital surgical procedures, or treatment of psychiatric conditions.
4. Review of all allergies and medications.
5. Consultation with primary care physician regarding patient's general health and ability to undergo desired surgical procedure.
6. Electrocardiogram (ECG) (recommended for patients over age 40 or with a previous history of cardiac abnormalities). A history of cardiac disease mandates a rather thorough evaluation before considering elective cosmetic surgery. Patients who have had a previous myocardial infarction run a significantly increased risk of reinfarction during surgery for up to 2 years. Purely elective surgery should probably not be considered during this time. This is especially true if the patient has symptoms of angina or heart failure.

Patients with congestive heart failure have decreased myocardial reserve, a problem that will be exacerbated by anesthesia. Therefore, any suggestion of failure should be evaluated and treated, if necessary, before surgery. In many cases, the patient may then be an acceptable candidate for surgery. However, this is a decision that must be individualized and, of course, be influenced by the opinion of the physician managing the cardiac disease.

Coronary bypass has become a common procedure. Patients who have had this operation will commonly be seen for consideration of facial plastic surgery. There is no contraindication to elective surgery if a patient is asymptomatic after bypass. Again, however, this consideration is individualized and should be with the approval of the patient's cardiologist.

On all but the most minor procedures, patients should be monitored for ECG and blood pressure variations, and an intravenous line should be in position. Adequate resuscitation equipment should be readily available for use in emergency situations.

PREOPERATIVE MEDICATIONS

Various preoperative regimens are employed by physicians to produce analgesia to relieve anxiety before injection of local anesthetics. Narcotic regimens have the advantage of sedation and euphoria, but nausea and cardiorespiratory depression may be problems. Neuroleptic analgesics and tranquilizers may also be useful for sedation but must be administered with discretion.

Twilight Anesthetic

The following regimen for "twilight" anesthesia is utilized by me and has been found to be safe and effective in an outpatient environment:

- Diazepam: 10 mg orally 5 hours before surgery
- Diazepam: 20 mg orally 2 hours before surgery
- Dimenhydrinate: 200 mg orally 2 hours before surgery
- Scopolamine: 0.4 mg sublingually 1 hour before surgery
- Diazepam: intravenously in 1 to 2 mg increments during surgery

These medications' mechanism of action is well-known to the average physician. Their effects can be reversed (to a large extent) by anticholinesterase drugs, such as physostigmine (Antilirium). They are effective orally, thus avoiding parenteral injections and allowing for patient sedation before starting an intravenous line. Most important is the fact that diazepam (Valium) used as a preoperative medication has been shown to elevate the toxic threshold of local anesthetics, such as lidocaine (Xylocaine) and cocaine. If diazepam is given in doses of 0.10 to 0.15 mg/kg, increased amounts of local anesthetics may be used. This becomes important when multiple cosmetic procedures such as blepharoplasty are performed at the same surgical setting.

Diazepam

Diazepam is an anxiolytic agent and is one of the most commonly prescribed medications in the world. Diazepam acts at the limbic and subcortical levels of the central nervous system and has been shown to shorten stage IV rapid eye movement (REM) sleep. Route of administration is extremely important. If given orally, diazepam may take up to 2 hours to induce anesthetic effects. Although it is not readily absorbed when given intramuscularly, diazepam can be extremely effective with a quick onset of action (1 to 5 minutes) when administered intravenously. Diazepam has also been noted to cause transient analgesia for several minutes following intravenous administration—a highly desirable effect for a preoperative medication. Caution must be exercised when the intravenous administrative route is chosen. Pain and thrombophlebitis can develop when diazepam is administrated by this route. Administrating diazepam slowly (1 minute for each milligram) and through a larger caliber intravenous catheter may help to reduce this potential problem. Diazepam is also reported to adhere to the plastic of intravenous bags or tubing. Thus, not all of the medication administered intravenously will reach the bloodstream and produce a therapeutic effect.

Initial plasma levels are high when diazepam is given intravenously, but they quickly drop as the medication redistributes itself within the body tissues. Although diazepam may have a long half-life, somewhere between that of digoxin and digitoxin, this does not appear to be a significant factor because the medication redistributes itself so quickly. The duration of action of diazepam is thus approximately 15 to 60 minutes in the average patient. Therefore, there is little concern that patients would still be affected by the medication regimen the day following their surgery. The exception to this rule is the chronic diazepam user. This person has already "filled" his tissue storage capacity, and redistribution of the medication is markedly reduced. The resultant elevated and persistent plasma levels mean that chronic diazepam users may show quick onset of actions and prolonged effects at reduced dosage levels.

Diazepam is contraindicated in patients with acute narrow-angle glaucoma, with untreated open-angle glaucoma, and those taking monoamide oxidase (MAO) inhibitors. Caution must be exercised when diazepam is used in conjunction with barbiturates or narcotics, so that the amount of narcotic is reduced by at least one third, and small incremental doses are given.

Dimenhydrinate

Dimenhydrinate (Dramamine) is commonly used for treatment of motion sickness. Its mechanism of action is by decreasing the cholinergic stimulation of vestibular and associated pathways. It is quite effective in decreasing nausea and also produces a sedative effect. Its duration of action is 4 to 6 hours.

Scopolamine

Scopolamine is an anticholinergic alkaloid of belladonna. Many over-the-counter sleep aids, such as Compoz, Sominex, and Nite Rest, contain small doses of this medication. It is beneficial as a preoperative medication because of its sedative, tranquilizing, and amnestic effects. It also inhibits secretions of the salivary, bronchial, and sweat glands, but has a less pronounced effect on the heart, intestinal, and bronchial muscles. Peak effects are obtained 20 to 30 minutes after sublingual administration.

Physostigmine Salicylate

Physostigmine is a reversible anticholinesterase. It works by increasing the concentration of acetylcholine at the cholinergic synapses. Given intravenously, it has an onset of action of approximately 5 minutes and a duration of action of 30 minutes to 5 hours. While excretion is not fully understood and the metabolism is not definitely known, the medication appears to be largely hydrolyzed and inactivated by cholinesterase; little is excreted in the urine. It can be used to reverse the central nervous system toxic effect of scopolamine and dimenhydrinate and to antagonize the central nervous system depressant effects of diazepam.

Physostigmine is given slowly intravenously in doses of 0.5 mg and can be repeated every 5 to 10 minutes up to a maximal dose of 2.0 mg. Too rapid administration can precipitate a cholinergic crisis (muscle cramps, hypertension, respiratory depression, nausea, and vomiting).

Other Preoperative Medications

Hydroxyzine

Hydroxyzine (Vistaril) is effective only when given in adequate amounts (1.5 mg/kg). It does have a beneficial bronchodilating effect but intramuscular injections are noted to be painful.

Hydromorphone Hydrochloride

Hydromorphone (Dilaudid) is is eight times more potent than morphine. Although it does have a rapid onset, its duration of action is shorter than that of morphine. It should be administered carefully when used in conjunction with diazepam because of diazepam's potentiating effect.

Lorazepam

Lorazepam is an effective antianxiety hypnotic agent. It is utilized as a preanesthetic medication due to its excellent amnestic action when given parenterally. Its administration is much less painful than diazepam and it is noted to have a reduced incidence of associated thrombophlebitis. Many surgeons feel that the medication produces an amnesic effect after 20 minutes that may persist up to 8 hours. Doses of 0.05 to 4 mg/kg have been recommended 15 to 20 minutes before surgery. If narcotic analgesics or tranquilizers are used in conjuction with lorazepam, the question should be exercised. A prolonged sedative effect may evolve. When lorazepam is used in association with scopolamine, hallucinations, erratic behavior, and increased depth of sedation have been reported.

Lorazepam has a short elimination half-life (5 to 15 hours). It is metabolized to inactive glucuronide metabolites. For this reason, accumulation is less likely. Since no metabolically active products are formed, the pharmacokinetic parameters of lorazepam are not significantly altered by liver disease.

Ketamine Hydrochloride

Ketamine is a rapid-acting phencyclidine derivative that acts on the cortical and limbic systems. This accounts for the occasional postoperative effect of disagreeable dreams and hallucinations. Ketamine produces "disassociative anesthesia," in which patients describe a feeling of separation from their surroundings. Ketamine has a rapid onset of action (30 or 40 seconds) when given intravenously and a duration of action of approximately 40 minutes. Intravenous doses range from 1.0 to 4.5 mg/kg.

Innovar

Neuroleptic analgesia can be obtained with Innovar, a combination of the short-acting analgesic fentanyl citrate and the long-acting cyclotropic drug droperidol. Little nausea and vomiting are associated with Innovar, but the degree of sedation is often unpredictable.

Droperidol is a neuroleptic and antiemetic medication that decreases anxiety and motor responses without inducing sleep. Its onset of action is 3 to 10 minutes, and its duration is approximately 3 to 6 hours. Hypertension and tachycardia are occasional side effects. When droperidol is used, postoperative narcotics should be used with caution. Their dose should often be decreased to 25 to 30% of the usual dosage.

Fentanyl citrate is an analgesic whose effect is similar to that of morphine but whose onset of action is much more expeditious and whose duration is much shorter. Fentanyl is 80 times more potent than morphine.

Injectable Local Anesthetics

Injectable local anesthetics play a vital role in outpatient cosmetic surgery. Their use is so widespread that many surgeons never give a second thought when using them. A more thorough understanding will allow the more appropriate use of injectable local anesthetics, avoidance of complications, and more effective coping with complications should they occur. In this chapter, we will review various types of injectable local anesthetics and analyze their pharmacokinetics. We will outline drug schedules and applications for the more commonly used injectable local anesthetics. We will discuss the complications associated with the use of injectable local anesthetics and how to deal with these complications.

It is important to remember that every milligram of injected local anesthetic eventually reaches the bloodstream. An adverse reaction frequently results from a toxic concentration of the drug profusing an affected organ system. The common practice of prescribing limits on the amount of drugs injected is useful but fallacious. The amounts of injectable local anesthetics that are tolerated depend on the pharmacogenetic scenario present in a given patient at a given time. For example, it is common to see a reaction to local anesthetic agents at one half to two thirds the usual dosage in patients with congestive heart failure. Therefore it is important to have a thorough understanding of the agents being used.

In general, local anesthetics work by preventing the sodium ion movement necessary for depolarization and propagation of an action potential, in essence preventing the conduction of nerve impulses. Local anesthetics act by interfering with the ionic exchange at the nerve cell membrane and stabilize the membrane against generation of an action potential. Some researchers theorize that this interaction takes place within the membrane approximately one third of the way into the sodium pump.

Local anesthetics consist of three parts: an aromatic lipophilic group, an intermediate chain (either an ester or an amide), and a hydrophilic group. The terminal hydrophilic group combines with an acid to form a water-soluble salt. The base (un-ionized form) is lipid soluble and penetrates the neuromembrane, producing anesthesia by the mechanism previously described. The pH of the tissue affects the ratio of salt to base (Henderson-Hasselbalch equation) and therefore the amount of the drug that is pharmacologically active. When the tissues are acidotic, a larger portion of the drug is in the inactive (salt) form. This accounts for the decreased activity (or effectiveness) of local anesthetics when used in infected or abscessed areas.

Most local anesthetics are absorbed rapidly into the bloodstream. Blood levels attained 3 to 5 minutes after applying local anesthetics to mucous membranes will equal 30 to 50% of the level attained if the drug were given intravenously. It should be noted that the addition of epinephrine to local anesthetics does not affect the absorption rate of agents when they are administered topically. Epinephrine does tend, however, to slow the absorption when combined with local anesthetics that are used parenterally.

It is essential to look at what happens to agents after they are absorbed and to know the process of their degradation. In general, amides are metabolized by the liver. Esters, on the other hand, are hydrolyzed by cholinesterase in the liver and in plasma. The degradation process appears to be greatest in plasma because of the presence of plasma pseudocholinesterase. Both processes, however, depend on enzymes synthesized in the liver. Thus, we may see problems in patients with liver disease or in patients with decreased hepatic blood flow, such as in congestive heart failure. It should be noted that many of the end products of catabolism of both esters and amides are water soluble and are subsequently excreted in the urine.

Adverse reactions resulting from local anesthetics are not common, but when they do occur, they can be disastrous. In general, there are two types of toxic or adverse reactions to local anesthetics: local toxicity and general toxicity.

Cocaine acts by blocking the reuptake of norepinephrine at the adrenergic nerve terminals and by preventing the uptake of exogenously administered epinephrine. These two effects result in increased levels of circulating catecholamines. This can result in increased sympathetic stimulation and sensitization of such tissues as myocardium, bronchial lobes, and blood vessels. This can result in the side effects of tachycardia, hypertension, and excessive vasoconstriction.

Cocaine's onset of action is immediate. The duration of effect varies from 45 minutes to 2 hours. Toxic levels, while not precisely known, range from 2 to 3 mg/kg, according to most authors. One must be extremely judicious, remembering the aforementioned mechanism of action, when using cocaine in association with MAO inhibitors, physostigmine (used to reverse effects of diazepam), and epinephrine-containing compounds; in patients with glaucoma (if cholinesterase inhibitors such as echothiophate drops are used); and in myasthenia gravis patients. Each of the aforementioned medications alters catecholamine levels and could, thus, precipitate a hypertensive crisis or result in other adverse sympathomimetic effects when used in association with cocaine. This is the reason that reactions have been reported with as little as 10 mg of cocaine.

Cocaine is used topically in the form of crystals or in solution. To discourage illegal use and for identification purposes, solutions are often tinted with dyes (such as methylene blue) that also inhibit mold growth in the solution. Great care should be taken to assure that cocaine is never administered intravascularly because death can result from direct toxic action on the myocardium.

Procaine Hydrochloride

Procaine (Novocain) is also an ester and a weak local anesthetic that is not active topically. Its onset of action is 2 to 5 minutes, and its duration is 45 to 60 minutes. The maximal dose is 1000 mg. Procaine is hydrolyzed intravascularly by cholinesterase; thus, procaine may prolong the effects of succinylcholine (Anectine), which is also catabolized by cholinesterases.

Tetracaine Hydrochloride

Tetracaine (Pontocaine) is also an ester, but its toxicity is 10 times greater than procaine. It has a prolonged onset time (6 to 12 minutes), and its duration is 1½ to 2 hours. The maximal dose is 80 mg (only 4 ml may be given if 2% pontocaine is used).

Amides

Lidocaine Hydrochloride

Lidocaine (Xylocaine) is an amide with excellent diffusion properties. It is effective by all routes of administration. Topically, 4% lidocaine is used; 1% to 2% is used for infiltration. It has an almost immediate onset and a duration of 1 hour. The maximal dose is 3 to 5 mg/kg when it is used alone and 7 to 8 mg/kg when used with epinephrine. Barbiturates can decrease the effectiveness of lidocaine activity through enzyme induction.

Mepivacaine Hydrochloride

Mepivacaine (Carbocaine) is an amide with a duration of action longer than that of lidocaine.

Bupivacaine

Bupivacaine is also an amide with a long duration of action (2 to 4 hours). It is approximately four times as potent as lidocaine and can produce seizures in patients at one fourth the blood levels. The maximal dose is 2 mg/kg, or approximately 11 ml if 2% bupivacaine is used.

Other Agent

Dyclonine Hydrochloride

Dyclonine (Dyclone) is an alternative to use when the patient is allergic to both esters and amides. Its onset of action is 3 to 10 minutes, but its duration of action is brief, only 30 minutes. Topically, a 0.5% solution is used. The maximal dose is 300 mg.

AVOIDING ANESTHETIC PROBLEMS

Some basic guidelines should be observed when using anesthetics. First, anticipate problems in patients who fit in class III, IV, or V of the American Society of Anesthesiologists' risk categories. The patient classification is as follows:

- Class I Normal, healthy patient
- Class II Patient with mild systemic disease
- Class III Patient with severe systemic disease that limits activity but is not incapacitating
- Class IV Patient with incapacitating systemic disease that is a constant threat to life
- Class V Morbid patient not expected to survive 24 hours with or without operation

Second, be very familiar with the anesthetic agent used and avoid excess medication. Third, if an extensive procedure is planned, be sure an intravenous line is in place and have resuscitation equipment available. Fourth, maintain verbal contact with the patient. Fifth, use epinephrine when possible. Sixth, aspirate frequently during injection and stage injections when this is appropriate.

The spectrum of a local anesthetic reaction is a continuum that has a beginning but an unknown end. Once a reaction evolves, it may be compressed into a few seconds or may continue on to cardiovascular collapse. It is imperative that the surgeon respond quickly and appropriately at the first sign of any anesthetic reactions to prepare for those reactions that might progress to life-threatening stages.

Most anesthetic reactions with local anesthetics are really manifestations of epinephrine toxicity. Faintness, sweating, pallor, and tachycardia are usually caused by epinephrine. If a patient states that he has had an anesthetic reaction and describes the aforementioned symptoms, the patient's true sensitivity or nonsensitivity to the anesthetic can be determined by an intradermal skin test injection, much like a tuberculosis skin test. If after 24 to 48 hours there is no reaction, one may safely assume that the patient's reaction was, in fact, a result of epinephrine and not a true allergic reaction to the local anesthetic.

The maximal effect of most local anesthetics injected into the skin is seen in approximately 40 minutes. Thus, it is most likely that a reaction will manifest itself within that time. It is important to be alert for the initial signs of toxicity, such as nervousness, excessive talkativeness, slurred speech, complaints of a taste "like a penny in my mouth" (intravascular injection!), and confusion. When these signs are noted, oxygen should be given immediately. The antidote for local anesthetic seizure and overdose is oxygen. Death from anesthetic reactions is usually a result of hypoxia. The reason for this is that oxygen demands on the brain are increased 300% in a seizure. Thus, cerebral hypoxia ensues and results inevitably in death. One should also be prepared to give diazepam in increments of 2.5 to 5.0 mg or thiopental in 50 mg increments. The patient should then be watched closely for progression of the reaction, and appropriate treatment steps should be initiated.

Later signs of anesthetic reaction include somnolence, muscular twitching, convulsions, cardiovascular collapse, and respiratory and/or cardiac arrest. Oxygen should be started at the slightest suggestion of a reaction.

If the patient begins convulsing, oxygen under pressure should be administered as well as diazepam in 2.5 mg increments or thiopental in 50 mg increments. The surgeon may use succinylcholine (60 to 80 mg intravenously) if he is prepared to intubate the patient. This will terminate the seizure and facilitate more vigorous ventilation of the patient.

Seizures can recur and progress to cardiovascular collapse. For cardiovascular collapse, oxygen under pressure should be administered along with intravenous fluids and intravenous epinephrine in 12.5 mg increments. Calcium chloride in 300 to 500 mg increments may be used if the first dose of epinephrine is not effective. If there is no pulse or blood pressure, cardiopulmonary resuscitation must be started immediately.

Malignant hyperthermia is a very uncommon but highly lethal complication of anesthesia, both local and general, which is characterized by a syndrome that includes some or all of the following: rapid development of high fever, tachycardia, arrhythmias, and unstable blood pressure. Patients tend to develop an acidosis which is both metabolic and respiratory with an associated decrease in oxygen tension. Additional laboratory findings include a decrease in serum sodium with a rise in serum levels of potassium, calcium, lactate, CPK, LDH, SGOT, and myoglobin.

Malignant hyperthermia can carry a mortality rate as high as 70%. This has been claimed to be reduced to levels of approximately 30% with adequate, aggressive treatment instituted immediately on recognition of the syndrome. Paramount in the treatment is the rapid use of the drug dantrolene sodium (Dantrium), which is a direct-acting skeletal muscle relaxant. Additionally, equally important therapeutic measures include discontinuation of the anesthetic, hyperventilation with 100% oxygen, aggressive cooling, treatment of the arrhythmia with procainamide, and correction of the acidosis and hyperkalemia with bicarbonate.

Although the syndrome seems to be endemic in certain areas, it can occur anywhere. The history of certain vascular or musculoskeletal disorders might be suggestive of the possibility of this hypermetabolic condition occurring in response to anesthesia. However, practically speaking, this type of screening is of little help in lieu of the rarity of the condition.

It is advisable that patients be monitored for temperature changes, in order that this rare entity be detected very quickly. This is of even more importance when a general anesthetic agent is utilized.

The manufacturer and sole distributor of dantrolene (Norwich Eaton) recommends that 36 vials of the medication be kept on hand for immediate use should the need for treatment arise. At a cost of approximately $40.00 per vial, this obviously represents a considerable investment. The shelf life of the drug is approximately 36 months.

Some outpatient surgical facilities have elected to transfer patients immediately when the aforenoted condition is detected. Due to their close proximity to a hospital, such centers feel that it is unnecessary for them to have dantrolene in their facility. Other centers have elected to maintain an initial dose (approximately four vials) for immediate treatment before transferring the patient to a neighboring hospital. Other centers have preferred to maintain a full treatment regimen of 36 vials in their facility. Obviously, the treatment of malignant hyperthermia, although rare, is a very real entity and a predetermined protocol should be established in every surgical center. Additional information can be obtained by contacting the Hyperthermia Hotline at 209-634-4917. Additional information concerning Dantrium can be obtained from Norwich Eaton Pharmaceuticals, 17 Eaton Avenue, Norwich, NY 13815.

MISCELLANEOUS

One may increase the amount of local anesthetic used by pretreating the patient with 0.10 to 0.15 mg/kg of diazepam. This should be avoided if intravenous barbiturates are to be employed. Superimposing diazepam on barbiturate use can result in significant degrees of respiratory compromise.

Calcium antagonists can result in marked peripheral vascular dilation. Patients who have this complication can easily become volume depleted with a minimal blood loss. Thus, one should remember that patients taking calcium antagonists may require increased fluids and that a reaction during a local anesthetic procedure may be, in part, caused by hypovolemia and not entirely a local anesthetic reaction.

Arrhythmias must be differentiated as to site of origin. Atrial arrhythmias are generally more benign. At any rate, they should be evaluated and treatment initiated if indicated. Ventriculatory arrhythmias are potentially dangerous and frequently are exacerbated during surgery. Although occasional unifocal premature ventricular contractions might not be a contraindication to elective surgery, frequent or multifocal beats are of significant concern and represent a potential hazard that demands careful consideration before embarking on elective surgery.

BIBLIOGRAPHY

Aesthetic Surgery of the Aging Face. Beeson WH, McCollough EG. St. Louis: CV Mosby, 1986.

Drug Evaluations, 6th ed. Chicago: American Medical Association, 1986.

"The Otolaryngologic Clinics of North America," Vol. 20/No.4/November 1987. Tobin HA. Rhinoplastic-operative setting and anesthesia. Otolaryngol Clin North Am 20:1987.

Tobin HA. Facial Plastic Times. Washington, DC: American Academy of Facial and Reconstructive Surgery.

4 Equipment and Facilities*

This chapter discusses the basic points related to establishing an office surgical facility. These points comply with standards of the Accreditation Association for Ambulatory Health Care (AAAHC), and all are aimed at providing a high-quality environment, for patient safety is of paramount importance. There are numerous guidelines, rules and regulations that apply to office surgical facilities, many of which vary from state to state. Before establishing an office surgical unit, it is advisable that you contact your local health care authorities and state board of health for appropriate guidelines. The AAAHC offers additional information. The Centers for Disease Control, the Office of Architecture and Engineering Health Care Facilities Service of the U.S. Public Health Service, and the National Fire Protection Association can also provide information pertinent to constructing your facility (see box for addresses).

Accreditation Association for Ambulatory Health Care, Inc.
9933 Lawler Avenue
Skokie, Illinois 60000-3702

American Society of Outpatient Surgeons
3960 Park Boulevard, Suite E
San Diego, California 92103

Centers for Disease Control
1600 Clifton Road, NE
Atlanta, Georgia 30333

Office of Architecture and Engineering Health Care Facilities Service
U.S. Public Health Service
5600 Fisher's Lane, Room 9-45
Rockville, Maryland 20852

National Fire Protection Association
600 Batterymarch Park
Quincy, Massachusetts 02269

DESIGNING THE SURGICAL SUITE

Office surgical facilities have a variety of forms and designs. Some are extremely sophisticated and closely resemble hospital surgical suites. Others serve as combination office, examination, and surgical procedure rooms. Whatever design one chooses, it is important that a great deal of thought be put into establishing a surgical facility that will provide patient safety and quality of care representative of national standards. If adequate standards are not met, the medical malpractice liability that can be incurred far outweighs the advantages of performing office surgery.

SIZE

The sizes of surgical suites vary. Many feel that a room 20 by 20 feet is the best size because it allows the physician and surgical personnel ease of movement within the room during surgical procedures. Additional equipment, such as lasers or liposuction units, can be easily added without restricting the functional movement within the room. In some localities, room sizes are regulated by local and state statutes. In others, no statutes apply.[†] The most commonly noted complaint by surgeons of their own office units is that the room is too small. If one is to err, it is recommended that the error be on the side of making the room too large.

In considering operating room (OR) size, remember to subtract the area taken up by cabinets. It is unobstructed OR space that counts. Also, remember to count the space taken up by wall thickness, additional structural support, plumbing, air-conditioning, etc. It is amazing how a room can shrink from the original planned size.

Take into consideration where the door to the OR is located. There must be adequate space to quickly evacuate a patient on a stretcher in case of emergency. A 4-foot doorway is ideal, but with newer narrow stretchers, one

---

*Portions of this chapter were adapted with permission from Beeson W, McCollough EG. Aesthetic Surgery of the Aging Face. St. Louis: CV Mosby, 1986.
[†]Consult appropriate sections of the 1981 edition of the Life Safety Code (NFPA 101) before building or remodeling an office surgical suite. National Fire Protection Association, Quincy, Massachusetts.

could get by with less. The important point to consider is how you evacuate a patient from the OR to the outside of the building in case of an emergency or disaster.

To provide adequate patient safety, one must be able to conduct full emergency code procedures in the OR and, if necessary, transport the patient out of the office to the nearest hospital via unobstructed hallways and exits.

WALL COVERINGS AND CEILING

Materials used in the construction of an office surgical facility should be easily cleaned and sanitized. A perforated dropped ceiling allows dust to collect and is not easily cleaned. However, a smooth, vinyl-covered drop ceiling, such as the type used in food preparation areas, can easily be cleaned and sanitized. Solid ceilings composed of drywall or plaster are somewhat more expensive but provide a more desirable ceiling for the office surgical area.

Various types of wall coverings can be used in the office surgical area, but the finish must be washable and meet certain standards for flame spread and smoke production. Some states and municipalities have regulations for interior finishes of surgical suites. The state department of health and the local building code authority should be contacted early in the planning and design state to identify requirements. When in doubt, reference should be made to the appropriate NFPA codes.

Because explosive anesthetics are no longer used, expensive conductive flooring, special electrical outlets, and other safety equipment are usually not necessary. Vinyl flooring and seamless epoxy drywall are appropriate selections. Drywall is easier to clean than ceramic tile because there are no joints. It is also repaired more easily and quickly, whereas matching broken or cracked tile can be difficult or even impossible.

While installation costs for ceramic tile are higher than those for painted or vinyl-covered walls, many feel that the tile is better able to withstand frequent cleaning and maintains a more attractive finish. Tile, however, will crack or chip if banged by a heavy object. Cracked or chipped tile must be replaced promptly because the exposed interior can generate dust and entrap microorganisms.

COLOR

In designing your surgical suite, it is important to remember that color can be used therapeutically. The choice of color to be used should not be based on one's personal preferences but rather on the psychologic and biologic effect colors can create. Red, orange, pink, and other warm colors tend to make us feel welcome. Therefore, one might assume these colors would be the most appropriate colors for an office surgical facility. However, studies have shown that environments in these colors cause patients to overestimate time, whereas colors such as blues and greens actually cause people to underestimate time. Additional studies have revealed that tasks requiring concentration and precision are best performed in rooms with cool colors. For this reason, cool colors are probably the best choice for waiting and operating rooms.

When the eyes change position after concentrating on a colored area, such as blood red, an afterimage of the color continues to be seen. Most surgical suite walls are painted bluish green, because it was thought that these colors tend to absorb or neutralize the afterimage associated with red blood. Some operating room designers have recommended that a blue field of color be placed under the table and extended 3 to 4 feet around the perimeter. It was thought that this color not only helped to neutralize the afterimages, but also enabled detection of needles and other objects that may have been dropped during or after a surgical procedure. Recently, some controversy has arisen over using bluish green colors in the operating arena. There are some who feel that the neutralizing effect is fallacious and that warmer, more welcoming colors would be appropriate to use in the surgical suite.

Some surgical centers have successfully used murals of outdoor scenes or other wall paintings to enhance the appearance of the operating room and recovery areas and to provide contrast to the usual hospital operating room environment.

Many persons believe that windows are highly desirable in the surgical area. They feel that lack of windows causes a high degree of sensor deprivation that results in increased fatigue. They point out that windows provide a welcome change to the environment, in addition to supplying natural lighting. If windows are incorporated into the surgical suite, it is important that they be placed in such a manner as to neither distract the surgical staff or compromise the privacy of the patient.

LIGHTING

General

Lighting should provide sufficient illumination so that even the most delicate procedures can be performed. This is a highly individual item. Many physicians feel that 6 to 8 banks of fluorescent lights provide sufficient lighting to their tastes, whereas others prefer more costly and more sophisticated lighting instruments, such as overhead ceiling-mounted units.

Light standards for surgical suites have been recommended by Health Care Committee of the Illuminating Engineering Society (IES). This committee suggests that general illumination should have the potential of 200 footcandles throughout the operating room. The minimum light delivered to the surgical field should be 2500 footcandles when the surgical field is 42 inches from the lamp cover and light covers an area 78 square inches or larger.

White light is a combination of colors and actually may contain a variety of source color. As the temperature rises, the color will change from red to yellow, then to white or even bluish white. The temperature is expressed in degrees Kelvin for reference purposes. Studies have shown that most surgeons prefer light at approximately 5000°K. This approximates the color of noon sunlight. Most surgical lighting ranges from 3500° to 6500°K.

Light produces heat in two ways. One is by producing invisible infrared rays, and the second is by energy transformation of the illuminated object. Heat-absorbing filters or heat reflectors remove most of the infrared rays from the beam. The IES defines the maximum amount of energy recommended at the wound level as 25,000 W/cm^2. The lighting manufacturer should supply certification that this energy level is not exceeded. For small light sources, Braubaker has suggested a simple test that is easily applied. A 1 cm circle is blackened on the flexor side of the wrist with a felt-tipped marker. The light source is held against this blackened mark, and, if no discomfort is felt in 60 seconds, the light energy is presumably less than 25,000 W/cm^2. This test is good for evaluating fiberoptic lamps.

Monitoring of heat production from lighting is important to avoid increased warming of tissues. If heat production is below 25,000 W/cm^2, even prolonged exposure to operating room light will result in less than 2°C increase in tissue temperature.

Emergency Lighting

If one does not have some type of auxiliary power supply, such as an inverter or generator that can supply power during a power outage, it is extremely important that some alternative light sources be available. This may be as simple as securing emergency power lighting that can be tied into the circuitry of the office. When a power outage occurs, the battery-powered light sources are triggered automatically. In addition, this basic light source can be augmented by placing battery-powered flashlights at strategic locations within the surgical area. To facilitate emergency closure in a prolonged power outage, the surgeon may wish to purchase a battery pack and headlight that directly illuminates the immediate surgical field during a power outage. Many of these units can be secured at a minimal cost.

ELECTRICAL CIRCUITRY

Electrical circuitry in an office surgical facility is extremely important. The more complex the electrical equipment being utilized in the operating room, the greater the possibility of a complication relating to its use.

Macroshock, the most common complication, results from electrical current entering into the body through the intact skin. This is a result of inadequate grounding or insulation defects that cause the surgeon or patient to act as the pathway to the ground. Microshock, on the other hand, occurs if the current is applied directly to the heart, bypassing skin impedence. Thus, much smaller voltages may be lethal because they can cause cardiac fibrillation.

In some geographic areas, electrical circuitry of an office surgical suite is regulated closely by state codes. In some areas the office surgical facility must be on a separate circuit from the rest of the building or office. Other areas have no restrictions. If one is building a new office, it is advisable to contact an electrical engineer to produce an electrical floor plan for the facility. If you are moving into an existing facility, it is wise to have the ground checked to be sure that the green wire (ground) has been pulled and that the operating suite is actually grounded. In some other buildings the ground wire might not have been pulled through the conduit, but only attached to the metal casing. This may result in inadequate grounding. This is easily checked by a technician from the hospital or a local electrical contractor who plugs in a special unit to check the ground. This is important because if your electrically run instruments, such as bipolar cautery and bovies, are not adequately grounded to a ground wire that runs to a ground stake in the building structure, your patient could suffer a serious burn. Proper grounding brings parts of equipment that are not components of the normal electrical circuit to the same potential as ground and provides a preferential path along which any faulty current may be harmlessly conducted. Thus, in theory, anyone in contact with the equipment, even under faulty conditions, would not be exposed to dangerous electrical potentials.

If flammable gases are to be used, complex electrical circuitry must be employed. The AAAHC requires that if flammable agents are in an operating room, the room must be constructed and equipped in compliance with standards published by the NFPA (code 56A, 1978), as well as applicable state and local codes. A significant reduction in costs associated with electrical wiring of an operating suite occurs if flammable anesthetics are not to be used. If only nonflammable agents will be used, consult the NFPA 566 code published in 1980.

EMERGENCY POWER

Auxiliary power units are a sophisticated but much more expensive means of ensuring that a power failure will not impair the safety of your patients during a surgical procedure.

Electrical generators are available that will supply power to an entire office or surgical area during a power failure. Gasoline or diesel generators tend not to be as reliable as natural gas generators. The gasoline and diesel generators tend to require more maintenance. In addition, fuel lines will clog if they are not run frequently, fuel can gel in the lines during winter, and water can settle in the line. All in all, natural gas generators appear to be more reliable and require far less maintenance. If one has natural gas lines, the generator can be placed outside the facility. If natural gas is not available, the same type of generator may be powered by natural gas from a propane tank.

In a preexisting building a generator sometimes cannot be placed in the building. In other circumstances, the physician may not wish to incur the considerable expense of a generator. In this case an electric inverter is an excellent alternative. The electric inverter converts AC from DC and provides an alternative 60-cycle 117 volts. It also provides a modified sine wave and this provides the type of current needed to preserve memory on computers. The inverter also monitors line voltage so that when there is a change, it activates in one fortieth of a second (switch-on time). This is fast enough to prevent memory loss in computers and computerized typewriters. Generators will not activate this quickly. Inverters are about the size of a shoe box and are run off four 6-volt batteries. These are not the typical care-type batteries but they are marine-type or golfcart-type batteries. The only maintenance required is placing water in the batteries every 3 or 4 months. With other auxiliary power generators, one must be extremely careful because they are not grounded. Inverters, however, are grounded. Special hydrocaps should be used with an inverter. These caps condense them back into water, thus preventing fumes and a possible explosion from the rapid recharging of the inverter.

An inverter can be retrofitted into an existing facility by the following steps:*

1. Run a heavy-duty extension cord from the inverter into the room (there are special hospital cords with six to eight outlets).
2. Mount red outlets on the operating room wall and have an electrician fit these outlets to an inverter. When the power goes off, plug the units into these outlets.
3. Have an electrician wire the inverter into existing outlets in the operating room (obviously the best solution, since there is no changeover time needed and power outflow is always constant). This is much more expensive and does require a substantial electrician effort.
4. The power needs for the average operating room are 500 W for 4 hours or a total of 2000 W-hr. For example, power requirements for typical components are as follows: oscilloscope, 50 W; light, 150 to 175 W; bipolar cautery, 50 W surge and 7 W on idle; suction 300 W (90 W surge); defibrillator, 100 W; power table,

1000 W; microscope, 50 W. Five hundred watts of constant draw are needed with 1000 to 1500 W surges expected. Usually, an inverter will provide five times its running capacity as surge power.

Sample Calculations

One thousand watts would be able to supply five times this amount, or 5000 W, of surge energy. In deciding how many watt-hours are needed, multiply volts times amp-hours to obtain watt-hours. For example, 6 V times 200 amp-hr equals 1200 W-hr. Four 6-V batteries would thus give 4000 W-hr. This would give over 9 hours of 500 W-hr rates, the recommended amount for a single operating room. Four golfcart-type batteries in this type of hookup would give approximately 9 hours of operation. If more power or longer operating time is needed, additional batteries are added. Thus, eight batteries would give 18 hours at a 500 W-hr rate.

Inverters are available from several manufacturing companies and range from approximately $3,000 to $5,000.

LAYOUT

In designing the surgical unit, one of the most important factors to consider is patient flow. In planning the location of the surgical unit, it is vital to consider ease of access to instrument cleaning, sterilization, and surgical supply storage areas. These clean and soiled areas should be located adjacent to the surgical suite, and all three areas should be away from the flow of general office traffic. This not only decreases contamination in the sterile areas, but also provides more privacy and less distraction for the patient and the surgical staff.

In addition, the surgical suite should be located close to your postoperative recovery rooms. It is advisable that the doors of both the surgical and recovery rooms be wide enough to admit stretchers or emergency carts in the rare event that an emergency requiring transportation should arise. Both areas should be large enough that a full emergency code procedure could easily be conducted in the area. The OR and recovery areas should be designed so that nurses can easily monitor patients in either area. Many facilities have windows or television cameras that allow supervision of the OR and recovery areas from the central nurses' station or surgical work area. This greatly increases the efficiency and productivity of the office surgery nursing staff.

The physician should create a work flow diagram to show patients, staff, and surgeon activities before laying out the rooms with the designer or architect.

Many surgeons will desire to incorporate additional functional elements into the office surgical center. Nurses' stations, large recovery areas, scrub areas, patient

---

*Material obtained from the annual meeting of the Society of Office Based Surgery, Los Angeles, California, January 1983.

dressing rooms and restrooms, nursing staff dressing room and lounges, central dictating coves, and physician dressing rooms are often all incorporated into this unit. Other office surgical centers consist of only an operating room and sterile and soiled work areas. It is important, however, to be sure that soiled and clean areas are separated from clean storage.

It is vital that the surgical area be designed so it is uncluttered. The use of compact modular and hidden storage areas helps keep the operative area as a whole clean. Sterile instruments and supplies should be stored in dust-free cabinets. Many facilities incorporate cabinets in the operating room suite, which allows supplies to be efficiently stored in the area where they are used.

Considerable thought and planning are necessary in devising an efficient and productive office surgical unit. It may be helpful to visit other office surgical facilities. Professional consultants with a medical architect or consultant with experience in designing office and ambulatory centers (not just hospitals) can be invaluable. If the surgeon plans to seek Medicare certification, the state department of health should be contacted regarding review of plans and applicable codes.

VENTILATION

It is imperative that surgery be performed in a clean and appropriate environment. Ventilation of the operative suite is important for both the comfort and the well-being of the patient, as well as the surgical staff. Obviously, marked extremes in room temperature, toxic accumulation of anesthetic gases, and significant concentrations of airborne bacteria do not constitute a desirable operation room environment. Just how important ventilation is and exactly what constitutes "good" ventilation are points widely debated. At a time when all costs relating to the delivery of health care are being scrutinized, the scope of this debate is sure to widen. Obviously, if body cavities are opened, a more sterile environment is needed than if only soft tissue surgery is being performed. There are a variety of opinions as to what constitutes a safe and appropriate environment for facial plastic surgery.

Most states have precise guidelines for hospital operating room ventilating systems. These standards may vary, but they usually correlate closely with the Federal Hill-Burton program recommendations. These guidelines state that air entering an operating room must be filtered by a mechanical filter with at least a 95% efficiency rating on particle size of 1 to 5 μm. A prefilter is required to be upstream of air conditioning equipment and must have a 25% efficiency rating. Air in the operating suite should be exchanged at least 25 times per hour, and five of those exchanges should be fresh air. In addition, a positive-pressure atmosphere should exist in the OR environment. The Hill-Burton program also recommends that the temperature range be 70° to 76°F and the relative humidity range from 50% to 60% to prevent generating static electricity.

Costly laminar flow, ventilation, and filtration systems may be indicated to reduce sepsis associated with total hip replacement surgery, but less sophisticated systems are more appropriate and cost-effective for facial surgery. Numerous surgeons can document infection rates in office surgical areas that are much lower than those of hospital operating rooms, even though these office units contain no sophisticated equipment. Hospitals and surgeons have long recognized that the degree of air filtration needed to prevent wound sepsis can vary greatly with the type of procedure being performed. Soft tissue surgeries can be performed in more conventionally ventilated areas, such as in emergency rooms and modified outpatient areas. The AAAHC has also recognized that the type of ventilation appropriate for a surgical environment can vary significantly and can be achieved in a variety of ways. Their guidelines for accreditation of ambulatory health care facilities state that appropriate ventilation must be provided. Appropriate ventilation is defined as each operating room being designed and equipped in such a way as to assure the physical safety of all persons in the operating area during surgery. A safe environment for treating surgical patients must include safeguards to protect the patient from cross-infection, and environmental controls must be implemented to assure a safe, sanitary environment.

The conventional operating room has been implicated as a source of bacterial contamination of the operative wound, leading to the development of postoperative wound sepsis. Wound sepsis is a result primarily of direct contaminants and secondarily of airborne contaminants. Appropriate ventilation of operating rooms is aimed at reducing infection arising from the latter. Although no firm data have been established to provide a direct correlation between the level of airborne bacterial contaminants during surgery and the development of wound sepsis, we do know that an important relationship does exist.

A multitude of sources can give rise to airborne bacteria. Alexakis et al point out that airborne bacteria can arise from the following sources: (1) desquamation of skin from the operative team or patient (the average person emits 1000 epithelial scales per minute along with any bacteria found on the body surface). The convection currents secondary to body heat tend to carry these particles upward, facilitating dissemination into the surgical field; (2) microbes are constantly exhaled from the respiratory system; (3) bacteria can become airborne from fomites and horizontal surfaces such as the floor. These sources of contamination may be affected by the position and clothing of the operating personnel; by movement of personnel; by talking; and by the type of air current, air exchange, and air filtration in the operating suite.

Numerous studies have clearly demonstrated that a totally clean environment becomes more difficult to maintain once humans are introduced into the space. The more human activity, the greater the amount of particulate matter that will exist in that space. Schonholtz showed that infection rates are proportional to the duration of the operation and the number of personnel in the room and they are inversely proportional to the number of air exchanges per hour. For these reasons, it is best to limit the traffic in office surgical areas and to refrain from entering the operating room unless one is appropriately attired. This would dictate that the office surgical suite not be used as an examination room in the morning and then as a surgical suite in the afternoon.

Conventional ventilating systems in many office facilities may not be able to deal adequately with the potential problem of airborne contamination in the operating suite. Studies have shown that prefiltered air may contain over 1 million particle levels per cubic foot and microbial levels up to 200 viable particles per cubic foot. In addition, many conventional office ventilating systems employ recycling of air for reasons of energy conservation. This could result in dissemination of contaminants from other areas in the facility. If the facility is a multispecialty office complex, this could result in airborne contaminants from the abscess being treated in the general surgeon's office across the hall being introduced into your operating suite via the common ventilating system. Gundermann reported on the spread of microorganisms by air conditioning systems that had not been properly constructed or maintained. Reports of bird nests in air intake ducts and insects in ventilating ducts have occurred in hospital settings. If this can occur in such strictly regulated environments, one must theorize that an even greater chance of occurrence would exist in a general office today.

The use of general anesthetics in the operating suite will constitute an additional need for ventilation to avoid toxic accumulation of these gases. This problem has long been noted by anesthesiologists, and efficient scavenger systems to remove such gases have been developed. These systems usually utilize the clinical suction or a separate exhaust duct and are independent of the main operating room ventilating system.

The type of environment you plan to create must take into account the rules and regulations existing in your state and city, as well as the type of surgical procedures you plan to perform. If you do wish to have a sophisticated ventilation-filtration mechanism, the service of a mechanical engineer with experience in the design of medical facilities should be obtained. Specific units can be designed for your office that will provide not only maximal filtration, but also exact climate and humidity control. However, the cost of such units may range from $15,000 to $25,000.

Portable ventilation-filtration systems are available that provide a positive-pressure operating room atmosphere, give over 25 air exchanges per hour, incorporate fresh air into exchanges, and utilize sophisticated ultrahigh-efficiency particulate air (HEPA) filters to provide 99.9% filtration efficiency. These systems provide clean air to the entire operating room and can be easily incorporated into most existing facilities.

Smaller portable filtration units are available commercially that supply filtered air to limited areas, such as the surgical wound. These systems are small and very mobile. Operating with a small HEPA filter and blower system, they can be positioned in the room to supply clean air on the surgical field. On the other hand, electrostatic units placed in air ducts and repositioning air ducts to provide a more positive-pressure environment may be sufficient.

Regardless of what system one obtains, it is important to remember that air conditioning should be designed to keep air in the operating room at higher pressure than in adjacent spaces and to keep clean work areas at an intermittent pressure. This will allow airflow from the sterile area toward the contaminated, general use areas.

In general, an appropriate ventilating-filtration system for an office surgical area should provide the following: (1) sufficient exchange of air to eliminate odors and buildup of toxic fumes; (2) sufficient filtration and exchange of air to reduce the chance of wound sepsis secondary to airborne bacterial contamination; (3) a positive-pressure atmosphere to reduce the flow of outside contaminants into the operating room; and (4) a comfortable environment (temperature and humidity) for both patient and surgical staff.

A ventilating system that is appropriate for one office surgical facility may not be adequate for another. In designing an appropriate office surgical suite, one must take into consideration both the type of surgery to be performed and the possible sources of air contamination. The method of achieving these goals may differ markedly from facility to facility.

If properly installed, filters will perform in accordance with the manufacturer's rating information. In general, there are four categories of filters. *Roughing filters* (also called furnace filters) are used in window air conditioners and household furnaces and are easily recognized by their rectangular design and 1- to 2-inch thickness. They are useful in keeping insects and large debris from entering a system, but they provide only 20% efficiency in removing airborne microbial contaminants. They may, however, be useful in prolonging the life of more effective filters and are often incorporated into sophisticated filtration systems as prefilters. *Medium-efficiency filters* consist of a filter frame 12 inches or more in depth filled with glass or synthetic fiber wound back and forth on the framework. Approximately 60% to 90% efficiency in removing airborne microbial contamination may be realized with these filters. *High-efficiency filters* work on the same principle as medium-efficiency filters, but they provide 90% efficiency in removing airborne microbes. HEPA filters are approximately 12 inches or more in depth. They provide efficiencies of 99.99% for removal of airborne microbial contamination. These filters require powerful blower units to force large volumes of air through this fine filtration system. HEPA filters are often used on laminer flow systems.

Electrostatic precipitators are approximately 80% to 90% effective in removing airborne microbial contaminants. They can usually be adapted to most existing facilities and require connection into the electrical system. These units must be cleaned periodically. If debris collects on the precipitator plates, loud thunderlike clapping noises can be created by electric arcs. *Air washers* and *scrubbers* remove only 50% or less of airborne microbial contaminants and are not often used in office surgical facilities.

Although appropriate ventilation and filtration systems are an important component of the office surgical facility, they play a secondary role in direct contamination as the leading cause of wound sepsis. Many studies have shown that adherence to strict aseptic technique is more significant in reducing infections than use of complex filtration systems alone. Schonholtz points out that there are no firm standards for allowable levels of contamination of air, solid objects, or personnel except for materials that are considered sterile. He further states that the control of postoperative infections is a multifacted problem with many variables. Attention to a multitude of details including meticulous aseptic technique is required for maintaining acceptably low infection rates. No single technique, no piece of apparatus, and no germicide alone can solve the problem.

MUSIC

Music may be as important a component in establishing an appropriate office surgical environment as the structural facility. Music therapy is commonly used in medical institutions and can have a dramatic effect when used appropriately in the office surgical facility. Pastorek points out that the goal of music during surgery is to induce a sense of serenity in the patient to complement local anesthesia. He points out that soft light music is most appropriate, and nonclassical music is best when it is almost of a meditative quality. Pastorek feels that heavy metal, disco, or rock and roll is totally counterproductive to the purpose of music in the office surgical arena and should not be used, even if requested by the patient.

MacClelland states that, in general, high-register notes have more of a calming effect. Tempo also appears to influence anxiety levels. Slower, steadier rhythms are more conducive to relaxation and feelings of well-being than rapid, dramatic compositions. MacClelland agrees that soft, soothing, orchestral selections seem to be most appropriate for the operating room. She points out the following benefits for music in the operating room: (1) music creates a warmer, more pleasant environment for both patient and staff; (2) it provides a diversion, distracting the patient from strange sites and treatments; (3) the patient undergoing regional anesthesia becomes less restless because discomfort from positioning muscle strains is lessened and time passes more quickly; (4) the use of head sets can muffle extraneous noises and may also keep the patient from overhearing inappropriate conversation; (5) members of the surgical team work in closer harmony because of decreased levels of tension and fatigue; (6) appropriate rhythms may stimulate rapid and coordinated movements; (7) the monotony of preparation and cleanup procedures is reduced, contributing to staff morale and efficiency; and (8) music in the recovery room can reduce the feeling of pain, discomfort, apathy, and sadness resulting from the lack of cerebral occupation. In addition, music may make the time spent in the recovery area seem shorter.

EQUIPMENT

To provide high-quality patient care, an office surgical facility requires a considerable investment in medical equipment. However, as with any endeavor, the surgeon has a wide range of choices in outfitting the surgical area. There are, nonetheless, basic pieces of equipment that are a necessity.

Monitors

Monitoring equipment should include means of determining pulse, blood pressure, electrocardiac activity, and blood, oxygen, and saturation (pulse oximetry). There should be a means of determining temperature. These data need to be recorded, either by attending personnel or by automatic recording devices.

Crash Cart

It is imperative that the appropriate medications are available to treat acute emergency medical conditions, such as cardiopulmonary arrest, anaphylactic reaction, and seizures related to anesthetic reactions. A list of medications for your office surgical crash cart may be obtained by asking your local hospital for a list of supplies used in their emergency drug carts. It is advisable to be sure that your drug cart contains all the medications recommended by the American Heart Association for treating acute cardiopulmonary disorders. These medications, however, will probably be included in your hospital drug cart list. It is important to remember that medications do expire and that they must be checked frequently and replaced as needed.

In addition to medications, the crash cart should contain equipment for administering emergency intravenous fluids and medications and for establishing an emergency airway. This should include Ambu bags, an appropriate

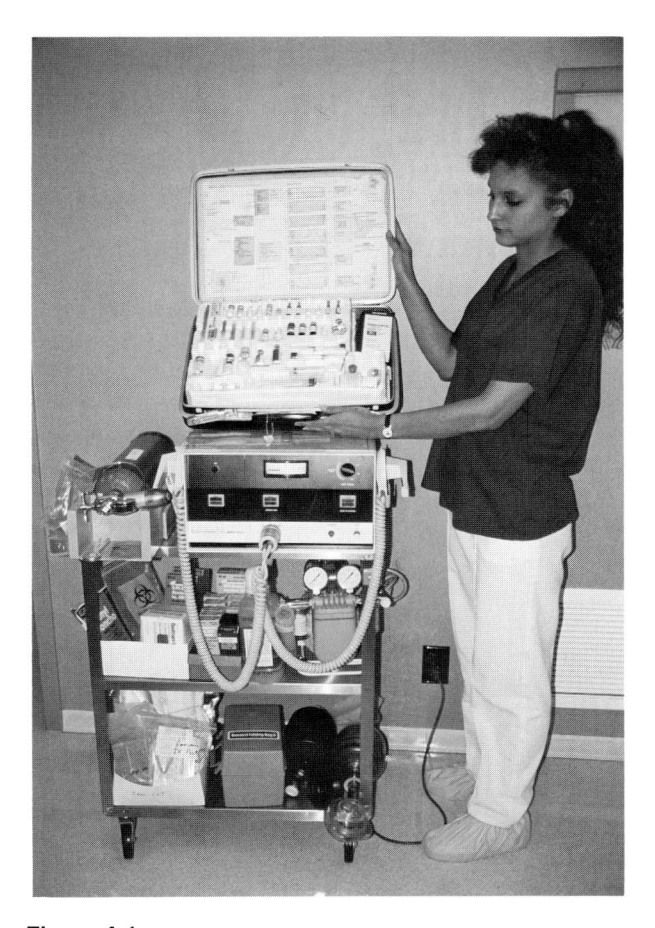

Figure 4-1.

range of endotracheal tubes, a laryngoscope with extra batteries and bulbs, and possibly a tracheotomy and cutdown set. Again, the thoroughness of your crash cart may vary with the type of surgical procedures you perform in your office and with the supplies recommended by your local hospital and ambulatory care facilities.

Hospital crash carts can be extremely expensive. Many physicians have found that a Sear's Craftsman tool chest can easily be converted into a serviceable crash cart that can be locked between surgeries. Many physicians have found that commercial crash carts, such as the portable suitcase-type kits available from the Banion Company, are useful in their office surgical area.

Medical Gases and Suction

Oxygen, nitrous oxide, nitrogen, and compressed air are the usual gases to be considered for an ambulatory surgical suite. Suction, although not a gas, should be considered with the gases, since the construction goes hand-in-hand. It is not absolutely necessary to have a central source for any of these, but in many cases it will be highly advantageous.

Arguments for central gases include economy in the purchase of the gases, since larger tanks will be used, neater working environment, and less frequent servicing needs. On the other hand, disadvantages include the cost of construction and servicing as well as the difficulties that can result from hidden leaks in the plumbing.

An adequate central source of suction is far preferable to individual suction units. It is much quieter and far more convenient. If portable units are to be utilized, one of high capacity should be chosen. The small portable suction units, such as the standard Gomco (which are so familiar on hospital wards), are usually inadequate. With the advent of liposuction surgery, much more powerful units are now on the market, which would serve nicely. The central suction is installed in the OR; two outlets are desirable, since one can be used by the surgeon, leaving one for the anesthetist. Similarly, it is frequently desirable to have one suction source for suction drainage, leaving another for general use.

There is relatively little need for compressed air. It can be handy for cleaning instruments, and with proper filtration, it can be used to power ventilators on anesthesia machines.

Operating Room Tables

A variety of operating room tables are available for office surgical use. These vary from sophisticated electric chairs that move to a variety of positions and have accessory equipment, such as lights and stands, to simpler hand-adjustable units. The type of table or chair used depends on the surgeon's preference. However, it must be remembered that a comfortable, well-designed chair will be greatly appreciated by your patients and may eliminate strenuous movements caused by patient discomfort during long facial surgery procedures. Many surgeons have found that an electric or hydraulic dental chair is a well-constructed, reliable unit and may be a fraction of the cost of the currently marketed surgical chairs. Dental chairs are usually designed for easy access to the head and neck area and are often ideal for the facial plastic surgeon. In addition, maintenance on such chairs is usually available at a much lower cost because of the large number of dentists in metropolitan areas.

Sterilization Equipment

A variety of sterilization equipment can be obtained for office surgical use. These vary from large, sophisticated steam-powered autoclaves to gas sterilizers. It is important to install a unit that will quickly sterilize the instruments used in your procedures. A unit that is too small requires several cycles to sterilize all the equipment needed for a large surgical case. It is more efficient and, in the long run, much cheaper to purchase a larger sterilization unit.

In addition, a gas autoclave is very useful. This unit is

Figure 4-2.

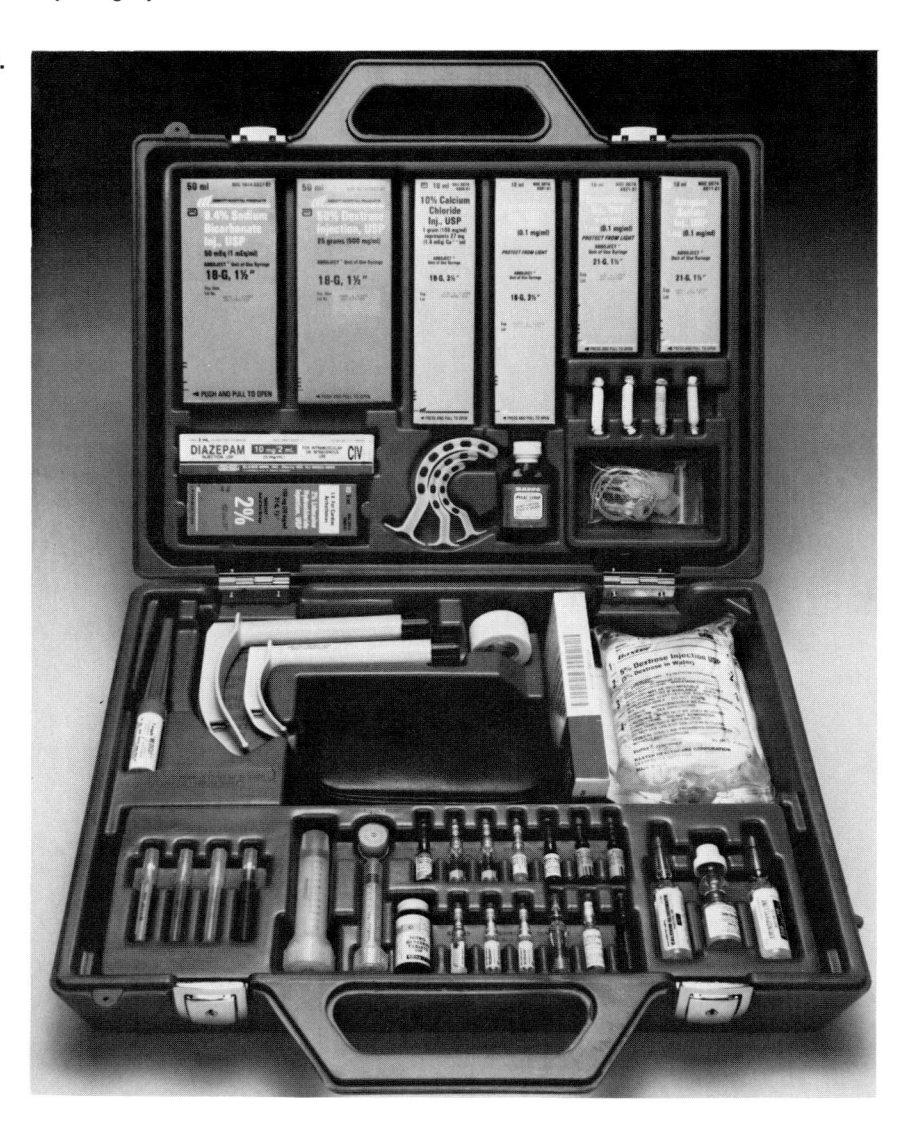

available in small sizes and utilizes ampules of ethylene oxide. It has proven indispensable for sterilizing many items that do not tolerate steam. Through the use of heavy plastic bags, these units control the escape of the ethylene oxide and are quite safe and effective. A ventilating system to the unit is available which meets the Occupational Safety and Health Administration requirements.

Whatever type is selected, it is essential that the equipment is checked periodically to ensure proper functioning. Culture sterilization checks should be performed at least monthly, and the test documented in office records.

Maintenance and Repair

To reduce liability and ensure that equipment is available in an emergency situation, it is recommended that the physician make periodic maintenance checks on the equipment. These checks should be recorded on the appropriate equipment and records maintained in the office.

Recovery

Space dedicated in the recovery area can be conservative, depending on the anticipated case load. Individual cubicles may be used to provide privacy, although in many cases, it proves more convenient to have all postoperative patients in one area where they can easily be watched by one nurse. The important principle to adhere to is that you must have adequately trained personnel in the immediate vicinity of the recovering patient until he or she is fully awake and alert. A nurse call system can be installed so that you can leave the patient under the temporary care of a family member who, in turn, can summon the staff if needed. Although it is perfectly acceptable to have a family member to sit with the recovering patients, it does not relieve the surgeon of his responsibilities to attend to the patient during recovery. Video monitoring can also be used in the recovery room to allow observation of the patients, even if you are not physically present in the recovery room area.

Bathroom Facilities

A bathroom should be located close to the operating room and recovery area. It would be very helpful to have a wide door with uncluttered space around the commode, since the patient will frequently need help after surgery. Supporting rails should be installed on the walls adjacent to the commode and a "call-for-help" alarm switch within easy reach is recommended.

Storage

It has often been said that there is never enough storage space. This is certainly true in most office surgical facilities. Roughly speaking, a storage area equal to the size of the operating room or 20% of your entire office area would be desirable. However, few facilities incorporate such space allocations. Cabinets are helpful and can significantly increase the storage capacity in your office. Such cabinets can be placed high on walls to allow work spaces underneath the cabinets. When designing your office surgical facility, storage is an important component that cannot be overemphasized.

Cleaning

Procedures must be devised to sanitize the room before and after a surgical procedure.

An appropriate surgical environment is more easily maintained by restricting clean operating room shoes with impervious soles or impervious shoe covers to the operating room or associated areas. This will help to maintain low levels of floor contamination. Various studies have shown that tacky mats do not significantly reduce general microbial contamination of floors in operating rooms. Thus, the most effective means of controlling floor contamination appears to be limited traffic flow and adequate housekeeping procedures.

Properly used, disinfectants are far more effective than detergents and water alone in reducing microbial contamination. Because using a detergent and then a disinfectant in a two-step procedure is expensive, disinfectant-detergent combinations are commonly used. A phenolic iodophor or quaternary ammonium product provides satisfactory results. The Office of Presticides Programs of the United States Environmental Protection Agency has been registering disinfectant products. These registration procedures require that products pass standard laboratory tests. For this reason, a registered product is preferred over a nonregistered product.

Under the Federal Insecticide, Fungicide and Rodenticide Act, the Environmental Protection Agency has the responsibility for licensing or registering all pesticides marketed in the United States. To obtain registration for disinfectant products, the EPA requires the manufacturers to submit detailed and specific information concerning the chemical composition of their product, toxicology data to document the composition of their product, toxicology data to document the hazards associated with the use of their product and the effectiveness data to support their claims against specific microorganisms. As of December 1991, forty chemical sterilants were registered by the Environmental Protection Agency. While validation of all sterilants is ongoing, the following is a list of products that had successfully completed preliminary tests for efficacy and validation as of December of 1991:

- Cidex Aqueous Activated Dialdehyde Solution
- Cidex Formula 7
- Cidex Plus 28-day Solution
- Actril
- Renalin

For information regarding testing on liquid sterilants, which is an ongoing process, individuals can contact the EPA's National Pesticides Telecommunication Network Hotline (1-800-858-7378).

Dirty mops and other cleaning utensils, combined with dirty mop water, can result in significantly greater floor contamination after cleaning than before. For this reason, a thoroughly dry, freshly laundered mop should be used.

Studies have shown that there is little epidemiologic significance to wall contamination unless the walls are touched or the soiling is visible. Therefore it is unnecessary to decontaminate the walls of the operating room between surgical procedures. Obviously, grossly soiled or touched areas should be cleaned immediately. Lamps and overhead tract in operating rooms become contaminated more quickly. In addition, they do present a hazard for the fallout of microorganisms onto sterile surfaces during operative procedures.

Detailed procedures on cleaning equipment, floors, and walls should be devised and closely followed. Assistance in this regard may be obtained by contacting your local hospital.

REFERENCE

Indiana State Board of Health, tele-conference 2:00 p.m. 12-13-91. Dialcom Facsimile Service Hotline.

5 Marketing

HOWARD A. TOBIN, M.D., F.A.C.S.

Several years ago, it would have been unheard of to include a chapter on marketing in a book such as this. Nowadays, however, it seems that everywhere you turn you are faced with the need to consider this subject. Actually, marketing a medical practice is not really new. Everyone has been doing it in one way or another since the inception of the private practice of medicine. It just was not called "marketing."

When I first went into practice, I kept hearing the old adage: "The most important things in developing a practice are affability, availability, and ability—and their importance ranks in that order." What was being taught, of course, was the concept that you built up your practice by putting on a good appearance to your colleagues. Of course, in those days, practices were almost entirely built up through doctor referral. Therefore the primary marketing effort was directed toward your fellow physicians. Marketing to patients was much more subtle because of the taboos and restrictions made by organized medicine.

Much of this was based on the notion that physicians knew what was best for the patient, and it was inappropriate for the latter to question the former. Based on that supposition, who would be best suited to recommend a doctor but another doctor?

Nowadays, consumers tend to make more decisions for themselves, and this includes choosing a doctor. Therefore marketing is appropriately directed not just to your colleagues but also to your patients and prospective patients. There is nothing wrong with this. Advertising, in its purest sense, is just a type of education with an element of persuasion. If you are attempting to persuade a patient to do something that you truly know to be in their best interest, it is nothing to be ashamed of.

MARKETING AND MEDICAL ETHICS

Before getting into a discussion of marketing and advertising techniques, we must remember that all physicians are bound by certain ethical codes that limit all marketing efforts. These standards are usually defined by either state or local medical societies, and, of course, will vary to a certain extent, depending on the location in which you practice.

In Texas, the State Board of Medical Examiners has passed guidelines for ethical advertising which state that physicians should not provide information that is either deceptive or misleading, nor should they make claims of superiority that would not be readily subject to verification. This seems to be very similar to what many state organizations have defined as the guidelines for ethical advertising.

The American Academy of Facial Plastic and Reconstructive Surgery has also established guidelines for ethical advertising that include the following:

> Advertisements should include only information that a reasonable person might regard as relevant to selecting a surgeon, such as physician specialty, board certification, description of services, ranges of fees for specific services, payment plans, and so on.
> Advertisements will exclude statements or photographs that promote relief unobtainable by the average patient, testimonials that do not reflect the typical experience of patients, and claims that take improper advantage of a person's fears, vanity, anxiety or similar emotions.

What that means is that physicians should present information that is essentially complete and accurate and should avoid statements that might lead a patient to draw a conclusion that is not supported by fact. Stated in another way, it is fine to emphasize your best features, but stick to the truth and be prepared to back up everything that you say.

There is no reason to feel shy or bashful about advertising your services. We have all now come to realize that it is truly in the public's interest to be exposed to advertising. Advertising allows patients to have a choice. It provides access to services that might not otherwise be available. It stimulates competition, which should lead to a general improvement in the level of care.

Of course, we all realize that advertising can be abused. There is no question that substandard practitioners may gain patients simply through advertising. Nevertheless, we must also recognize the fact that for many years, these same substandard practitioners flourished without the benefit of advertising. There is plenty of room to criticize the old way as well as the new. The "good old boy" system in which patients were referred to golf partners and buddies regardless of their skills can be criticized just as much as a slick, sophisticated marketing program.

It must be our hope that as advertising becomes more accepted, the public will learn to recognize that advertising must be only one step in the process of selecting a surgeon. Patients must learn that they have a definite responsibility to learn about the credentials and abilities of a prospective surgeon. This is also true in regard to marketing an ambulatory surgical facility. Although we are well within our rights to emphasize the advantages of our facility, we still have an obligation to avoid any misleading information that would overemphasize the scope of the services that we can offer.

By advertising our services, we can increase our practice or utilization. Is this something to be ashamed of?

Remember, the highest quality of care is only useful if there are a sufficient number of patients to take advantage of it. McDonald's hamburger chain serves as a great example. When you go into a McDonald's restaurant, the facility is always clean. The food is consistently of high quality. Employees are friendly. Recipes are carefully developed to cater to the mass taste of modern America. Even so, McDonald's success still largely rests on its advertising. It is constantly in a struggle to attract more customers than its rivals. Quality and service are important, but the message must be constantly delivered in one form or another. Unfortunately, the consumer often has a short memory.

Suppose you did a rhinoplasty on a patient who had a friend who had accompanied her to your office. The friend was quite impressed, but was not thinking of that type of surgery at the time. Ten years later, she decides to have a face lift. She really liked you, and would tend to choose you as her surgeon, but unless your name is in front of her in some way, she may just end up at the office of another doctor whose name is simply more "current." Sounds silly? Think of your last purchases, or the last time you sought professional help. How carefully did you analyze all of the choices? Did you not pay more attention to current information?

With this in mind, we will proceed to a discussion of the marketing and advertising techniques that are available to your practice and your surgical center, which may help to keep your name in a prominent place for patients who would benefit from your services, and actually like to choose you over your competitors.

Much of the following information is drawn from lectures given by Price Womack, president of Womack, Griffin and Claypool, an advertising agency with expertise in medical marketing based in Odessa, Texas.

Mr. Womack points out that marketing is no substitute for quality in any product. As we have just stated, if you claim to have a very good product, be sure that when the patients begin beating a path to your door that they find the product to be as good as you assert. He also warns against overconcern about what your peers may feel about your advertising. Your colleagues will not change their feelings about you simply because you advertise. If they liked you before, they will probably continue to like you. If they disliked you before, this will merely serve as an additional reason for their dislike. As Oscar Wilde said, "there is something about your success that displeases even your closest admirers."

The five P's of marketing
Product—Before you begin to advertise, you must have a product to sell. In the case of a surgical center, define your area of interest. Decide exactly what you are hoping to accomplish through your marketing effort.
Pipeline—Plan for a route into your practice. Just what about your marketing plan is going to attract the patients? Specifically, how will they be brought to the practice? Will it be through the referral of other doctors or will they be attracted directly to your own private practice?
Price—Be sure that your prices are competitive. If you plan to position yourself above the average prices in the area, be sure that you present a reason for the higher prices.
Promotion—How will you promote your practice? Will it simply be through advertising or will you use additional marketing techniques such as personal appearance, direct mail, brochures, etc.
Planning—The overall strategy that ties your marketing program together.

Marketing actually begins with your own personal selling skills. This is especially true in a private surgical center where patients will be coming to see you as much as they will the center itself.

The way you dress, the way you relate to patients, and the way you teach your staff to respond to patients all constitute the fundamental essence of any marketing program. As we have mentioned in other chapters within this monograph, an individual's staff will either make or break him. Therefore, in marketing, it is important not only to select the best possible staff, but also to train them properly and to set the highest example for them to follow. A marketing program must be consistently carried out by the entire staff, not just by you alone!

Another important marketing tool is *promotion*. Promotion means that you take a certain aspect of your practice and use it as an example of your overall services in an effort to attract other people. For example, if you have operated on a celebrity or an important person who might be willing to "go public," this can be promoted as an example of the type of patient who would choose to use your services. A newsletter is a very good example of a means of promotion. In a newsletter, you can select topics that will highlight your major interests. These can be written in a newslike fashion, yet will call attention to aspects of your practice that you feel are important. You can feature new services that are added to the surgical center, discuss new types of equipment that you may purchase, introduce new members of your staff, emphasize expanded hours, and talk about recognition that you may have received through appointments to committees, publication of papers, and so on.

Public relations is another important aspect of a marketing program. In essence, public relations can be considered as synonymous with access to the media. This can really be a two-edged sword. When you have a message that you wish to deliver to the media, it must first of all be related to something that they consider newsworthy. This implies that the subject might be controversial. Unlike paid advertising, public relations and press coverage offers no assurance that the final message will be the one that you wish to deliver. There are countless instances in which press releases have backfired and resulted in adverse publicity.

When you bring your message to the media, you must be prepared to deliver it in a succinct and effective manner. You must also be prepared to answer questions that may be provocative or challenging. Finally, you must be prepared for the publication of information that may be out of context and, frankly, exactly the opposite of the message that you chose to deliver.

Regardless of this threat, public relations can be an extremely important part of an overall marketing program.

Finally, in considering a total marketing plan, we come to the consideration of paid advertising. Prior to embarking on an advertising program, the first step must be to target the audience. Give considerable thought to who are your potential patients. Consider their socioeconomic status, where they live, what newspapers and magazines they might read, what television shows they are likely to watch, or which radio stations they are likely to listen to. Another important consideration is the age group of your target audience, since different forms of media will appeal to different age groups. Finally, you must consider whether you are targeting primarily women or whether you wish to address both men and women, or perhaps men alone. Basically, what you are trying to decide at this point is to whom you are trying to talk.

In arriving at these decisions, it is worthwhile to carry on an analysis of your practice. You may be surprised to find that the work you are actually doing is not exactly what you had perceived. Although certain patients may stick out in your mind, you may find that the vast majority of your patients come from an entirely different socioeconomic level. Of course, an equally important decision is whether you wish to begin targeting a new area or remain in the same pattern that has been developed by your past practice.

Once you have satisfactorily carried out an analysis of your present situation, you then begin to make plans for your advertising program. To do this, you must decide where you want to position yourself in the market. Advertising must have a specific purpose. It must be designed to get across a certain message. Remember that you cannot tell everything in an advertisement. Positioning is the most important initial decision in an advertising campaign. It sets the pace for where you are trying to go, who you are trying to reach, and what you are trying to accomplish.

Try to decide what the basic message is that you are trying to impart. You want to do more than simply list your name and address, of course. You have to have some idea that will catch the audience's attention. There should be some special message that you are trying to provide. Obviously, this is not a simple task. Most doctors who are just getting into advertising tend to feel that they have to include everything in their ad. This is impossible. The purpose of the ad is not to provide your audience with total information about yourself and your facility. This will come later when you succeed in bringing the people to your door, or at least get them to look for complete information.

To get ideas, of course, you may depend on a professional ad agency. Even so, you will have to direct these individuals since there are still relatively few people who have experience in medical advertising. Do not be afraid to obtain ideas from other sources. Look at other advertisements and keep the ones that you think are effective, attractive, or catchy. Try to extract the essence of these examples to be used in your own. This does not mean that you can copy an ad or other type of advertising material. Often this material is protected by copyright. Nevertheless, the basic idea is not subject to copyright, since every idea is actually a modification of some previous idea.

Once you have decided on your basic message, then you will make a decision as to how extensive your advertising program will be. Usually, this will be determined by a budget that is established. Unfortunately, this is where many physicians become disillusioned. Somehow, they seem to have the idea that a single advertisement will bring the public beating a path to their doors. This unfortunately is not the case.

Advertising must be looked on as a long-term investment. It is very unusual for a single ad or even a single short-term advertising campaign to produce dramatic results. Most of the effect of advertising is accumulative. This should not be surprising when we consider the fact that people are constantly bombarded with advertising messages. Most of these messages are quickly ignored. For the advertisement to be effective, therefore, it either must hit the right person at exactly the right time, or it must occur with enough frequency that it begins to make an indelible impression on the audience.

Considering these factors then, it is easy to understand why it is important to remain true to your basic message. If your ads are varied constantly, the audience will not come to recognize the compaign at all. For these reasons, it is important to establish reasonable objectives and ensure that you have provided for adequate exposure to meet these objectives.

To a certain extent, your advertising will be determined by what your competition is doing. You may decide to meet the competition head on, or you may choose to make an end run. An excellent example can be seen in the case of two cosmetic surgeons from the eastern part of the United States. Both of these individuals practiced away from large urban areas. Both were attempting to attract patients from a moderately large surrounding geographic area. The two areas of interest overlapped.

One of the doctors had already embarked on an extensive advertising program featuring svelte models in ads with a sophisticated approach. The second doctor recognized that he was not prepared to embark on as extensive or expensive a campaign as the former. His answer was to develop a campaign that was more homey in style and emphasized the personal relationship that he had with his patients. Both doctors have found their campaigns to be highly successful. They are competing in the same market, but they are targeting different groups.

In addition to pointing out how you must target your audience, this example also serves to demonstrate that just because you are facing an individual who has a larger advertising budget, that does not necessarily mean that you can't carry on your own much more modest but successful advertising program.

In emphasizing the importance of repetition in advertising, we must not overlook the fact that somewhere along the line you have got to evaluate the results of your program. There is no simple answer as to how long this should be. Part of it will be dictated by your own economics. Part will be dictated by the type of media you are using and the frequency with which you are using it. Nevertheless, you need to keep track of the results of your advertising program. A good way to do this is to survey your patients and ask them how they heard of you and what brought them to your facility.

As an extreme example, if after 2 to 3 months of advertising, none of the patients indicated that the ad had brought them in, then obviously there is something wrong. On the other hand, you may find that initially only a very few patients are responding to the ad but that the number is slowly increasing. This may then encourage you to continue for a while to see if the advertising will ultimately be worthwhile. The main point is that you have got to keep on tracking its progress so that you can decide whether your campaign is working.

SPECIFIC TYPES OF MEDIA

Yellow Pages

The decision regarding advertising in the Yellow Pages is not if, but how much. Virtually every physician lists himself in the Yellow Pages. Prior to the late 1970s, it was generally considered unethical for a physician to put more than his name or specialty. Now, this has all changed. A physician may advertise his services or his facility as long as he follows the normal guidelines for ethical advertising. Once the decision has been made to extend a marketing program beyond the traditional means, Yellow Page advertising deserves serious consideration.

If a prospective patient is seeking you out as an individual physician, he is unlikely to consult the Yellow Pages. If, on the other hand, he is seeking a type of service without a definite decision made as to the choice of provider, he is very likely to use Yellow Pages advertisements as a source of general information.

More than any other media, Yellow Pages advertising has "staying power." It lasts a full year and is targeted toward a select audience.

The disadvantages of Yellow Pages are largely related to the fact that an individual book may not cover your entire targeted audience. For that reason, you may have to use multiple listings. In addition, since deregulation of the telephone system, there are now competing directories for many markets. Finally, space in Yellow Pages can be very expensive, especially in the larger markets.

All things considered, Yellow Pages probably represent one of the best media to allow you to advertise not only your practice but your surgical facility.

In planning your ad, remember that the individual who looks at the Yellow Pages is already seriously contemplating the type of services listed. The main thrust of your ad should be to encourage the patient to call for further information. Although the ad should be informative, avoid the temptation to include too much text. Instead, emphasize the fact that a telephone call will bring additional information.

Additional sources of Yellow Pages advertising include referral ads such as those that are organized by The American Academy of Facial Plastic and Reconstructive Surgery. These consist of advertisements placed by the parent organization, which offer each member of that organization an opportunity to include a listing in the ad. Costs of the advertisements are shared by the members who choose to participate.

Television

Television penetrates nearly every home in America. The average family has their television set on for 2000 hours per year. Therefore television offers the opportunity to reach a very large audience with a very high emotional impact because of a combination of sight and sound. It also offers an opportunity for a very personal type of advertising because of the ability to provide "one-on-one" contact. All of these factors make television advertising very attractive.

There have been a number of companies that have recently specialized in the production of medical ads for television. Some doctors have reported excellent results with this type of advertising. On the other hand, it is interesting to note that many of those same doctors subsequently drop this type of marketing. When looking at cost factors, it is not hard to see why.

The one major disadvantage to television advertising is the fact that it is very expensive. Another possible disadvantage is that many people in the viewing audience may still consider television advertising for physicians to be inappropriate, somewhat unethical, and indicative of a lack of quality. To a large extent, this will depend on the given area and also the sophistication of the ad. There is no question that any of these objections could be overcome by a properly produced ad.

This emphasizes the point that in television, more than any other media, the ad must be of high quality. People have become accustomed to highly professional advertisements on television. Anything less is likely to have a negative impact. The standard to which your advertisement must reach is essentially the standard of the high-quality network ad. This will add even more to the expense of such an advertising campaign. This high quality is important, for the viewing audience will judge the quality of your work by the quality of your ad.

Again, as we have mentioned before, it takes more than a single ad to have an impact. How long do you need to run the ad? Again, there is no simple answer. Although repetitive advertising is important, it should be noted that you need not constantly run the ad. Consider running in clusters. Run the ad fairly frequently for a few weeks, and then stop for a few weeks. The viewing public does not notice that your ad has stopped for a period of time. Also, remember to target your ad. Decide when you want to run the ad. What type of television show do you want your ad to accompany? You will certainly reach a different audience when you are running your ad during the Donahue show as contrasted to the evening news, or a weekend news program.

In summary then, television offers a great opportunity to reach a large market effectively, but is probably the most demanding in terms of investment of expense and requirement for sophisticated expertise.

Radio

Radio offers an inexpensive way of potentially reaching over 98% of the homes in America. The problem is that the market is very sharply segmented, with different types of people listening to distinctly different stations. Added to this is the fact that people are generally involved with other activities as they listen to the radio, and so your message may not have the same degree of penetration than it would have in other media.

Nevertheless, the advantages are significant. The low cost allows much greater frequency, and the elective audience allows you to pinpoint your market. Obviously, if your primary interest is to attract patients interested in face lift surgery, you would tend to stay away from a rock station, preferring perhaps an easy listening or adult contemporary station.

In choosing your station, you will have to depend on your own judgment, since every station will try to convince you that they are number 1 in its own particular area.

Magazines

Magazines are becoming a very popular medium for medical advertising. Very likely, one of the major appeals is the fact that you can contain a great deal of information in a magazine advertisement. Because of the fact that magazines tend to be read by several people and passed on a number of times, they can offer a great deal of exposure. Magazine readers are often willing to spend time reading a rather lengthy advertisement if it contains information that is of interest to them. This can be very appealing to physicians who feel uncomfortable with the idea of running a flamboyant or glitzy ad. An ad in a magazine can be tastefully laid out and yet contain primarily information and text.

Since magazines, unlike television, are voluntarily brought into the home, many physicians feel more comfortable with this type of advertising since they do not feel that they are imposing their message on an unwilling public.

Considering all of the factors just mentioned, it is easy to see why the choice of a particular magazine is very important. Here is where you actually target your audience. Every magazine is geared toward a certain segment of the population and each magazine has its own personality. All of these things must be taken into consideration.

Equally important is the editorial policy of the magazine. You certainly would not want to run an ad for cosmetic surgery in a magazine that basically has a negative attitude toward this type of work.

One possible disadvantage of magazine advertising is that many magazines have a wider geographic distribution than you may choose. Consider the possibility that the magazine may have regional editions. This is especially appealing, since your prestige will be enhanced when readers assume that your ad is reaching a much larger geographic segment. This gives you high credibility.

Advertising in a prestigious magazine imparts some of the magazine's prestige to you. Surprising as it may seem, some people seem to feel that magazines are quite selective in who they will allow to advertise. Many times people will remember your ad and not remember whether you were actually written up in the magazine.

As we have said before, you must not feel that a single advertisement will have a great deal of impact, regardless of how prestigious the magazine. As is always the case in advertising, repetition becomes the most important factor. In a magazine, repeated advertising eventually leads to readers associating you with that magazine. If the magazine is held in high repute, you are also likely to be viewed in that light.

Newspaper

Newspaper advertising offers the most rapid and flexible penetration of the print market. It also offers a tremendous degree of flexibility because of the speed with which the ad can be developed, changed, or placed.

On the one hand, newspaper advertising can be used to make an immediate announcement, such as a change in office hours or the announcement of a new associate or the inauguration of a new service. In contrast, one can develop a long-term strategy of continued newspaper advertisement to present an ongoing image of a facility. This can be done much the same as one would do with magazine advertising.

Unlike a magazine, newspapers can offer much greater frequency with ads being placed daily or weekly, or at any desired schedule. The ad can also be subjected to periodic variation, although you must be careful to maintain sufficient continuity so that the reader continues to associate the advertisement with you. Along the same lines, newspaper advertising allows for the insertion of a large amount of text, although again you must be careful to avoid so much verbiage that the reader chooses to ignore the entire ad.

In this regard, an advertiser has two basic choices to make with all types of print media. He may choose a basic advertising format that has artistic impact which is designed simply to attract the reader's attention to the product or the facility. In this case, the message must be basic and succinct. On the other hand, you may choose to make your ad more informational. In this sense, you are counting on the subject's interest to be sufficient to draw the reader's attention to the ad. When this route is chosen, you must accept the fact that the lowered initial impact will cause many readers to entirely overlook the advertisement.

You should be aware that so-called advertising experts have taken both sides of this issue and either type of advertising may be appropriate to your individual goal.

Disadvantages of newspaper advertising are mainly related to the distribution limitations of the newspaper and the quality limitations of the layout and print.

Newspapers, by their very nature, are designed to appeal to a mass audience. This is becoming more and more true as competition results in fewer newspapers even for the major cities. Therefore you will be paying for your ad to reach a market that is far broader than the potential market for your services.

This limitation can be minimized by carefully selecting where the ad is placed in a newspaper. For example, ads for a cosmetic surgery practice might be placed in the Women's section or the Society page. Certainly you would tend to avoid the Sport's page. On the other hand, if your practice were primarily related to hair transplantation, the Sport's page may be exactly where you want your message to be. You may also choose to avoid the major daily newspaper in favor of a more selective regional type of newspaper such as the weeklies that are published for various areas in the larger cities. Additionally, selective newspapers can be used for expanding your practice into additional areas. This could be especially applicable if you are considering opening up a satellite facility.

Another disadvantage of newspaper advertising is the quality of the print. When designing your ad, you must realize that photographs will not have the same high quality that they have in magazine print. Therefore, the visual impact of your message may be lost and you are not likely to have as personal an appearance in a newspaper.

Outdoor Advertising

Although few physicians will choose to advertise on billboards, the subject should be considered for completeness. There are some circumstances that might be well served by this means. If your facility is hard to locate, a prominent sign might be placed for direction. As more and more hospitals choose to use this type of advertising, private facilities are likely to follow suit, and so the medium should not be ruled out entirely.

If you do decide on this type of advertising, the message should be kept simple, depending, instead, on the visual impact of the sign.

Along these same lines, it is worth emphasizing the importance of general signage—specifically the way you put your name on the door. A great deal of importance should be placed on this apparently simple concept, for it does have influence on your patients. A well-thought-out logo that is carried through in all of your communications will serve to make a definite statement about your overall operation.

Direct Mail

Direct mail marketing offers one of the most flexible means of getting a message to a select audience. The effectiveness of direct mail advertising depends on utilizing a mailing list that is custom designed to reach the market you are seeking. This indeed can become a sophisticated art. Mailing lists are constantly being developed, refined, bought, and sold. The list can be as simple as everyone in a chosen geographic area or as sophisticated as selecting a given age group, sex, and lifestyle preference based on shopping habits, religious preference, membership in organizations, etc.

For the most part, owners of private surgical facilities will use one of two sources. The first would be a local mailing list that may be narrowed down to relatively broad socioeconomic levels. The cheapest way to obtain such a list is simply to base this on geographic distribution, assuming that your target audience would live in certain defined neighborhoods. This type of list can readily be obtained from direct mail sources in your local community. It is unlikely that you would choose to go to the additional expense of the more selective types of lists, but these can be obtained from your local vendor.

The second type of list that you can use is one that is developed personally. In essence, you would be using your own patients and your own personal contacts. This can include members of organizations to which you belong, your trade vendors, members of your local Chamber of Commerce, members of your own religious organization, and any other contacts that you may develop.

Firms that offer mailing lists are usually easy to find. They may be listed in the Yellow Pages either under direct mail, mailing services, or list processors. All of these firms offer a variety of services. In addition to supplying you with lists, they will compile lists for you from others such as outside brokers, they will keep your own lists on computer and provide sorting services. For example, the lists can be sorted by zip code to allow cheaper mailing under bulk rates. They also can be sorted under any chosen category to give you better insight as to the constitution of your lists. Finally, the services will also provide direct mailing for you, addressing and stuffing envelopes and even printing material for you.

Although all of this work can be done by outside sources, in this era of home computers with desktop publishing, more and more facilities are finding that the job can be done just as well and more economically in-house.

6 Quality Assurance and Risk Management

HOWARD A. TOBIN, M.D., F.A.C.S.

It is indisputable that any conscientious surgeon establishing his own ambulatory surgical facility would want to provide his patients with the optimum care that he can provide. Quality assurance (QA) is simply the sum total of the efforts that have been expended in this realm. Quality is difficult to assess, although most people have a feel for it in one way or another. General George Patton, in a letter to his son, stated that "The most vital quality a soldier can possess is self-confidence, utter, complete and bumptious."[1] We also face a soldier's challenge to have the same assurance that we are doing everything possible to provide our patients with the best service possible. Although we may be convinced that we are making the maximum effort, it still behooves us to demonstrate this effort to others both within and outside of our organization.

In the following discussion, I will deal with the two basic elements of an ongoing QA program. The first is what we shall call QA activity, and the second, QA studies.

QA activity comprises a wide range of endeavors that should, in effect, deal with every aspect of a surgical practice. In its most basic form, all of our efforts to maintain or increase the quality of care given comprise QA activity. What I am talking about here are some of the ways in which a practice can measure or demonstrate this ongoing commitment. I would emphasize the fact that quality assurance must involve the *entire staff of an organization*. This can be difficult for a surgeon to understand when he is used to having complete control over his own practice.

It is common to see either one of two extremes when surveying the QA program of a facial plastic surgical center. On the one hand, we might see the attitude of the take-charge surgeon who feels that he, alone, must be in control of every aspect of the practice. His response to most questions regarding QA is that he is sure it is going well, because he has checked or supervised that aspect of his practice. For example, one very common QA activity is to survey patient satisfaction. In this case, the surgeon's response might be that he always makes himself available to the patients and responds to their complaints and suggestions. Although this would certainly be indicative of a personal concern, it does not ensure that patients are being encouraged to voice complaints or make suggestions. Furthermore, it does not provide for the involvement of the rest of the staff in the QA program.

On the other hand, we often see the opposite situation, wherein the responsibility for the QA program is delegated to a key staff person. In this scenario, one might expect a response such as, "I know that it is being done, but Mary takes care of that, and I'm sure she has the information somewhere." Simply delegating a job does not mean that it is necessarily involving the staff of the facility.

In summary, then, the primary characteristic of QA that must be established is that it must become a team effort. Although every staff member may not be involved in each component of a QA program, at least a significant number of people must be involved, and ultimately, the information must filter down to all staff levels, so that each individual develops a commitment to the concept of ongoing QA. How all of this is carried out will vary according to the way the surgeon chooses to run his facility, but eventually it boils down to communication.

How often do we look back on problems that have developed only to bemoan the fact that it was "simply a problem of communication." Whether it be communication with patients, colleagues, family, friends or coworkers, communication defines our ability to work effectively as a team. In some cases, much of our interaction may be understood through experience, but even this is a form of communication, although it is not verbal or written. These clearly understood, although unwritten, types of procedures are quite acceptable, although it is imperative that everyone be aware of and clearly understand them as established protocol. In a very small organization with only a few employees, many of whom have been together for a long time, this unwritten code may constitute the bulk of the procedures that define the ongoing activity of the organization (see Policy and Procedures, pp. 77–84).

Unfortunately, as a practice grows, things become more complex. New employees are added. Staff changes. Responsibilities change. All of this growth leads to an inevitable need for more formal methods of communication and the dreaded addition of paperwork. Years ago, one of the blessings of office-based surgery was freedom from paperwork, and although it is still true that paperwork can be lessened, it is an unfortunate fact of life that documentation is the hallmark of an effective risk-management program, and we are unfortunately faced with the demand to protect ourselves from outside threats of alleged malpractice.

Notwithstanding, there are positive aspects to documenting QA activities in that we use this to establish overall quality of our practice to outside observers, whether it be through accreditation, licensure, or satisfaction of the requirements of third-party payers. Furthermore, documentation serves as an important risk-management tool. Risk management is a concept that is growing in importance and will be discussed in more detail later in this chapter.

The task of documenting our QA activities need not be as burdensome as it might appear on the surface. At the Facial Plastic and Cosmetic Surgical Center, nearly all of the documentation is carried out by recording minutes of our periodic office meetings. It is at these meetings that the staff reviews the QA activities that have taken place. The minutes are a part of our permanent record and are distributed to the entire staff, thus assuring us, as well as outside observers, of compliance with the requirement of staff participation in QA activity.

QUALITY ASSURANCE STUDIES

QA, in general, is the means by which a facility looks at itself to see if it is doing a good job and seeks ways to improve itself. QA should really permeate all of the activities in the surgical center. By constantly thinking of QA, the staff and governing body will place itself in a posture of constantly seeking problems and correcting them before they can lead to patient harm. When an accrediting or certifying organization comes to inspect a facility, they are largely trying to assure themselves that the facility has an ongoing QA program. QA studies are merely ways of demonstrating this activity.

Since most facial plastic surgeons who seek accreditation will look to the Accreditation Association for Ambulatory Health Care (AAAHC) for certification, I will use the format required by them as a model for explaining the development of a satisfactory QA study. This format proves to be quite confusing at first, but really is quite simple once it is understood. The standards of AAAHC basically state that an acceptable QA study has the following components: (1) the problem is identified; (2) the frequency or severity of the problem is analyzed; (3) correction or improvement is carried out; (4) a reassessment is done to see if the problem has been effectively addressed; and (5) the results of the study are written up, reviewed by the staff, and reported to the governing body.

Let's go through a simple example. Your secretary comes to you complaining of frequent interruptions when she is trying to do her dictation—*1. Problem identification*. You ask her, "Well, how often do you really get interrupted?" She decides to keep a log on her desk to jot down exactly how many times people come into her office and interrupt her while she is doing the dictation. She does this for 2 weeks—*2. Analysis of frequency*. You discuss this and decide that maybe she should keep her door shut while typing—*3. Correction*. A follow-up evaluation is carried out for another 2-week period indicating that the interruptions are much less frequent—*4. Reassessment*. At the next staff meeting, all the above is reviewed. It is explained that the secretary will routinely close her door when doing dictation and the staff should respect her privacy at this time whenever possible. The study is written up with a note to carry out another reassessment evaluation in 6 months to see if the improvement continues—*5. Reporting*.

Remember, not all studies have to be medical or scientific. QA studies can deal with all aspects of the practice, such as medical records, cost containment, staffing, utilization of equipment, patient comfort and convenience, and marketing, to mention some of the possibilities that exist. Plans should routinely be made for periodic reassessment in a reasonable period of time, after which the study is fully closed out. The studies should be carried out by different members of the staff to ensure that everyone is involved with QA. Getting different members to participate will also help to develop an understanding that the governing body (which in most cases will be the owner-surgeon) is committed to the concept of ensuring and improving quality.

Try to make your studies relatively simple and straightforward so that they are easy to document. Pick something that can be evaluated in a quantitative rather than a qualitative way. Report your studies in a summary fashion that follows the specific requirements of the accrediting organization. If you are faced with a complex problem in your practice, it may be important to examine it thoroughly and analytically, but it may not be the best topic for a formal QA study. Remember that these studies are only an example of the total ongoing effort that a facility makes in the area of QA.

Until now, we have discussed the general concepts of QA. With all of this in mind, let us proceed to a review of some of the most important components of an overall QA program.

Credentialing

"I'm the only one who operates here, and everything that I do, I have privileges to do at the local hospital. Isn't that enough?" That's a common statement made by owners or operators of solo or small group surgical facilities. When you look at it closely, it's easy to see why this kind of attitude really defeats one of the fundamental reasons that surgeons choose to work in their own facilities: the desire to regain some independence and control over their practices that had been conceded to the hospital over a period of time. With these rights must come responsibilities.

In 1984, the House of Delegates of the American Medical Association adopted a policy regarding criteria for delineating clinical privileges, which stated that "delineation of privileges shall be determined on an individual basis, commensurate with an applicant's education, training, experience and demonstrated current competence." That means that any surgical facility has the responsibility of determining whether or not a surgeon is properly trained and experienced to carry out a specific procedure. In formulating this policy, the Delegates further emphasized that "in implementing these criteria, each facility shall formulate and apply reasonable, nondiscriminatory standards for the evaluation of an applicant's credentials, fee of anticompetitive intent or purpose."[2] That statement was obviously intended to prevent the members of one group or specialty from unfairly hindering an individual from another group or specialty from receiving credentials simply because he came from another background.

Mainly, facial plastic surgeons have fallen back on this statement to protect their rights in disputes over credentials in hospitals. Again, however, the statement not only points out rights, but it also denotes responsibility. A similar directive is emphasized in the policy statement of the American College of Surgeons, which stated that "eligibility to perform hospital surgical procedures as the responsible surgeon must be based on an individual's education, training, experience and demonstrated proficiency."[2]

The Joint Commission of Accreditation of Hospitals (JCAHO) requires that regardless of the method of granting privileges, it be "based on the individual's demonstrated current competence."[2] These guidelines are in conformity with the standards of the AAAHC, which emphasized the importance of independent credentialing.

In a larger facility, all of this should be quite straightforward. All that is needed is a committee of doctors who individually evaluate prospective staff members. Of course, protocols must be in place to protect the rights of individuals who are denied requested privileges. Most important, there must be a mechanism to ensure that doctors are not denied privileges simply because another doctor sees a competitive threat. Facial plastic surgeons are all well aware of the fact that such obstacles have frequently been raised in hospitals and ambulatory surgical centers by members of other specialties who have been dedicated to protecting their "turf" in areas of overlapping interest.

It is not surprising, then, that facial plastic surgeons might be reluctant to establish rules that would limit privileges, but this is clearly a responsibility that must be taken seriously if fair and impartial credentialing is to succeed. None of us wishes to see ambulatory surgical centers simply become hideouts for doctors who wish to engage in practices that they are not qualified for. A willingness to judge our competitors fairly is essential if doctors are to live up to their primary responsibility to police themselves. Certainly, if we don't do it, someone else will.

How about the solo physician operating in his own office? Does he still have a responsibility to carry out credentialing? Of course he does. In this case, he should clearly delineate the procedures for which he can document that he is trained and experienced to carry out. This should be stated in his bylaws. If he should decide to undertake new or different procedures, he should authenticate the way in which he has gained the knowledge and experience required to perform the procedure.

As is the custom in a hospital, he should periodically review his privileges. Furthermore, he should establish some criteria whereby his privileges are reviewed by his peers. Peer review is a complex and controversial issue, but it is worth mentioning in this context that, in all aspects of QA, it is important to involve at least one or two other physicians in the review process.

One final word on credentialing. It is not enough to simply credential the medical staff. You must also be sure that other health care providers have the necessary and appropriate training, as well as sufficient skill, to deliver the services that are called for in their particular job description. In some cases, such as for nurse anesthetists, specific credentialing may be required. In other cases, such as medical assistants, it may suffice to document that they have received adequate on-the-job training and are supervised adequately. In the case of nurses, one must demonstrate that they are currently licensed as well as being adequately trained for their specific jobs.

You must also be certain to document compliance with standards that you may have set for your individual facility. For example, it is common to require cardiopulmonary resuscitation (CPR) proficiency by all members of the staff. This is laudable, but if such a requirement is established in the bylaws, it becomes your responsibility to adhere to the rule. Therefore there must be documentation of CPR adequacy for each employee.

From the previous discussion, you may come to the conclusion that it would be simpler to avoid such requirements, but as we stated at the beginning of this chapter, the essence of QA is the demonstration to others that we are expending an adequate effort to assure our patients of high-quality medical care.

Policy and Procedures

Every organization must have rules by which it operates. A private surgical center is no different. Of course, every physician abhors red tape and paperwork. One of the reasons to have your own surgical center is to provide flexibility as well as the prerogative to make your own rules and regulations. There is nothing wrong with this, and in fact it is one of the great advantages of having your own facility. On the other hand, it is important that the staff of the facility have an understanding of their responsibilities. In a small organization, most, if not all, of the policies and procedures may be verbal. As we discussed before, however, it is often difficult to remember policies when they are not written, and as an organization grows, it becomes more important to have a written set of policies and procedures.

It is tempting to simply boilerplate a procedure manual from the hospital. It is better, however, to develop your own policy and procedure manual, which is relatively simple and suited to your own needs. If you do begin with someone else's, at least be sure that you go through it and discard any rules that you feel would be inappropriate for your own organization. Furthermore, remember that it can be written in plain English rather than legalese.

Although a policy and procedure manual may seem like an onerous chore, it can be helpful in your defense. If there is some question as to whether a certain procedure was appropriately carried out, it certainly would be helpful to be able to show that it was the standard procedure in your facility as designated by the policy and procedure manual. For example, suppose an infection resulted from an operation and there was a question as to whether adequate prep was carried out before surgery. In most cases, this would not have been documented in the operative or nursing notes. If it were the standard procedure to carry out a certain routine, and this was documented in the policy and procedure manual, this would serve as evidence that it was carried out in the particular case in question. Especially if the appropriate staff person could testify that he or she was aware of the procedure at the time in question. (Note, however, that you must adhere to the procedures in your manual. If a physician's staff fails to do something required by the manual, a lawyer may argue that the physician violated his own procedures and therefore is negligent.)

The medical record is obviously the way in which we document quality care of the individual patient. Physicians have traditionally been quite lax in their attention to necessary detail in completing medical records. Years ago, medical records were simply a way in which the doctor reminded himself of the salient features of the care of his patient. Of course, this has now completely changed. The medical record is now often thought of as simply a legal document that can save you or, more likely, hang you in court. Of course, as is so often the case, the answer is somewhere in between.

Let us, for the sake of this discussion, try to put the legal ramifications behind us, and simply think of the medical record as our way of demonstrating quality care. What, then, are the essentials of treatment that should be documented in the chart?

First of all, it should be established as to why the patient has sought your care. In the area of cosmetic surgery, one might be tempted to say that it is obvious. Certainly, the patient just wants to look better. Unless it is so stated, somewhere in the record, there is no way for an outside observer to recognize it. I am reminded of an accreditation survey in which I participated a few years ago wherein we were inspecting the facility of a very busy and prominent cataract surgeon. Because of the volume of his practice, he had developed techniques of streamlining his medical records. Unfortunately, he had become so efficacious that there was never a mention on the chart that any of his patients had come to see him because of difficulty with their vision, let alone a desire to have their vision surgically improved. Although this individual had an impeccable reputation, he exposed himself to the possible criticism of performing unnecessary surgery since there was no way for him to demonstrate that his patients were actually seeking the surgery that he offered.

The record should also demonstrate that you have carried out an adequate evaluation of the problem with which the patient presented and that the assessment has led to an appropriate diagnosis.

From that point, you should record your plan of action. This should include both your recommendations, as well as the specific treatment that you have provided. Included in this entry should be any discussion of alternatives, as well as some form of documentation that you have reviewed potential risks and limitations. It is always helpful to demonstrate that you have encouraged questions and responded to them.

Since a medical record is a very individual thing, it is recognized that there are many ways in which a physician can accomplish these goals. At the Facial Plastic and Cosmetic Surgical Center, we have found the following techniques useful, and you may choose to adopt some or all of these for your own personal use.

Patient Registration Sheet

When the patients register, they are asked to fill out an information sheet (see Figure 6-1). The form initially inquires as to why the patient has come in for consultation. A check sheet focuses on the problems that are most common to our practice. In a sense, this serves as a marketing tool, since it may remind patients that we perform additional services that may be of interest. For example, one of my major interests is malar augmentation, an operation that not many patients are familiar with. It is surprising how often, however, the patients will check "cheekbones" on the form. When asked about it, they usually reply that they didn't actually know that surgery could be done to enhance cheekbones, but they were interested in the idea.

Beneath the checklist is an area for patients to elaborate on their request. In most cases, a member of the staff will talk to the patient before their consultation, and this forms the basis for the initial discussion.

The form also asks, briefly, for history related to any general illnesses that the patient may have had. We ask in two ways: first by the direct question "Do you have any illnesses?" "What operations have you had?" "To what

FACIAL PLASTIC & COSMETIC SURGICAL CENTER — PATIENT REGISTRATION FORM

The following information will help us to serve you better. Please make every effort to fill out the information fully and accurately. Please be sure to complete both sides of the form. Your responses are held strictly confidential.

PERSONAL INFORMATION

NAME _____
DATE OF BIRTH _____ AGE _____ SEX _____ S S # _____
HOME ADDRESS _____
    city _____ state _____ zip _____
    TELEPHONE home (___) _____ work (___) _____
Single ( ) Married ( ) Separated ( ) Divorced ( ) Widowed ( )
Where employed? _____
Occupation? _____
Education *highest year completed* _____
Name of spouse if married _____ how many children _____
    Spouse's occupation _____
    Spouse's employer _____
In case of emergency, contact: _____
    Relationship: _____ phone (___) _____
Who is responsible for charges? _____

Please circle below the type or types of surgery you are interested in discussing
NOSE FACE EYELID NECK MOUTH EARS SCARS CHEEKS
CHIN WRINKLES
    OTHER _____

INSURANCE INFORMATION

Although insurance usually does not cover the cost of cosmetic surgery, there are many instances in which coverage is applicable. If you feel that your treatment might be covered, please fill in the following:

Primary Policy
Company _____
_____
Address _____
_____
Insured's Name _____
_____
Gp # _____
Policy # _____

Secondary Policy
Company _____
_____
Address _____
_____
Insured's Name _____
_____
Gp # _____
Policy # _____

Please use this space to give us any other information you feel would be helpful for your consultation.

WHY DID YOU SELECT OUR CENTER   Please indicate all that apply   ( ) General reputation or recommendation
( ) Patient referral. May we ask who? _____ May we acknowledge referral? ( ) yes ( ) no
( ) Doctor referral. May we ask who? _____ May we acknowledge referral? ( ) yes ( ) no
( ) Speaking engagement. Where? _____ ( ) Magazine. Which? _____
( ) Newspaper ( ) Yellow pages Which book? _____ ( ) Other - (please indicate below)
_____

The medical history is an extremely important part of your consultation. It helps to alert us to any potential problems that might interfere with your surgery. Please take the time to fill this out completely and accurately. If you need some help, the staff will be glad to assist you.

List all prescription drugs you are taking: _____
List any nonprescription drugs you take (i.e. aspirin, cold tablets, etc.) _____

_____

Figure 6-1.

Please tell us about any serious illnesses you have had in the past for example, heart disease, blood pressure problems, pulmonary disease, kidney disease, diabetes, thyroid trouble, stomach ulcers, etc. _____

Please list any operations you have had (including cosmetic surgery) give aprroximate dates _____

Describe any difficulties you have had with anesthesia _____

Describe any injuries you have sustained include dates _____

Are there any hereditary disorders in your family that might be of significance ? _____

List any drugs to which you are allergic _____

Do you smoke? _____ If so, what form and how much?_____

How much alcohol do you drink? ( ) none   ( ) occasional   ( ) moderate   ( ) heavy

How is your general health? _____ **Are you under a doctor's care?** _____

Please review the list below and check anything applicable. You may use the space to the right for any explanation that you think would be helpful. Please be as complete as possible.

( ) Severe dryness of the eyes
( ) Glaucoma or blurry vision
( ) Recurrent severe dizziness
( ) Severe headaches
( ) Chronic sinus problems or nasal blockage
( ) Recurrent fever blisters
( ) Paralysis of the face
( ) Asthma or emphysema
( ) Chronic hoarseness
( ) Shortness of breath
( ) Chest pain
( ) Heart disease or high blood pressure
( ) Chronic abdominal problems
( ) Kidney or bladder problems
( ) Blood in bowel movements
( ) Blood in urine or trouble urinating
( ) Bleeding disorders (you or anyone in your family)
( ) Easy bruising
( ) Menstrual disorder
( ) Abnormal lump or node
( ) Problems with bones or joints
( ) Unexplained weight loss
( ) Cancer
( ) Emotional problems
( ) Chronic skin condition
( ) Complications after surgery
( ) Bad surgical result or unsatisfactory medical care

Height _____

Weight _____

Date this form completed _____ Signature _____

are you allergic?" etc. We then list a series of symptoms for the patient to check, after which we ask him or her to elucidate. Some of the more important questions are asked in more than one way. For example, in the narrative section requesting information about illnesses, we specifically mention hypertension. It is also one of the questions that can be checked off at the end of the form. When the questions are too general, the responses tend to be inadequate. We specifically ask patients if they have ever had any difficulty with anesthesia. During the consultation, these positive responses are reviewed in detail and set the stage for the remainder of the workup.

A pertinent review of symptoms are then listed on the form, and the patients are asked to review them and check the pertinent questions.

In addition to the medical aspects of the Patient Registration Sheet, we also ask for insurance information, as well as general information about the patient, his or her employment, family information, etc. There is also a section that deals with how the patient learned about us and what made him or her select our Center. This helps us to evaluate our marketing and is discussed further in the previous chapter of this book.

After the patient has completed the form, he is asked to sign it. This serves as a permanent part of the patient record, and the signature verifies that the patient has answered the form to the best of his ability. This is further emphasized on our surgical permit, which contains a statement indicating that the information on the Patient Registration Form is complete and correct.

Consultation Notes

During the actual consultation notes are made on a consultation sheet. The form has various anatomic diagrams (see Fig. 6-2), which facilitate the notation of physical findings. There is also a large area for general notes. This, to a large extent, represents the initial physical examination. The form is also used to annotate briefly unusual aspects of a case, or particular complications that were pointed out.

If computer imaging was used, it is noted on the sheet. In most cases, an actual hard copy of the imaging will be placed in the chart, although we do retain the images on disk. Computer imaging has become widely accepted. Initial concerns of implied warranty have not proven to be a problem, and we are aware of no suits over this issue. It is important, however, to have a record of the fact that the patient was forewarned that the computer images represent goals of surgery rather than an indication of what the patient may expect to be an infallible result of the operation.

Actually, the surgeon who offers this service will, at some point, become as proficient at imaging as he is at operating, so that he can actually give the patient a true idea of the *anticipated* result of surgery. In this sense, the imaging system is probably more precarious in the hands of the novice surgeon than in the one with experience, for it is the latter who is more likely to have a reasonable idea of the result of his operation.

Returning to our consultation sheet, you will see a small list at the lower left hand corner of the form. This represents a summary of the written information given to the patient at the time of consultation. Specifically listed are such items as our general information booklet which is given to nearly all patients. This booklet contains general information, including reference to common complications, about most of the procedures offered at our Center. There is additional space to list other items, such as our patient newsletters or reprints of scientific articles written about topics that are pertinent to the patient's desired procedures. We feel that it is important to document that the patient received this information, since it forms a part of what is generally considered to be informed consent.

Ideally, the surgeon should document *all* of the discussion between himself and the patient. Unfortunately, in a busy practice, this is not practical. The previously mentioned shortcuts can assist in establishing the fact that a complete discussion was carried out. As is always the case, reality is a compromise and I feel that time is better spent in genuine interaction with the patient rather than simply in documentation. Attorneys may argue, but I still feel that overly defensive medicine can destroy the bond of confidence that will usually exist between the surgeon and a properly selected patient. That is not to say that we ignore the importance of documentation, but we try to keep it in perspective.

One technique that we use serves to help document our consultation as well as firming the bond developed during the initial interview. This is our "follow-up letter" which is sent to all new patients.

Follow-up Letter

After each new consultation, a letter is sent to the patient. An example is shown in Figure 6-3. It is worth spending a little time reviewing this letter, since it forms an important part of the medical record.

The initial paragraph is a personal note that indicates our appreciation that the patient has chosen us for consultation. In that paragraph, I review my recommendations and indicate the procedures that will provide the aesthetic improvement that the patient desires. The phrasing in this sentence is important, since you must not indicate that you are guaranteeing a result. Nevertheless, there is certainly nothing wrong with expressing your opinion as to the suitability of the recommended treatment. After all, if you didn't think it was going to work, you had no business suggesting it.

The next paragraph states the following: "I hope that I have answered any questions that you had about the operative procedure that you are considering. You will

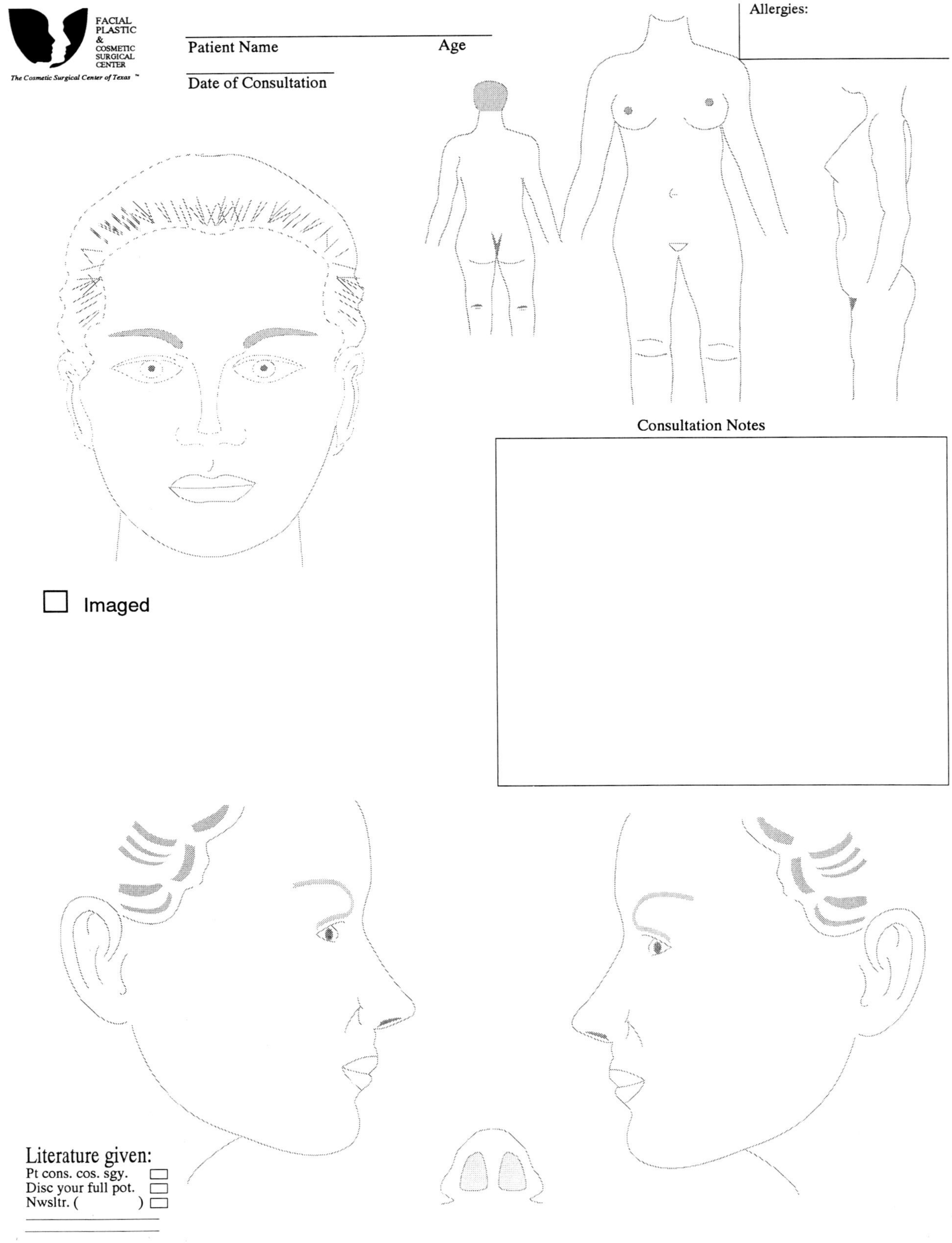

82   Developing a Practice in Ambulatory Surgery

FACIAL PLASTIC & COSMETIC SURGICAL CENTER
The Cosmetic Surgical Center of Texas

Patient Name _____ Age _____

Date of Consultation _____

Allergies:

☐ Imaged

Consultation Notes

Literature given:
Pt cons. cos. sgy.   ☐
Disc your full pot. ☐
Nwsltr. (   )   ☐

Figure 6-2.

FACIAL PLASTIC & COSMETIC SURGICAL CENTER

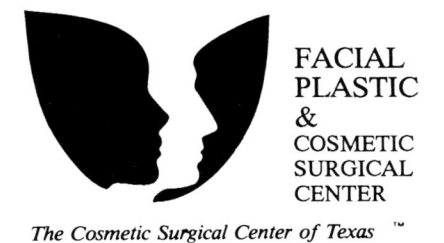

The Cosmetic Surgical Center of Texas ™

Howard A. Tobin, M.D., F.A.C.S.
Certified American Board of Facial Plastic & Reconstructive Surgery
Certified American Board of Cosmetic Surgery

Jane Doe
P.O. Box 888
Abilene, TX

Dear Jane:

I enjoyed visiting with you and discussing your interest in rhinoplasty surgery. Based upon my evaluation and your desires, it appears likely that the operation would lead to a result that would meet reasonable expectations for improvement.

I hope that I have answered any questions that you had about the surgery you are considering. Please be sure to read carefully the written material that was given to you during your consultation. If you have any other questions or require any additional information, please don't hesitate to contact me either by phone or in person.

When you are ready to schedule your surgery, please get in touch with Dena, at the Center, and she will help you to make the necessary arrangements. We appreciate your interest in our Center and look forward to being of service to you.

Sincerely,

Howard A. Tobin, M.D., F.A.C.S.

HAT/wl

6300 Humana Plaza, Abilene, TX 79606, (915) 695-3630, 1 (800) 592-4533 FAX (915) 695-3633

Figure 6-3.

find additional information in the literature which we gave you, and I would suggest that you refer to it. If you require additional information please don't hesitate to contact me either by phone or in person." I feel that this paragraph forms an important part of our informed consent and is therefore a valuable risk-management tool. It clearly states that the patient is expected to familiarize himself with the information that was given at the time of consultation. Again, this works hand in hand with the notation as to exactly what information was given. It also serves as an open invitation to the patient to voice any additional questions.

When patients later sign their operative permit, they acknowledge two statements that are intended to confirm and endorse the phrase that appears in the letter. These statements are:

- *I have been given an opportunity to ask questions about my condition, alternative forms of anesthesia and treatment, risks of nontreatment, the procedures to be used, and the risks and hazard involved, and I believe that I have sufficient information to give this informed consent.*
- *I agree to follow the instructions given to me by Dr. Tobin to the best of my ability **before**, during and after the above mentioned surgical procedure, and will notify Dr. Tobin of any problems following my surgery.*

Although these statements are no substitute for an adequate briefing of the patient, they do serve to emphasize that an effort is being made to be responsive to the questions of the patient.

If computer imaging has been carried out as a part of the consultation, the following paragraph is included in the letter: "The computer imaging which we carried out during your consultation gives an approximation of the goal of surgery. Of course, this cannot be taken as a guarantee of what the actual result of the operation will be, but it does give an estimate of the result that we will be seeking."

Although much of the information in the letter consists of standard phrases, of course, each letter is individualized, and a copy kept in the patient's record.

Fee Quotation

So many disputes ultimately rest on disagreement about money. When surgery is urgent or of an emergency nature, of course money must not be the primary element. In ambulatory surgery, however, most of our work is elective, and it is vital that both the patient and the surgeon have a clear understanding of the monetary factors involved. Regardless of who discusses the fees, there is likely to be some misunderstanding unless there is a written agreement. We have developed a form that we feel covers all of the potential costs of the surgery (see Fig. 6-4).

Although our particular form is computer generated for each patient, a similar form can be developed that allows you to simply fill in the blanks. The following are the elements of the form that I think are worth having.

First of all, the form should have the patient's name and the date. It is surprising how long people will hold on to this type of form. We have had patients come back several years later expecting us to adhere to a fee quote made long ago. For that reason, we also stipulate the length of the agreement, in our case 2 months. Although we will generally honor a quote longer than that, even if we have raised our fees, there is no reason to commit yourself to that. It is quite possible that, in the interval, you may have received your new malpractice policy! When our premium went up from $40,000 to $70,000, I can assure you that fee adjustments were made!

We then stipulate the fees for the individual surgical procedures that will be carried out. We separate these in most cases, citing a fee for each procedure. If we give a discount for combined procedures, as is our normal custom, we show this as a special credit.

The next section deals with operating charges. Our policy is to charge for time and supplies as used. Therefore, we can only make an estimate of the operating expense. Of course, with experience, we get pretty good at judging the cost, but we can never be sure of the exact amount. For that reason, in cases where there is no insurance coverage, we will usually guarantee a maximum of one or two hundred dollars above the estimate.

Finally, we address the anesthesia charges, which, in our clinic, are paid directly to the anesthetist.

After the form is completed and reviewed with the patient, we ask them to sign one copy, which we keep in the chart. Another copy is given to the patient. It is very helpful to have a signed form, since it can later be shown to the patient to remind them that they have agreed to the terms and stated fees.

Patient Instructions

Quality care requires that patients be adequately instructed in the proper care required both before and after surgery. Although much of this information may be verbal, it has been demonstrated over and over again that patients remember little of what is explained to them. This is especially true in the case of postoperative patients. It would be foolish to think that a recovering patient would remember much of what he is told before leaving the recovery room. Therefore it is important to provide patients with written pre- and postoperative instructions.

Of course, there are many ways of doing this. Many surgeons have developed different forms for each surgical procedure in their armamentarium. Since so many of our operations consist of multiple procedures, we have developed a general sheet of postoperative instructions that covers most of the important points related to the most

FACIAL PLASTIC & COSMETIC SURGICAL CENTER

The Cosmetic Surgical Center of Texas ™

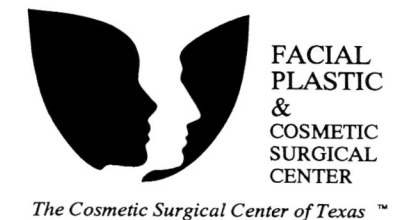

Fee Quotation

Mary Largenose
6402 Anystreet
Abilene, TX   79606

This fee quote is prepared for Mary Largenose. It is valid until 05/04/92. Surgery scheduled beyond that time is subject to rate change.
Please note that operating room charges represent our best estimate based on past experience.

Operation

Rhinoplasty $2800.00

Estimate of operating room expense $700.00

Please note that the operating room fee is an estimate. Any charge in excess to the estimate will be billed, while any charge less will be credited to your account. The operating room fee is guaranteed not to exceed $900.00

Total due to Cosmetic Surgical Center $3500.00

A $200 non refundable deposit is required upon scheduling. The entire balance is due ten days prior to surgery, and is non refundable after that time.

The above quotation does not include fees for general anesthesia. This payment is to be made directly to the anesthetist and is due on the day of surgery.

Anesthesia fee   ——— $325.00

Total estimate   ——— $3825.00

I have read the above quotation and, if I choose to have the surgery, I agree to its terms.

March 5, 1992   Mary Largenose

6300 Humana Plaza   •   Abilene, Texas 79606   •   (915) 695-3630

Figure 6-4.

common surgical procedures. This form is reproduced in Appendix 8 for general reference, and it can be modified for an individual's own unique practice.

As a responsible part of your risk-management program, it is also essential that the fact that you gave the pertinent information to the patient be recorded on the chart.

It may seem, as we review this abundance of paperwork, that we are essentially duplicating one of the most onerous chores of the hospital. Unfortunately, to a degree, this is the case. When one decides to direct his own surgical center, there is no way to avoid much of the responsibility that was previously delegated to the hospital staff, and basic risk management demands sufficient documentation. The only advantage is that in the private surgical center, a good deal of this can be streamlined, and it is my hope that in this chapter, you will find a few hints that will achieve this goal without sacrificing quality.

Operative Permit

There is certainly no unanimity of opinion as to what should be placed on an operative permit. Traditionally, standard hospital forms have been quite simple, stating that the patient gives the surgeon broad latitude to use his judgment when unusual circumstances arise. There is usually a general statement to the effect that the patient has been advised as to the nature of the operation as well as the alternatives and risks. How much should you include on your own permit that you use in your surgical center? There is no clear answer. Lack of informed consent in past years was one of the more common grounds for suit. It is proportionately less used now, but that is probably simply related to the fact that there are many more fertile grounds for suit. It does not mean that the surgeon can ignore adequate documentation of informed consent. This is especially true in a private surgical center.

Several years ago, the state of Texas established some guidelines in this area. They determined the common risks for a number of procedures, and the Texas Medical Association has strongly recommended that these particular risks be written out on the operative permit. That does not serve as a substitute for adequate consultation regarding risk and complications, but it does provide a baseline.

Some surgeons choose to have a separate permit for each of the more common procedures that they perform. This is certainly a possibility, but can get a little complicated if you combine procedures. We have attempted to combine the most common risks related to all of our most common operations on one form, which is reproduced in Appendix 7. Actually, we don't call the form a *permit*, we refer to it as an agreement related to the patient's request for surgery.

In addition to listing common risks and complications related to surgical procedures, there are a number of other important areas that we touch on:

1. We have the patient acknowledge the higher risks involved with smokers. This is an area of common knowledge, but is worth emphasizing to the patient.
2. We caution female patients as to the risk of anesthesia to the fetus and have them affirm that they are not pregnant at the time of surgery.
3. We obtain release for use of photographs.
4. We have the patient affirm that they have had an opportunity to review the form and ask questions.

At the time that the form is given, the patient is instructed to take it home and read it carefully. They are advised that they will be given an opportunity to ask any questions they might have prior to signing the form on the morning of surgery. A note is made in the chart indicating that the form was given to the patient. We feel that it is important to give the permit to the patient well in advance of the surgery, since it refutes the possible argument that the patient was asked to sign a form that they did not have the opportunity to study or question, or that they were already committed to proceeding with the operation when the form was presented. The form is written in plain language, and just above the signature it carries the admonition: **"DO NOT SIGN THIS FORM UNLESS YOU HAVE READ IT AND FEEL THAT YOU UNDERSTAND IT. ASK ANY QUESTIONS YOU MIGHT HAVE BEFORE SIGNING."**

Finally, on the morning of surgery, after the form has been signed and witnessed by the patient and a member of the family or one of our staff, I again review the form and ask if there are any questions, at which time I also initial the form. No form is perfect, and, admittedly, attorneys will always look beyond the form, but this one covers many of the possible pitfalls and also serves as a reminder of some of the crucial areas of informed consent.

In the final analysis, informed consent relates to communication between the patient, the surgeon, and the staff.

Physician's Orders

In the hospital, there is a mandated system of ordering treatment and medication. All of us have disdained the medical records librarian for the multitude of entreaties and warnings about delinquent records. When first beginning a career in office-based surgery, one of the surgeon's greatest joys is the absence of a requirement to document every decision or instruction on a formal order sheet. While it is true that a formal order sheet is not a necessity, there is a need to document, in some way, the surgeon's orders. Obviously, in most cases, the orders are verbal, and the documentation will be reflected in the notation regarding the execution of the order. Nevertheless, the

Quality Assurance and Risk Management 87

Patient: _____
Date: _____
Operation: _____

Facial Plastic & Cosmetic Surgical Center
Abilene, Texas
Howard A. Tobin, M.D.

FACIAL SURGERY WORK SHEET
both sides same unless indicated
Photo shows tissue removal

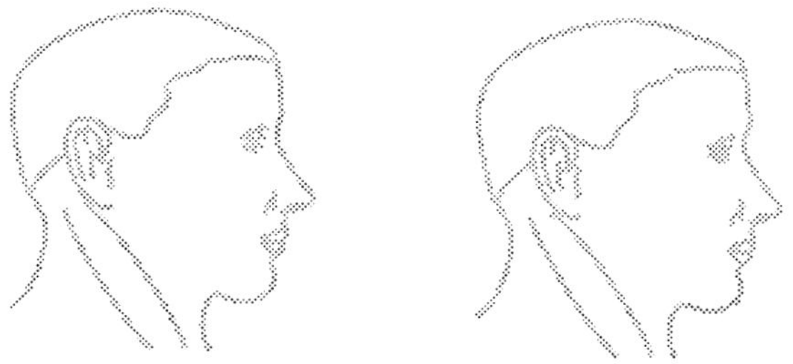

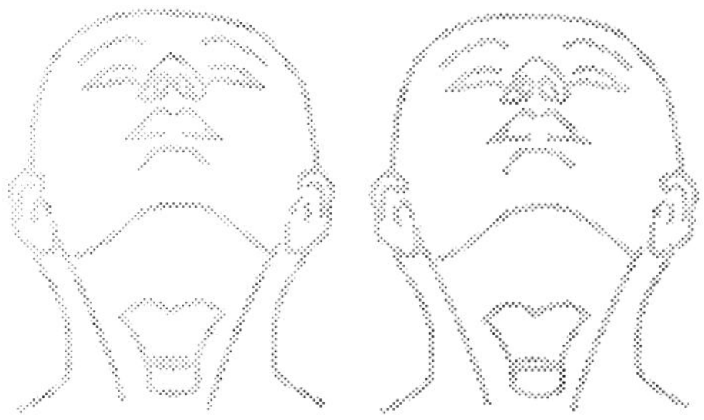

LIPOSUCTION
Cannula _____
Fat Return _____
Open l.s. _____
l.s. = lo suction
n.s. = no suction

UNDERMINING
Bleeding _____
Suction Drains_____
Dressing: Cotton__ Kerlix__
Kling__ Coban__ _____

INCISIONS
Blade _____
Bovie xxxxx

CLOSURE
Sub Cut _____
Skin: Staples xxxxxx
    Suture ------- (   )

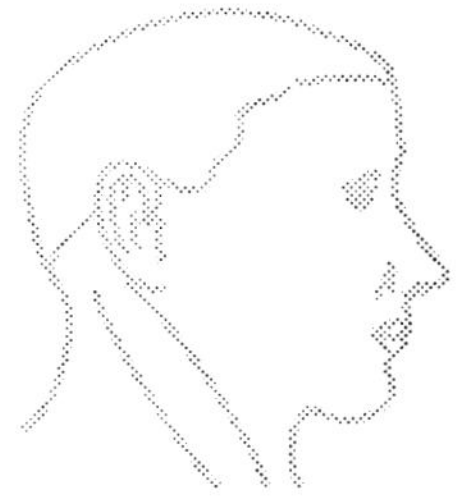

PLATYSMA - PAROTID FASCIA
___ Parotid fascia flap
___ Undermine platysma
___ Cut lower border platysma
        suture _____

___ Plicate fascia
___ Plicate platysma

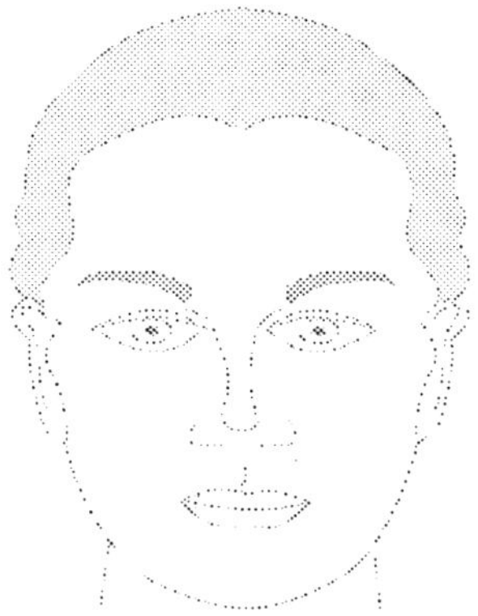

PEEL
Baker ___
TCA _____%

IMPLANT
Malar ___: Canine fossa incision,
#0 Chromic pull out, close 4-0 chr.
Implant _____

Chin ___: Submental incision; sub-
periosteal dissection; close 4-0 chr
& 6-0 plain
Implant _____

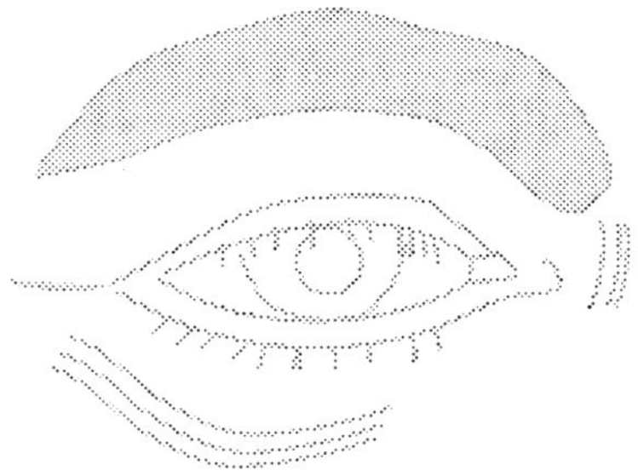

Eyeliner___
Color_____

← direction of pull
▥ undermined area
▨ skin excision

Blepharoplasty
__ Electrosurgical incision
__ Close upper lid running 6-0 plain
__ Close lower lid 6-0 plain interrupted, lat. only
__ Lower lid - skin flap ☐ muscle flap ☐
__ Coagulate fat - upper lid ☐ lower lid ☐
__ Muscle excision = skin on upper lid

Figure 6-5.

88 Developing a Practice in Ambulatory Surgery

Facial Plastic & Cosmetic Surgical Center

Patient Name _____ Age _____
Date of Surgery _____ Operation _____
Anesthesia _____
Surgeon Howard A. Tobin, M. D.

Incisions
☐ Open Rhinoplasty
☐ Intercartilagenous
☐ Transfixion
☐ Rim with delivery
☐ _____

Tip
☐ Cartilage excision (see diagram)
  ☐ Submucosal
☐ Divide at dome
  ☐ Sub mucosal
☐ Suture Medial Crura
☐ Suture Lateral Crura
☐ Tip Graft (see diagram)
☐ Strut (see diagram)
☐ Excise soft tissue
☐ Morcelize (see diagram)

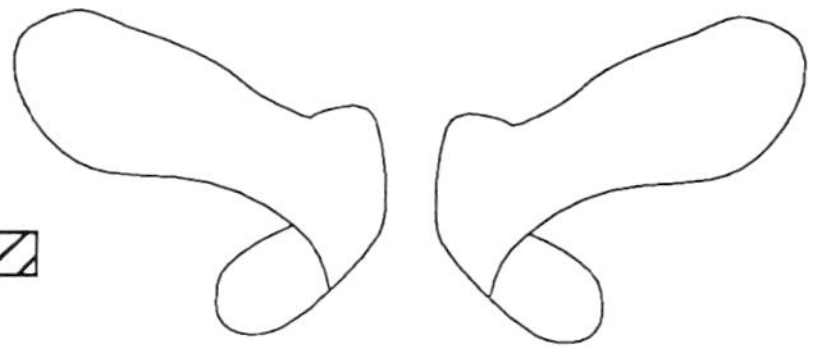

Profile
☐ Lower dorsum with osteotome
☐ Lower dorsum with scissors
☐ Lower dorsum with rasp
☐ Smooth with rasp
☐ Lower septum (see diagram)
☐ Trim caudal septum (see diagram)
☐ Dorsal Graft _____
☐ Gelfilm on dorsum

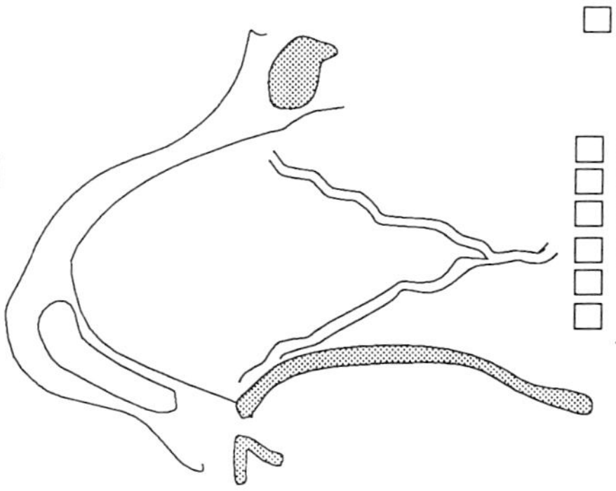

Upper Lateral Cartilage
☐ Divide from septum
☐ Trim dorsum
☐ Trim caudal

Osteotomies
☐ Medial
☐ Lateral
  ☐ Parkes
  ☐ Micropuncture
  ☐ Multiple
_____

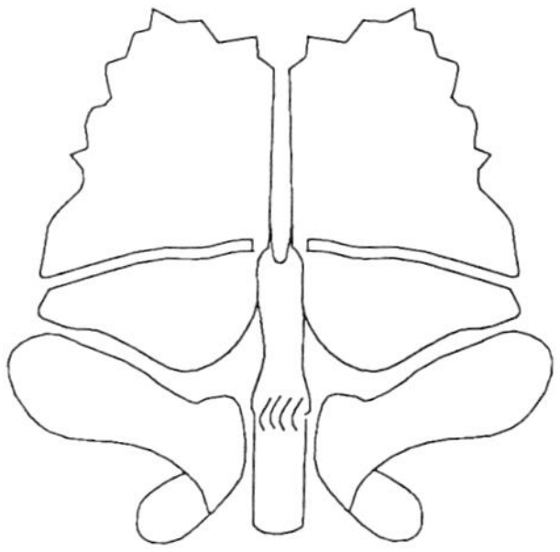

Alar Base
☐ (see diagram)
☐ suture _____

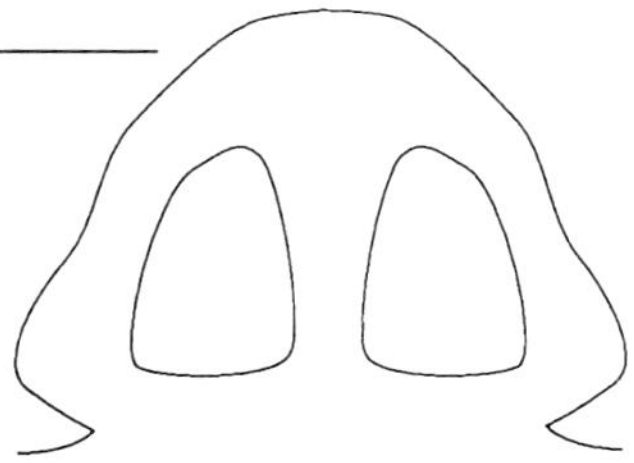

Septum
☐ Obstruction: ☐ R ☐ L
☐ Elevate mucosa ☐ R ☐ L
☐ Remove cart/bone (see diag)
☐ Replace cartilage ☐ crushed
☐ grid (see diagram)

Turbinates
☐ Outfracture
☐ Crush
☐ Partial resection
☐ Electrocoagulate
_____

Closure
☐ Cart. approx. _____
☐ Incisions _____
☐ Quilting suture _____
☐ Matress base columella _____
☐ _____
☐ _____

Dressing
☐ steristrip tip
☐ tape dorsum
☐ cast
☐ pack _____
☐ gelfoam pack
☐ splint with plastic
☐ _____

Additional Notes:

Figure 6-6.

surgeon must not neglect to establish criteria for recording this information. Combining the order itself with a notation as to its execution on a single form, or in a specific area of the chart, is one way of managing this problem.

At this point, we must interject that not every surgical facility will be subject to the same regulations. For example, various accrediting or licensing bodies will have specific requirements that will have to be fulfilled. In some cases, this may result in requirements that approach those of the hospital and may almost defy streamlining. In my role as surveyor for the AAAHC, I have had the unique opportunity of visiting Medicare-certified surgical centers in various states and have been rather astounded as to the variability in requirements for charting and documentation. In some states, such as Arizona, they appear quite reasonable, allowing concise and streamlined records, while in my own state of Texas, we struggle to keep our charts down to the size of a weekly magazine.

Operative Report

In the hospital, we become used to a formal report of surgery. Many surgeons who operate in their offices tend to omit this in favor of a simple note as to what was done. It is important to remember that documentation is just as important in your office as it is in the hospital, although the surgeon does have more flexibility in his own facility. In many hospitals, surgeons have used computer-generated operative reports for standard procedures. There is some question as to the legal validity of such a report. It certainly wouldn't look good in court if a lawyer could show that every one of your rhinoplasty reports was exactly the same. It would be far more desirable to have a brief but individual report of the procedure.

In our clinic, we tend to rely on standard forms, which allows the surgeon to write in the specific detail of a procedure, depending heavily on diagrams to depict findings and details of surgery. This certainly makes it convenient to review the details of an operation and would allow the surgeon to prepare a detailed narrative. These forms have been reviewed by malpractice attorneys who have felt that they would be adequate in the defense of a potential malpractice case, if there was adequate material on the form to document what was and was not done.

In recently reviewing these forms, James Scheper, a malpractice attorney from Hamilton, Ohio, commented on the fact that the operative record in a single surgeon practice need not be in a form that would necessarily allow anyone to be able to recognize all of the details of the operation, since, unlike the hospital, a number of physicians do not ordinarily have access to the medical records.[3] He also commented on the fact that it is common for a defense to be hampered by too much written information, when some of that information may be inaccurate or erroneous, such as could happen when narrative operative reports are written some time after the surgery, or based on a standard form.

Although this technique may be criticized as not conforming to the standard operative report format, it succinctly provides all of the required information. Two of these work sheets are provided for reference (see Figures 6-5, 6-6).

RISK MANAGEMENT

The surgeon spends all of his waking hours considering the risk to which he subjects his patients. He is constantly weighing risk against gain, advising patients, and helping them to reach a decision regarding treatment. Since no treatment is without risk for the patient, each decision takes on an air of liability for the surgeon. This is a concept of liability that each of us understands all too well. In fact, if we ask a doctor what risk management is all about, chances are he will tell us that it relates to reducing one's chances of being sued. However, there is much more to risk management.

Risk management relates to all of the risks that we face in running our practice, and they extend way beyond what is commonly referred to as "malpractice." Risk management has been defined as "the results-oriented approach to protecting the assets of a business so that its operations can grow profitably."[4] It relates to all the risks that we face in running our business, and, indeed, it is important that we recognize it as a business, especially when we increase the scope of our practice to include an ambulatory surgical center.

REFERENCES

1. Beck EM, ed: Bartlett's Familiar Quotations. Little, Brown & Co., Boston, 1980
2. Delineation of Hospital Privileges—The American Academy of Otolaryngology—Head and Neck Surgery & The American Academy of Facial Plastic & Reconstructive Surgery, 1985
3. Personal communication
4. Fifer WR. Risk management and medical malpractice, *Quality Rev Bull* 1979; 5:9–13
5. Charles SC, Kennedy E: *Defendant*. Vantage Books—Random House, New York, 1986
6. Crill JL: In Davis JE, ed: Major Ambulatory Surgery. Williams & Wilkins, Baltimore, 1986, p 428

CHAPTER 6 ADDENDUM

INJURY AND ILLNESS PREVENTION PROGRAMS

A risk management program includes not only activities directly related to reducing one's risk of exposure to medical malpractice, but also includes programs to decrease the incidence of injury or illness to both employees and patients in the medical work place. An appropriate risk management program is extremely complex. It should include employee training and operating new equipment, procedures on handling infectious medical waste, and systems to monitor potential hazards in the medical work place.

The California Medical Association has taken the lead in developing an outstanding injury and illness prevention program. Developed by the Technical Advisory Committee on Injury and Illness Programs, the California Medical Association has recently published several documents which are valuable instruction manuals for any medical practice. They include important information on establishing written programs for identifying hazards in the work place, developing safety procedures, developing employee training programs, and implementing periodic inspections. While these documents are specific for the state of California, they are important resource documents for any physician. They can be purchased by contacting the California Medical Association, 221 Main Street, P.O. Box 7690, San Francisco, CA 94120-7690. Request "Injury and Illness Prevention Programs for the Medical Office—Section I and Section II."

Legal Considerations of an Ambulatory Surgical Practice

E. SQUIER NEAL, J.D.

A surgeon is never far removed from the law. As a physician, he daily weighs the legal ramifications of life or death decisions, of disclosure of confidential patient records, of peer appraisals before credentialing committees and disciplinary boards.

As a business man, he regularly signs contracts for real estate, goods, and services.

As an employer, he is obliged to offer employees fair conditions under current labor law.

Hidden legal dangers exist in all of these aspects of practicing facial plastic surgery, and any surgeon who blithely goes about his practice in total legal innocence can expect frustration, even financial disaster, in this increasingly litigious society.

In this chapter, our intent is to alert surgeons to the basic legal principles that govern what they may and may not do as they practice medicine and manage that practice.

Of necessity, the chapter has limitations. In no way do we intend to provide the comprehensive legal advice that only your personal attorney can give. We skip entirely any discussion of laws related to such personal areas as estate planning, domestic relations, and tax law. We speak in generalities only—not only because specific legal principles can vary from state to state, but also because principles that apply to a solo practitioner may not apply to a physician in a group, hospital, or university practice.

There are five general areas of law, however, about which the surgeon may be expected to demonstrate awareness. These we cover: patient records, business contracts, employee policies, peer review, and malpractice litigation.

PATIENT RECORDS

Patient records can generate legal problems in two ways—when their contents are disclosed without patient consent and when they are inaccurate or incomplete.

Confidential Records

In general, the law regards the physician-patient relationship as sacrosanct. Most states accordingly grant the privilege of confidentiality to the patient. Unless the patient expressly consents, the physician may not disclose the contents of the patient's records or any information regarding the patient. Unauthorized invasion of a patient's privacy can have costly ramifications. This includes use of patient photographs without signed consent from the patient.

There are exceptions, and every medical practitioner should be aware of statutory reporting requirements that often circumvent confidentiality defenses in legal situations. For instance, physicians may discuss the content of patient records with consulting physicians or others in the rendering of patient care or in the interests of research, so long as confidentiality is maintained. Also, a court can order the disclosure of records relative to a pending case. Moreover, a patient waives the privilege of confidentiality with respect to records about injuries that he claims were the result of malpractice.

While statutes vary from state to state, most jurisdictions require the following disclosures to override the confidentiality privilege: births and deaths, controlled substances, child abuse (every state gives immunity for such reporting), suspicious wounds or injuries, and epileptic seizures and related disorders.

Complete Records

When the surgeon documents all care given, he has an important historical record. His patient files contain the information necessary to provide future care, to defend the appropriateness of past care, and to prepare retrospective medical reports required by disability and other patient claims.

The most insignificant fact during a patient visit should not go unrecorded, as it later may provide the basis to prove your own point or to disprove a patient's allegation. An unrecorded temperature or weight, for instance, may support the patient's contention that a procedure never was performed. An unreported telephone call from the patient, to the pharmacy or to a consultant likewise may serve to substantiate a negligence claim against you.

If your overburdened schedule tempts you to postpone recording such small details until you need to, dismiss the thought. Juries usually can recognize "doctored" records and are offended mightily by them. Updating records daily should eliminate the temptation to amplify them later on.

Records that lack objectivity also do you more harm than good. Entries involving petty items or personal

> **SAMPLE PATIENT CONSENT FORM FOR RELEASE AND USE OF PHOTOGRAPHS**
>
> The undersigned _____ is a patient of _____, M.D., and has been photographed during the course of treatment. The undersigned grants _____, M.D., and the American Academy of Facial Plastic and Reconstructive Surgery the on-going and unrestricted right to use the photographs of the undersigned for general information, education and public relations purposes.
>
> The undersigned acknowledges that he/she relinquishes all right, title and interest in these photographs, or any right to profit or gain directly or indirectly realized through the use of the photographs.
>
> This form and the effect of my consent have been fully explained to me and any questions I had are fully answered.
>
> Date: Signed:
>
> _____   _____
>
>   Witnessed:
>
>   _____
>
> *Source:* Larry D. Schoenrock, M.D.

criticism tarnish the image of a surgeon when his records are opened in court.

Your own use of patient records to write medical reports also depends on complete, accurate, and up-to-date notes. Requests for these documents have increased in recent years as patients try to establish entitlement or benefits under disability and workmen's compensation acts or as they try to establish injury in malpractice claims.

To safeguard yourself legally, your medical reports should contain certain elements: the patient's history, the date the history was obtained, and all relevant information as to what was *not* seen or said as well as the more obvious opposite. It is significant and should be reported, for instance, that the patient complaining of severe facial pain did not grimace or exhibit any other physical manifestations indicative of such pain. Impressions, findings, diagnosis, and prognosis should be stated with reasonable medical certainty. If further medical care is recommended, it should be so stated along with an opinion of the elective versus mandatory nature of the follow-up.

Medical reports that you write to help patients make claims against workmen's compensation or medical disability plans often require that you keep additional kinds of patient data. The American Medical Association, for instance, has guidelines on how to evaluate a level of impairment and thus establish a level of benefits under workmen's compensation. Likewise, the Social Security Administration has a comprehensive set of medical guidelines under which medical disability is governed. If certain medical signs, symptoms, or values are missing from a particular medical report, the report will be of no use to the patient—who then may file action against you.

BUSINESS CONTRACTS

Contract law regulates many aspects of all businesses, including the practice of facial plastic surgery. Your own employment contract, your invoices for the purchase of goods and services, and your lease agreement for office space are but a few of the documents you may sign that will be governed by contract law.

Generally, contract law applies to any document between two willing parties or entities dealing at arm's length with a mutual understanding of the purpose of the contract, as evidenced by the parties' signatures on the document containing the understanding.

Legal problems with contracts usually arise when not all terms and conditions of a contract are put in writing, or when one party to the contract fails to read or understand all of the contract's terms.

Without exception, a document signed as a contract should contain all of the terms and conditions to be part of the agreement. Verbal variations, such as "Don't worry about paying the balance until later," often are useless comments. While a contract may have been altered verbally, proving the verbal agreement may be difficult under the statute of frauds if the other party changes his mind or chooses to renege.

Your failure to read or understand all of the terms of a contract also is no protection against future charges of breach of contract. If you do not have time yourself to acquaint yourself thoroughly with the smallest type in the lengthiest document, be prepared to hire someone to review the contract for you. Never ask the other party to the contract to explain what some contractual term means.

Let's look at how these principles of contract law may affect three areas of your medical practice.

Employment Contract

If you sign an employment contract, it typically will contain certain restrictive provisions, in addition to details on your salary, benefits, and duties (hours, call schedule, patient scheduling, and assignment). Restrictive provisions are provisions that prohibit your engaging in similar employment following your termination (for whatever reason) from the contractual job.

State laws differ regarding the validity of restrictive provisions, but if the state where you practice admits their validity, then you must be prepared to have your practice of medicine governed by restrictive provisions of any contract you sign.

If a state recognizes the validity of restrictions on employment opportunity, it does so on the grounds that an employer has a right to the fruits of its employees' labor. Presumably, a medical clinic or corporate group attracts patients because of its reputation established through the years. The "clinic" or "group" cannot practice medicine, however; it is the employees who practice medicine. Patinets are loyal to the employees who treat them, not to the clinic or group. If an employee were to leave the clinic or group, he thus could take many of the patients with him, and to protect the employer, some states allow restrictive provisions on employment following termination.

Restrictive provisions must be reasonable in two respects, time and geography, if they are to be valid. A legitimate restriction might prohibit your practicing for three years, for instance, in the same area from which your former employer draws its clients.

Contracts for Goods and Services

Sales contracts are governed by the Uniform Commercial Code (UCC), a statute all states have incorporated in their own sales laws. Under the UCC, which regulates the conduct of and between contracting parties, when a purchaser obtains goods (accepts delivery) and the goods are defective, the purchaser and the seller have certain rights. The purchaser, for instance, has the right to return the goods, and the seller has the right to substitute conforming goods to avoid losing the sale.

Since the UCC governs the buyer's and seller's conduct at each stage necessary to complete the contract (manufacture, delivery, inspection, acceptance or rejection, substitution, payment), the contracting parties need to take cautious and deliberate actions. For example, holding non-conforming goods too long before notifying the seller of the defect may result in the buyer's implied acceptance of the goods and prevent their return.

Adhesion Contracts

Many real estate leases and purchase agreements—including the document pertaining to your own medical office—may contain standard provisions that the landlord or seller asks all tenants or buyers to sign. Such documents, called contracts of adhesion, usually are lengthy, preprinted forms and always favor the party who printed them.

Since contract law assumes that both parties to a contract are on equal footing and have negotiated the terms in the contract, the courts in some states may void adhesion contracts, if requested. They do so on the grounds that one party put itself unfairly in the position of dictating terms on a take-it-or-leave-it basis, giving itself an overwhelming bargaining position over the other party, who may or may not understand that contract terms are all negotiable.

EMPLOYEE POLICIES

Medical employers frequently are punished financially through ignorance of state and federal labor laws. For example, many do not realize that they can be held accountable not only for their own acts but also for those of their employees—and, in some cases, for those of their patients. One doctor, for instance, ignored the complaints of his medical secretary who repeatedly reported sexual overtures by a patient. The employee finally got the

AVOID MALPRACTICE CLAIMS BY FOLLOWING TEN BASIC RULES *

Malpractice claims seem to follow patterns. We believe you can avoid many such claims, if you follow these rules:

First, keep accurate records. Record objectively and clearly the symptoms and prescribed treatment. Be especially careful to include notations of drug allergies, instructions to the patient, any failure of the patient to show up for appointments or to follow prescribed treatment, and the "handing off" of the patient to another health-care provider who will become responsible for future treatment. (It is often a good idea to send a letter to the patient being "handed off" to record the termination of the relationship; keep a copy for your files.)

Second, do not alter records. It almost always looks bad to a jury when records have been altered, particularly after a suit has been filed. If accuracy requires a correction, draw one line through the incorrect language, and date and initial the correction.

Third, never assume anything. Many malpractice claims seem to arise from taking things for granted, particularly in surgery. The surgeon is often blamed, rightly or wrongly, for mistakes of others. An operation on the wrong patient or the wrong side of the body may stem from another's omission, but the surgeon will be a target defendant anyway. Double-check everything; never assume others have done what they are supposed to have done.

Fourth, take time to get to know your patients. Most people will look for reasons not to sue their doctor. It is much easier for a claimant to convince himself to sue someone he doesn't know than to sue someone who has taken the time to get to know him.

Fifth, don't venture outside your qualifications. Limit your practice to areas within your qualifications.

Sixth, do not encourage unrealistic expectations. Particularly in cosmetic surgery, patients should not be encouraged to believe that the treatment will effect radical improvements. All health-care providers should avoid overly optimistic prognoses.

Seventh, use a consent form. Before any surgery, the patient should sign an "informed consent" form. Such a form might also provide for the use of the patient's photographs in educational, professional and public relations efforts.

Eighth, maintain confidences. Do not allow your staff to discuss any patient's symptoms or treatment. Do not use a patient as a "reference" without checking with that patient first.

Ninth, cover absences. Make sure patients do not feel abandoned when you are unavailable. Arrange for a qualified person to take your calls during that time. If you plan to leave your practice or to drop part of your practice, write to patients you are treating to let them know your plans and how they can find care after you withdraw.

> **Tenth, be careful about billing.** Before letting an unpaid bill go into collection, think about whether the patient has any legitimate basis for dissatisfaction with his treatment.
>
> If you receive service of court papers naming you as a defendant, contact your insurance company immediately. The insurance company will appoint a lawyer to represent you and will provide you a defense, if you act promptly.
>
> ------------------------
> * The information is reprinted with permission from "Six Ideas for Health-Care Providers," published by Smith, Gambrell & Russell, attorneys-at-law, 2400 First Atlanta Tower, Atlanta, Georgia.
> Copyright 1986, Smith, Gambrell & Russell.

doctor's attention by naming him in a sexual harassment suit, a suit the doctor lost.

To avoid problems, develop an employee policy manual with the help of an attorney and then follow it scrupulously.

The key word to all policies is reasonableness. For instance, you should not expect employees to work beyond established office hours unless you are prepared to pay overtime (this is true even if the employee volunteers for extra hours). If you allow one employee three months off with pay for a medical problem, then the same option must be available to all other employees—including pregnant employees, since the courts now view pregnancy as a medical disability. If one employee is merely reprimanded for tardiness, another may not be fired for the same infraction.

Violations of the standard of reasonableness can leave you open to suit under state or federal legislation outlawing employment discrimination.

Another common source of discrimination allegations is employee dismissals, especially dismissals of senior employees. To avoid being sued for discriminatory dismissal, you will need to maintain personnel records that contain results of regular, formal performance evaluations. Each employee should be evaluated annually, and the written evaluation should be signed by both the employer and the employee.

PEER REVIEW

The medical profession often comes under criticism for failure to police its own ranks, and yet there is a good argument legally for refusing to criticize a colleague's professional skills.

According to Henry B. Alsobrook, Jr., an attorney quoted in an April 1984 *Medical Economics* article, a physician must take care that his criticism of a colleague does not so impair that individual's professional reputation that it could be considered defamatory. Defamation is a violation of civil law—it is called slander when done orally and libel if written.

Casual comments about a referring physician to the referred patient should be made most carefully.

In certain situations, criticism may be "privileged," that is, there is immunity from liability. Testifying as an expert witness in court is one such instance; peer review activities (medical staff credentialing, quality assurance, disciplinary proceedings) are another. The extent of immunity, however, varies from state to state even though all states demand that critical comments be based on fact, not innuendo.

An increasing number of physicians, if denied hospital privileges, are taking their cases to court—in the form of anti-trust suits. The impact on peer review is twofold. The courts make public the confidential records of hospital privileging committees, an act that in turn discourages many physicians from accepting offers to sit on peer review committees.

If you find yourself before a peer review committee, you should first avail yourself of whatever document outlines your rights in this instance.

Hospital bylaws usually contain this information, if you face a privileging or disciplinary committee. Disciplinary proceedings before state licensing boards usually follow a state administrative adjudication law that details due process requirements of notice, subpoena, access to information and files, legal representation, a hearing, and administrative appeal rights. Further, upon exhaustion of the administrative procedures, there is review of the state agency's action in state court.

MALPRACTICE LITIGATION

Probably the single most threatening legal situation for any surgeon is a malpractice suit. So quickly has the number of suits risen since the mid-1970s, and so great have been the well-publicized awards, that physicians today must look out equally for personal and patient welfare. A defensive posture, new to the practice of medicine, seems required for survival.

The cause of the escalation in malpractice claims, and the consequent increase in malpractice premiums, is hard to pinpoint. Depending on who is speaking, imprudent insurance companies sought investment capital when interest rates were high by insuring bad risks; the number of negligent physicians is growing; the public is avarice personified; or some combination of these possibilities.

Whoever is to blame, everyone is paying. Physicians pay, not just in high premiums, but in the personal anguish of claims and suits filed, especially if they are without merit. According to the 1985 American Medical Association Special Task Force on Professional Liability and Insurance:

"It is often not how physicians practice, but the fact that they practice ever closer to the edges of technological frontiers that places them at greater legal risk. Physicians are among the nation's best and brightest—highly educated, motivated for the most part by humanitarian concerns, yet held accountable for complex judgments made under pressure of life-and-death considerations . . . negligence does occur, physicians are too often sued for adverse events—bad results—beyond their control."

Patients pay for the costs physicians must pass along. They also pay for tests and procedures physicians might not have ordered if they had not needed to protect themselves from lawsuits. A third price for the patient is that the malpractice crisis encourages physicians to avoid high risk patients and high risk specialties.

Until the crisis blows over, surgeons had best know what could happen to them in court; for that reason, the remainder of this chapter details what to expect if you are sued.

Types of Suits

In civil law, the two most common legal actions are contract and tort, or civil wrong. Contract actions may allege breach of the contract itself or breach of a warranty under the contract. In tort actions, suit is filed to recover for a civil wrong. The most common civil wrong is negligence, a failure to abide by the standard of conduct of a reasonably prudent man.

Negligence consists of three elements: a duty owed, a breach of the duty, and the breach of the duty proximately causing the injury. For example: A motorist owes others a duty to observe all traffic rules, including stopping at a red light. If a motorist fails to stop, he has breached the duty owed. As a result of running the red light, if the motorist hits another vehicle that is passing through the intersection on a green light, the damage done is the proximate result of the motorist's breach of his duty. The motorist was negligent and is now liable for damage to the other vehicle.

Standard of Care

Malpractice is a form of negligent conduct. Because medicine is a science and not readily comprehended by the average individual, the law applies a somewhat different standard of conduct than that of the reasonable man. Known as the "standard of care," a physician's conduct is examined in the context of what reasonably prudent physicians would have done under similar circumstances. Because lay persons (jurors) need assistance in evaluating a physician's conduct, expert witnesses are necessary. Experts state the standard of care, and jurors assess whether a physician's conduct has met that standard.

When this rule of law was first adopted, the standard of care applicable to a physician was the standard of care of physicians who devoted particular attention to the ailment, in the same locality. The law recognized that specialists should be held to a stricter standard and should be "judged" by those who devoted special attention to the ailment, i.e., members of the same specialty as the defendant. Since the creation of the rule, much concern has centered on the qualifications of the experts who are called to evaluate the claim.

Is a general plastic surgeon who performs rhinoplasties qualified to evaluate a rhinoplasty performed by an otolaryngologist-head and neck surgeon? The question centers on whether the procedure or the specialty is the focus. Defense lawyers argue that specialty is the focus; plaintiff lawyers argue just the opposite, especially in cases where no otolaryngologist-head and neck surgeon can be found to state an opinion favorable to the plaintiff. Whether an expert can express an opinion depends on his credentials and qualifications, as assessed by the trial judge.

The Locality Rule

Another concern of the original rule was the restriction, "in the same locality." This clause gave the rule its name: the locality rule. Plaintiff's lawyers often complained that they were unable to find experts in the same community who were of the appropriate specialty or who would

> **IF YOU MUST GO TO COURT**
>
> When selecting an attorney, it is wise to look for a legal specialist. Someone with actual experience (and success) in defending malpractice claims will better represent you than would counsel who specializes in, say, tax matters. In many cases, insurance companies will designate qualified counsel in a malpractice suit.
>
> Most attorneys will provide some type of pretrial orientation. This is especially important in order to put you, the defendant, at ease so you can present the appropriate and best image to the jury. A defendant who does not know where to sit or who appears nervous on the stand (or worse, hostile) will not inspire professional confidence with the jury.
>
> If you are not able to visit the courtroom ahead of time, at least have a sketch drawn for your benefit. Be aware of who sits where, who the various court participants are, and the general court routine (jury selection, swearing-in procedures, interrogation and cross-interrogation, opening arguments and concluding statements, and so on).
>
> Be early for any court appearance. Judges consider their time and overburdened court dockets at least as important and probably more so than the schedule of a busy doctor-defendant. No matter your excuse, tardiness will only antagonize the court.
>
> Discuss with your attorney in advance how to sit (never informally), what to wear, how to hold your hands during the swearing-in—all designed to convey an aura of professional competence to the jury. Answer all questions correctly, but do not volunteer extra details. You may be asked if you discussed your answers with your attorney. Do not dissemble; it is expected that you have discussed your testimony in advance. What you want to avoid is giving the impression that you were coached.
>
> Speak audibly and, above all, never lose your temper—no matter how severe the provocation.

testify. The rule was changed to a "modified" locality rule, i.e., in the same or similar communities. This would permit plaintiff or defense lawyers to obtain experts from communities where the standard of care was the same as the community where the injury occurred.

With the advent of national specialty boards, inventive plaintiff lawyers argued that standard of care has risen above community levels and that members of the same specialty board, regardless of their location of practice, should be competent to express opinions. Very few states adhere to the locality rule; most operate under modified locality and a few have adopted the national standard. The decision to permit an expert to testify rests with the trial judge.

Some cases do not require expert opinion. If the court feels that a jury can reasonably understand the facts, the jury may assess the defendant's conduct without expert testimony. A jury can understand the amputation of the wrong limb or X-ray of the wrong extremity. It is equally clear that in complex cases where expert testimony is mandatory, the lack of an expert will be fatal to the plaintiff's claim.

Doctrine of Informed Consent

In addition to the duty of a physician to exercise reasonable care in treating a patient, a physician must reasonably inform each patient of the risks of and alternatives to a recommended treatment plan. Known as the doctrine of informed consent, the physician must provide a patient with sufficient information so that a patient can make an intelligent and informed decision. Whether the physician's disclosure to the patient is reasonable also is the subject of expert opinion. As with the standard of care, the lack of an expert opinion that the physician's disclosure did not conform to the relevant community standards is fatal to the plaintiff's claim.

Pretrial Discovery

Once suit is filed, the patient and physician become parties, *i.e.*, plaintiff and defendant. Attorneys are agents for their clients, and although the trial rules discuss the rights and duties of the parties, lawyers actually do the work.

Discovery is the investigative stage of a lawsuit. Unless there is real cooperation, information can be obtained only through a formal process. A party can issue interrogatories (questions); the answering party can either answer or object. A party can issue a request that another admit the truth of a certain fact (the surgeon was the only individual who used a scalpel on the patient). The answering party can admit or deny.

The deposition is another discovery tool. A deposition is a recorded question and answer session. It may be stenotyped and transcribed; it may be videotaped. Many states and prudent counsel require a simultaneous stenotype of videotaped depositions. The deposition of a party can be used to learn information, it can be used to challenge a party's later version of the same fact, and it can be used in lieu of live testimony in court. The same is true of interrogatories and admissions.

If you are a party, you may (and will) have your attorney present. If you are only a witness, you still may have an attorney present. All parties and counsel may be present at a deposition, and a party may have a consulting expert present to assist. Prior to the taking of a deposition, you should review the mechanics of a deposition with your attorney. There are a number of ground rules. A statement uttered is in the record, even if it should not have been uttered. Listen to your attorney. He may instruct you not to answer a question. You are paying him for his advice, so follow it.

Trial

The jury is the arbiter of fact. It is up to six or twelve persons to decide disputed issues. The jury is selected in a process known in English law as *voir dire, veritatem dicere* (Latin for "to see, to hear, to speak of truth," one of the protections derived from the oppressive and inquisitional Star Chamber days when a king's privy council alone could decide a man's fate based solely on rumor). Parties interrogate prospective jurors to assess their demeanor and learn their biases. Jurors can be challenged for cause (age, relationship, definite bias, infirmity) or dismissed ("preempted") for no cause stated (usually done based on gut feeling).

Once selected, civil juries usually are able to separate at the end of a day and travel home. Sequestered juries, a circumstance of highly prejudicial and notorious cases, are under court personnel surveillance twenty-four hours per day and are housed in a nearby hotel.

Following jury selection, the court instructs the jury on how and what evidence it is to consider. Counsel then present opening statements of what they expect to prove. The plaintiff presents evidence first, the defense presents defense and rebuttal evidence, the plaintiff presents any rebuttal evidence it may have, and counsel present closing arguments.

Settlement of a case can occur at any time: during initial contacts between lawyers, during discovery, trial, and while on appeal. Settlement terms always reserve and never concede the issue of liability. Settlement almost always is accomplished to avoid further expense. The time for discovery and trial has a cost. Economically, it is wise for the defense to settle for less than its anticipated cost to defend through trial, especially when the defense can preserve and not concede the issue of malpractice. When evidence is damaging to a party, and the chance of an excessive verdict, or no verdict, becomes apparent, settlement during trial becomes a reality.

Screening Panels

Twenty-eight states have some form of review process prior to the commencement of litigation in malpractice claims. The panel usually consists of physicians and functions under an informal set of guidelines. Parties submit evidence; the panel deliberates and renders an opinion. In most states the panel opinion is admissible at trial, though not conclusive on the issue of malpractice. In two states, only a unanimous opinion is admissible. Panel members may be called as expert witnesses to present oral testimony in addition to the written opinion.

Other features of state malpractice legislation may include a limitation on the total recovery, the maintenance of a state fund to pay a portion of any recovery, and a limitation on attorney fees payable out of state fund recovery monies.

7 Financing a Practice

STEVEN J. BECK

Lenders still consider good risks, but the days of financing your practice by the seat of your pants are over.

My experience collaborates that conclusion. However strongly physicians as a group have demonstrated their ability to generate good income, their interest in making other investments, and their reliability as solid customers, the fact remains: a doctor no longer can walk into a financial institution, present his medical degree, and expect the full amount requested on a loan application. This is as true for the physician who wants to extend an existing practice as it is for the physician who is only starting the practice.

With lines at the credit window longer than ever, physicians—along with everyone else—must convince lenders that loaned monies will be repaid. Detailed practice plans and financial projections must be developed.

Before we look at how to develop and present the practice in financial plans, it is wise first to discuss how much capital will be needed, where it will come from, and the various types of loans that might suit your purpose.

HOW MUCH MONEY IS NEEDED?

The average loan granted to a new surgeon varies a great deal. They range from $40,000 to $150,000, depending upon the location. In our area, the loans range from $100,000 to $175,000 depending on the specialty. Unlike the laws of science, there are no hard and fast rules on how to determine the amount of money that will be needed for a medical practice.

Loan amounts instead depend on such factors as geographic area and the purpose for which funds are requested. In one area, a bank may limit loans to equipment purchases for group practices. Elsewhere, new physicians may expect no help setting up solo practices, but might obtain a loan to help them buy into an existing group. Other banks, in yet other locations, work directly with local chambers of commerce to identify physicians who plan to locate there and to give them start-up loans. Some banks only make personal loans to physicians.

Determining which lending institution will be most responsive to your needs takes a bit of research.

CHOOSING A LENDING INSTITUTION

Both objective and personal facts should affect your choice of a lender. In other words, you should look not only for an institution whose lending practice fits your needs, but also for a loan officer whom you trust and respect. Remember you actually borrow money from the officer and not the institution. Key to both decisions: plan to establish a long-term relationship. You can only benefit from establishing yourself with an institution that offers a broad enough program to satisfy future as well as current borrowing needs, and with a loan officer who is as committed to your future success as you are. The following are the main sources of physicians loans.

Commercial Banks

Banks are the most traditional source of debt financing. They often offer the best rates on both secured and unsecured loans for working capital, equipment, and real estate. Some have special departments to attract and advise physicians and other professionals on loan needs.

You will want to explore both large and small banks, as each has its advantages. Large banks may be less personal and more cautious in making loans than small banks. On the other hand, they may offer more services and have greater financial resources.

If you have your personal accounts at a bank, it probably will be very interested in serving your loan needs as well. Your existing business with the bank also will give you leverage to negotiate terms beneficial to yourself.

Banks sometimes require that your net worth equal 25%–40% of the amount you request in a loan. This may sound difficult for a new physician to produce. They also may require a great deal of written information before they consider a loan, frequently place restrictions on the loan, and ask for periodic financial reports during the life of the loan. Our bank does not require this percent of net worth. We make loans to doctors based on future earnings and net worth.

Savings and Loans

With legislation having eased restrictions on the lending activities of Savings and Loan Associations, these institutions have become a viable alternative to commercial banks. They offer doctors debt financing terms similar to those of banks, whether the doctor is in the market for medical equipment or an entire medical practice. Like banks, Savings and Loans favor borrowers whose personal accounts, including mortgages, rest with them.

Small Loan Companies

Think of these companies as those who lend sums banks do not want to bother with to borrowers whom banks consider poor risks. Accordingly, interest rates are higher and the loan typically must be secured through the borrowers maintaining a cash balance in a bank account and/or his pledging personal assets.

Small Business Administration

This federal loan program is recommended whenever a potential borrower has some deficiency in the normal credit worthiness of his business, such as not having been in business long enough, or not having enough equity in his business. Through this program, the lender grants a loan of a certain amount, which the Small Business Administration guarantees up to 85%.

Life Insurance Policies

If you own a whole life insurance policy, you can borrow against its value, usually at below market interest rates. Insurance companies may lend as much as 95% of the policy's cash surrender value, especially to physicians interested in developing medical office facilities. Borrowing against the policy is better than cashing it in because you retain the right to the premium rate that applied to your age when you bought the policy.

Other Lending Institutions

The American Medical Association keeps a list of doctor-short communities that offers financing or free facilities to physicians who will relocate there. Also, the American Professional Practice Association, in conjunction with local lenders, offers new physicians and established physicians loans to start or expand medical practices. Family or friends may offer to lend you money; better yet, ask them to cosign the loan. As long as you make regular payments, the arrangement will cost your relative or friend nothing, and it will help you establish your own good credit rating.

Another source of funding, equity financing, is available to established physicians. Equity financing can take several forms: using your own after-tax profits to fund growth, forming a professional corporation, setting up a general or limited partnership, or undertaking a joint venture. You are best advised to consult your lawyer or financial advisor if you think you are ready for the legal complications of equity financing.

Established medical practitioners are your best source of information on who is a knowledgeable loan officer, or get recommendations from your local medical society, lawyer, or accountant. Ask for names of lenders who regularly deal with physicians, have an interest in the profession, can gauge the market for your services in the community, and know how much money it takes to establish a medical practice.

Then meet several times with each of your top candidates. If a long-term relationship is to develop, the loan officer has to be someone who has your best interests at heart, someone with whom you feel a rapport and to whom you can entrust the details of your personal financial situation.

A good loan officer will tell you if his institution is not your best source for one particular loan, knowing that such frank advice is convincing evidence that he or she is looking after your interests and therefore is likely to encourage your future reliance on them and their institution.

TYPES OF LOANS

Your lender will advise you on the types of loans and repayment programs available through his institution. Most loans fall into three categories, as will be described. Like most generalizations, these categories are arbitrary and simplistic, created primarily to give you a quick understanding. As you read them, beware if the categories overlap, that all terms are negotiable, that lenders are open to negotiation on business loans in a way they are not on personal loans.

Short-Term Loans

These loans, available through banks and Savings and Loan Associations, are good sources of working capital. Also called lines of credit, they typically work this way: a master note is signed for the full amount of the commitment. The interest is charged only on amounts you use when you use them. Usually, the note is deposited into your checking account, and you draw on the funds as you would on that account.

Interest rates usually fluctuate on short-term loans. They typically float two to three points (depending on your credit worthiness and the size of the loan) above "prime," the lowest interest rates banks charge to their best business customers. An advantage of short-term loans to new physicians lies in the repayment plan. A typical repayment program would require you to pay interest, on a monthly or quarterly schedule, during the first 12 to 15 months of the loan. This gives you the breathing room you need to build up your practice. During the next, say, 4 years, you would still make quarterly payments (which are much easier on your cash flow), but they would include some portion of the principal as well as interest.

Intermediate-Term Loans

Depending on the loan amount, intermediate-term loans may be available from banks and Savings and Loan Associations as well as small loan companies. They are, for the most part, "asset based," that is, they usually are used to buy equipment and the term of the loan is tied to the life of the equipment. The equipment serves as collateral to secure the loan.

Unlike short-term loans, the interest rate sometimes can be fixed, payments are monthly and include both principal and interest. Fixed rate loans can work to your advantage in two ways: (1) you will know exactly how much you owe each month and therefore can budget your debt retirement more easily; and (2) even if interest rates climb during the life of the loan, you are guaranteed your lower, original rate. The disadvantages are: (1) monthly payments can hamper your cash flow in the early months of practice; and (2) if the interest rates drop, you will find it costly either to continue paying the higher, original rate or to refinance the loan at the new rate.

Long-Term Loans

Real estate mortgages are the most common type of long-term loans. Since each real estate loan is based on the individual peculiarities of the property to be built, it is impossible in one paragraph to explain all the terms and conditions that will be involved. Conventional, fixed rate mortgages are just as available as adjustable rate mortgages today, with almost countless variations on either theme. Banks and Savings and Loan Associations offer both, alone or in conjunction with various federal guarantee programs.

Again, the terms of almost any loan are negotiable. The lender wants your loan to be structured in a way that increases the certainty of your repayment. Propose the terms most advantageous to your retiring the debt; the worst thing the lender can do is to say no and suggest something else.

DEVELOPING A LOAN PACKAGE

Lenders can evaluate your request for funds fairly only if they receive certain information. This information can be presented on standard forms that the lender may have available, or it can follow almost any other format as long as the required information is there.

Whether you choose to put together the information yourself or get professional assistance is up to you. Many people with all kinds of credentials are available—accountants, lawyers, financial planners, investment bankers, loan officers, and more. My best advice is to choose your advisors carefully, getting referrals from other practitioners, the local medical society, or local society of certified public accountants. You will want someone with a proven track record in financial planning, someone with enough initiative to give you new ideas, and someone sufficiently organized to keep you apprised of the reporting and filing dates.

Whoever prepares the loan package and however well it is done, there unfortunately is no guarantee that it will result in a loan. Be assured, however, that no credit requests will ever be considered without your giving considerable time and thought to what may seem like a lot of tedious questions. The bright side: the very documents that tell the lender whether you will succeed are the blueprint you will need to succeed. Here are the chief documents any lender will want to see in your loan package:

Your Resume

The primary concern of the lender is whether you will pay back the loan. His chief measure of this is his assessment of you, personally, no matter how solid your finanical history or brilliant your practice plans. The education and experience, the awards, and publications on your resume communicate this measure clearly.

Your Personal Financial Status

The lender will want to know your net worth, since that figure is often the basis for the sum of money the bank will lend. To calculate that quickly, add up your assets (cash, savings, stock and other investments, house, car) and subtract from the total all your liabilities (charge account balances, outstanding loans on cars, house, medical school). The result is your net worth.

The lender will want this information spelled out in detail on a form he will provide (Fig. 7-1). He will check your credit references. Do not omit anything, and if there is a potential problem you know of, let him know from the start; it may not be as serious as you think. If he is knowledgeable about physician loans, for instance, he

PERSONAL FINANCIAL STATEMENT

Important: Check the applicable block: As Used herein, the singular shall also refer to the plural if more than one signs.

☐ I am applying for individual credit in my own name and am relying on my own income or assets and not on the income or assets of another person as the basis for repayment of the credit requested.

☐ We are applying for joint credit and are relying on our combined income or assets as the basis for repayment of the credit requested.

☐ I am applying for individual credit, but I am relying on income from alimony, child support, or separate maintenance or on the income or assets of another person as the basis for repayment of the credit requested.

☐ This statement relates to my guaranty of the indebtedness of other person(s), firm(s), proprietorship(s), partnerships(s), or corporation(s).

☐ This statement relates to existing credit for which I have been requested to provide periodic financial information.

I hereby make application for ☐ Secured ☐ Unsecured credit.

Amount Requested: _____ Purpose of Loan: _____

Terms Requested: _____

APPLICANT INFORMATION	CO-APPLICANT OR OTHER PARTY INFORMATION
Name	Name
Address	Address
City, State / Zip	City, State / Zip
Date of Birth / S.S. #	Date of Birth / S.S. #
Occupation	Occupation
Home Telephone / Business Telephone	Home Telephone / Business Telephone

CONDITION AS OF _____ 19___

Leave no blanks. Insert "0" or word "NONE" where necessary to complete information

ASSETS	DOLLARS	LIABILITIES	DOLLARS
Cash on hand and on Deposit (Schedule 1)	$	Notes Owed:	
U.S. Government Obligations		Secured by Real Estate (Schedule 5)	$
Other Investments (Schedule 2)		Secured by other than R.E. (Schedule 6)	
IRA and/or Keogh Plans		Unsecured (Schedule 6)	
Notes Receivable:		Contract Accounts Unpaid (Schedule 7)	
Secured by Real Estate (Schedule 3)		Open Accounts Unpaid (Schedule 7)	
Secured by Other Collateral (Schedule 3)		Current & Unpaid R.E. Taxes	
Unsecured (Schedule 3)		Delinquent & Unpaid Interest	
Accounts Receivable (Schedule 3)		Current Year Federal Taxes	
Life Insurance-Cash Value (Schedule 4)		Any Other Indebtedness-Itemize	
Real Estate - Appraised Value (Schedule 5)			
Farm Implements or Machinery			
Autos Make Year			
Any other Property or Investments-Itemize (Market)		TOTAL LIABILITIES	$
		NET WORTH	
TOTAL ASSETS	$	TOTAL LIABILITIES AND NET WORTH	$

Contingent Liabilities

Liability as Guarantor or Cosigner for accounts and Notes of others	$
Liability for Leases	
Liability other than above - Itemize	
TOTAL CONTINGENT LIABILITIES	$

ANNUAL INCOME	APPLICANT	CO-APPLICANT OR OTHER PARTY	ANNUAL EXPENDITURES (exc. ordinary living expense)	APPLICANT	CO-APPLICANT OR OTHER PARTY
Salary, Wages, Commissions	$	$	Mortgage or Rent	$	$
Income from Business			Income Taxes		
Rents and Royalties			Insurance Premiums		
Income from Investments			Property Taxes		
Alimony, child support or separate maintenance income need not be revealed if you do not choose to have it considered as a basis for repaying this loan.			Alimony, child support or separate maintenance		
Other Income-Itemize			Other-Itemize (include installment payments)		
TOTAL INCOME	$	$	TOTAL EXPENSES	$	$

Please complete the schedules and sign on the reverse side of this statement.

Figure 7-1.

DETAILS RELATIVE TO ASSETS AND LIABILITIES (if space is insufficient, attach supplemental list)

SCHEDULE 1 - Cash on Deposit

Name of Depository	Type	Amount	Name of Depository	Type	Amount
		$			$

SCHEDULE 2 - Other Investments - Stocks and Bonds

Description	Preferred/ Common	Number Shares	Book Value	Market Value	Listed on Exchange	#Shares Pledged	Where Pledged
			$	$			

SCHEDULE 3 - Notes and Accounts Receivable - Secured and Unsecured

Maker	Cosigner or Guarantor	Maturity	Rate	Interest Paid to Date	Face Amount	Balance Due	List Security if Secured
			%	$	$		

SCHEDULE 4 - Life Insurance

Issuing Company	Beneficiary Name and Relationship	Kind of Insurance	Face Amount	Present Cash Value	Amount of Policy Loan	Annual Premium
			$	$	$	$

SCHEDULE 5 - Real Estate

Description & Location	No. Acres	Title in Whose Name	Purchase Amount	Date	Appraisal Value	Date	Mortgages Indebtedness
							$

By Whom Appraised? _____ When? _____

SCHEDULE 6 - Notes Owed "Unsecured and with Security other than Real Estate"

Owed To	Balance	Date	When Due	Interest Rate	Secured, Cosigned or Guaranteed By
	$			%	

SCHEDULE 7 - Contracts and Open Accounts Unpaid

Owed To	Amount	When Contracted	When Due	For What
	$			

OTHER INFORMATION

If no provision has been made for payment of Federal taxes for current year, state estimated amount.	$
Are you a partner/owner in any firms? If so, supply name(s) and interest.	
Are there any judgements unsatisfied or suits pending against you and for what amount?	
Have you ever declared bankruptcy? When?	
Do you have a will?	
Are you obligated on any leases not included in Liabilities above?	
Give details	
Are any of your assets, other than those indicated in the schedules, pledged or hypothecated in any way?	
Are any liabilities, other than those indicated in the schedules, secured, cosigned, or guaranteed?	

The information contained in this Statement has been carefully read by the undersigned and is provided to you for the purpose of securing credit from time to time in whatever form. I hereby certify it is a true and correct exhibit of my financial condition and may be treated by you as a continuing statement thereof until replaced by a new Statement or until I specifically notify you in writing of change(s) therein. In consideration of any such credit which you may advance to me, I agree if at any time this Statement shall prove incorrect, in your judgement, as a statement of my then condition, or if at any time by reason of insolvency, application for receiver, or any act or omission on my part in your judgement such credit is prejudiced or impaired, all or any of my obligations to you, whether direct, indirect, contingent or fixed shall stand immediately due and payable without demand upon or notice to me. I hereby authorize you to obtain a consumer report or reports to be used in connection with this application and to obtain and exchange credit information from and with other creditor grantors and consumer reporting agencies. I authorize you to retain all information and reports for your files.

Applicant Signature _____ Date _____

Co-Applicant or
Other Party Signature _____ Date _____

knows that most recent medical school graduates already carry an average $40,000 educational debt load; as long as you are steadily repaying the debt, it will not jeopardize an additional loan to start up your practice. Also tell the lender what your annual living expenses are so that he can structure a realistic repayment plan (Fig. 7-2).

Business Financial Status

Only established practices that want a loan to expand or buy equipment will be asked to provide this information. The purpose is to establish your past performance; 3 years of tax returns may suffice. In addition, the lending officer will want to be provided the last 3 years profit and loss statement and balance sheet that are prepared by your accountant.

Projected Earnings

If you are just starting your practice, the local medical society will have the information you need to calculate future earnings. Also, any accountant who specializes in medical practices will be able to help provide this information.

To figure potential gross income, multiply the estimated patient volume by the fee you will charge for each service. Be realistic. Next, deduct operating expenses. The result will tell you how much income you will have left to retire your debt.

To project expenses, rely on local medical society figures, since cost will vary widely from region to region. In its continuing survey on the cost of practicing medicine, for instance, *Medical Economics* reportes that office overhead is lowest in the Eastern states, higher in the Midwest, and highest in the West.

That same national survey reveals that office overhead costs have risen at five times the national inflation rate since 1981. In 1984, the medium overhead in a plastic surgeon's office (all board specialties) was $114,030. That figure represents 41.4% of the physician's gross income. The seven major expense categories studied were: payroll (nonphysician employees only), malpractice insurance, depreciation on medical equipment, office base, professional car, continuing education, and drugs and medical supplies (Figs. 7-3, 7-4).

Your Practice Plan

Do you have a name for your practice, such as The ABC Center for Facial Plastic Surgery? Who are the principals? At what location(s) will you practice? What competition might you expect? In fact, what is your marketing plan (size of your market, your share of the market, you plans to reach your clients)? What procedures will you perform? What personnel will you hire? What office space will you rent, buy, or build? What equipment will you need and how much will it cost? How much income can you anticipate a year from now? In 2 years? In 3 years?

The answers to these questions should be written up, in narrative form, to let the bank know you have well-thought-out, short- and long-term practice plans (Fig. 7-5).

Breakdown of Loan Proceeds

The information requested here will tell the bank how the loan relates to your practice plans. Basically, you will answer the questions, how much do you want to borrow, what will it be used for, and how long do you think it will take you to repay it? Remember, the primary thing that any lender wants to know is when will you be able to repay the loan.

Perform a Balance Sheet

Somewhere among your loan application documents, you will have to project assets (including those acquired with the loan), liabilities, and net worth to some date in the future, preferably the opening day of your practice.

Cash Flow Projections

You will also have to estimate cash flow projections. Since like most businesses, you will be in a position of granting credit (Medicare, Medicaid, and other insurance programs), you will need a realistic estimate of your cash receipts and cash dispursements. The cash flow projections will forecast over some time period in the future what those realistic estimates of your cash receipts and cash expenditures are. This will tell the lender and yourself of your ability to continue to repay any loans in the future (see Fig. 7-4 for an example of a cash flow budget).

HOW LOANS ARE REVIEWED

Your loan application will be treated like those of other businessmen. The lender will search it for answers to the same questions. First and foremost (again): is the application of a person likely to honor his debt? Is his work history strong? Is his credit good? Are his references solid?

Second, does sufficient business acumen show in the preparation of his loan package. Has he estimated a realistic sum of operating capital and equipment purchases? Does his marketing plan demonstrate knowledge of the competition? Are his projections for future earnings

COST-OF-LIVING BUDGET

(based on average month - does not cover purchase of
any new items except emergency replacements)

DETAILED BUDGET

REGULAR MONTHLY PAYMENTS

House payments (principal, interest, taxes, and insurance) or rent .... $ ____
Car payments (including insurance) .... ____
Appliance - TV payments .... ____
Home improvement loan payments .... ____
Personal loan, credit card payments .... ____
Health plan payments .... ____
Life insurance premiums .... ____
Other insurance premiums .... ____
Savings/investments .... ____

TOTAL $ ____

PERSONAL EXPENSE

Clothing, cleaning, laundry ...... $ ____
Drugs .... ____
Doctors and dentists .... ____
Education .... ____
Dues .... ____
Gifts and contributions .... ____
Travel .... ____
Newspapers, magazines, books .... ____
Auto upkeep and gas .... ____
Spending money and allowances ... ____
Miscellaneous .... ____

TOTAL $ ____

FOOD EXPENSE

Food - at home .... $ ____
Food - away from home .... ____

TOTAL $ ____

TAX EXPENSE

Federal and state income taxes ... $ ____
Other taxes not included above .... ____

TOTAL $ ____

HOUSEHOLD OPERATING EXPENSE

Telephone .... $ ____
Gas and electricity .... ____
Water .... ____
Other household expenses, repairs, maintenance . ____

TOTAL $ ____

BUDGET SUMMARY

A. INCOME: GROSS

MONTHLY TOTAL $ ____

LESS EXPENSE:

Regular Monthly Payments .... $ ____
Household Operating Expense ..... ____
Personal Expense .... ____
Food Expense .... ____
Tax Expense .... ____

MONTHLY TOTAL $ ____

B. MONTHLY TOTAL EXPENSES $ ____

SAVINGS (A-B) $ ____

Figure 7-2.

106 Developing a Practice in Ambulatory Surgery

PRO FORMA INCOME STATEMENTS

	1st Year - Months 1 2 3 4 5 6 7 8 9 10 11 12	2nd Year - Quarters 1Q 2Q 3Q 4Q	3rd Year - Quarters 1Q 2Q 3Q 4Q
Sales			
Less: Discounts			
Less: Bad Debt Provision			
Less: Materials Used			
Direct Labor			
Manufacturing Overhead[1]			
Other Manufacturing Expense (Leased Equip.)			
Total Cost of Goods Sold			
Gross Profit (or Loss)			
Less: Sales Expense			
Engineering Expense			
General and Administrative Expense [2]			
Operating Profit (or Loss)			
Less: Other Expense (e.g., interest, depreciation)			
Profit Before Taxes (or Loss)			
Income Tax Provision			
Profit (Loss) After Taxes			

[1] Includes rent, utilities, fringe benefits, telephone.
[2] Includes office supplies, accounting and legal services, management, etc.

Figure 7-3.

PRO FORMA CASH FLOWS

	1st Year 1 2 3 4 5 6 7 8 9 10 11 12	2nd Year - Quarters 1Q 2Q 3Q 4Q	3rd Year - Quarters 1Q 2Q 3Q 4Q
Cash Balance: Opening			
Add: Cash Receipts			
Collection of Accounts Receivable			
Misc. Receipts			
Bank Loan Proceeds			
Sale of Stock			
Total Receipts			
Less: Disbursements			
Trade Payables			
Direct Labor			
Manufacturing Overhead			
Leased Equipment			
Sales Expense			
Warranty Expense			
General and Administrative Expense			
Fixed Asset Additions			
Income Tax			
Loan Interest @ ___ %			
Loan Repayments			
Other Payments			
Total Disbursements			
Cash Increase (or Decrease)			
Cash Balance: Closing			

Figure 7-4.

Outline of a Business Plan

I. Cover Sheet
   A. Name of the business
   B. Names of the principals
   C. Address
   D. Telephone Number

II. Table of Contents

III. The Narrative Support
   This provides detailed information about the business, including:
   A. Description
   B. Market(s)
   C. Competition
   D. Location(s)
   E. Management
   F. Personnel
   G. Application of any expected funding

IV. Strategic and Tactical Plans
   A. Formal Statement of Business Purpose
   B. Strategic Objectives of the Business
   C. Tactical Objectives

V. Operational Plans
   A. Detailed Assumptions
   B. Income Statement Forecast
      1. One Year (by month)
      2. Two Years (by quarter)
   C. Balance Sheet Forecast
      1. One Year (by month)
      2. Two Years (by quarter)
   D. Cash Flow Forecast
      1. One Year (by month)
      2. Two Years (by quarter)
   E. Financing Plan

VI. Historical Analysis (for Established Businesses Only)
   A. Historical Financial Statements
      1. Income Statements (for the last 2 or 3 years)
         a. By division, department or profit center, if relevant
         b. By product
      2. Balance Sheets (for the last 2 or 3 years)
   B. Tax Returns (for the last 2 or 3 years)
   C. Ratio Analysis
      1. Liquidity ratios
      2. Leverage ratios
      3. Turnover ratios
      4. Profitability ratios
      5. Trading ratios
   D. Break-even Analysis (Margin Analysis)

VII. Sensitivity Analysis
   This demonstrates the impact on the financial forecasts and cash flow
   as a result of changes in the underlying assumptions.

VIII. Supporting Documents
   A. Management's Personal Resumes
   B. Personal Financial Statements and Financial Commitments of the Owners and Principals
   C. Credit Reports
   D. Leases
   E. Contracts
   F. Market Analyses
   G. Letters of Reference

Figure 7-5.

realistic? A good loan officer knows the answers to these questions.

Remember, you are not only a physician, you are also a business person. And like any other business, your practice must have a sound financial footing to ensure your continued success.

EXPECT RESTRICTIONS ON YOUR LOAN

Once you have obtained your loan, expect the lender to have as much interest in your success as you do. He will want you to follow your practice plan precisely and may put any or all of the following restrictions on your loan:

1. Require you to provide a copy of your lease.
2. Require that you use loan proceeds only as you said you would.
3. Require that you pay taxes when due.
4. Require life and disability insurance on you, and other insurance on the business.
5. Require you to provide collateral.
6. Require periodic financial statements by an acceptable certified public accountant.
7. Require that any other loans to your practice be subordinated to the lenders.
8. Require you to pay salaries at an agreed-upon level.
9. Restrict your borrowings from other sources without prior approval.
10. Restrict your freedom to sell or encumber assets without the lender's prior approval.

SIX Cs OF CREDIT

The six c's of credit are the criteria used by all lenders to decide whether or not they will risk granting credit to a loan applicant. They include:

1. **Character.** The single most important factor in any loan request is the individual who owns or manages the business. Regardless of how good the business looks on paper, unless the principal owner is of good character, the loan *will not* be approved.
2. **Capital (equity).** The second important factor is the ratio of the owner's money that is at risk to the lender's money at risk. As a rule of thumb, a lender does not want more than 3 or 4 dollars of his money in a project for every dollar that the owner-borrower has invested. This is because, whenever the debt-to-worth exceeds 3 or 4 dollars to 1, there is a significant increase in the failure of the business regardless of the type.
3. **Capacity.** Capacity is the ability of the borrower to repay the loan on a timely basis. Here, the lender looks for cash flow, profitability of the business, and other indicators of the borrower's ability to pay off the debt. As a rule of thumb, most lenders would like to see as a minimum, $1.25 in cash flow for every $1.00 in total principal and interest payments.
4. **Collateral.** Collateral is whatever assets a business may have that back up the primary source of repayment, which is the capacity. Collateral might include accounts receivable, inventory, equipment, real estate, life insurance policies, certificates of deposit, and so on. Lenders regard collateral as a "back door" to the borrower's assets if the loan is not repaid on a timely basis.
5. **Coverage.** Coverage refers to insurance coverages on both the business and principal owner. Lenders want to know that both are adequately covered.
6. **Circumstance.** Lenders like to keep aware of circumstances outside the business's control that would affect their ability to repay, such as the economy, heavy concentration of other facial plastic surgeons in the area, and so on.

8 Office Computerization

DOT SELLARS, C.M.A.-A., C.O.A.P.

Combining the methods of business with the ethics of professionalism is essential for the success of the medical practice. The effectiveness and efficiency of the medical office must be analyzed in an effort to decrease costs and increase earnings. Obsolete, inadequate, or unsuitable equipment in use is almost a guarantee that the office is not being run in an efficient or cost-effective manner. Internal disorganization also is a culprit that can compound many problems.

Since machines speed up the work process, a computer system is almost mandatory for managing the business side of the medical practice. Advanced technology should provide not only for better work and increased efficiency, but also for better internal control.

As a direct result of the major changes occurring in the health care industry, many administrative problems may be occurring within the medical office. Cash flow may be poor, accounts receivable may be high, paperwork may be voluminous, and there may be a need to implement a new information system.

Do you need a computer? A computer system can enhance your business operations if properly planned for and implemented. It is designed to perform the accounting functions, improve cash flow, reduce paperwork, and provide statistical reports for making better decisions.

ANALYZING YOUR COMPUTER NEEDS

A careful analysis of your own individual needs and priorities is essential before choosing a system or changing a system. What do you want the computer to do for you? Make a list as extensive as possible but divide it into three categories: (1) what you must have; (2) what you would like to have; and (3) what would be nice to have. For example, you "must have" a computer that will do your accounting, insurance claim processing, and billing. If appointment scheduling is not a priority, it could be listed with "like to have." It also may be "nice to have" a system that will allow specific research capability for writing scientific papers. Completing this process not only will help you learn what a computer can and cannot do for you, but also will help you to determine the cost of each feature for deciding whether or not the benefits can be cost-justified for your practice.

If your primary purpose for getting a computer is to do your accounting, insurance claim processing, and billing, an in-depth study must be done. Financial records are vital. So a thorough audit of all your areas of operation should precede any decision about acquiring a computer.

To assess the organization and efficiency of your office procedures, you must know how your current system operates. If you don't know the reason for every piece of paper and how it's handled by your staff—and for what purpose—how can you possibly evaluate whether or not a computer system would be adaptable to your practice? The reason this is so important is that a computer must work for you. Your staff should never have to work for a computer.

The more details you can provide about your practice, the better. Do you know your present practice characteristics? You'll need to provide the vendor with accurate statistical information about your practice, such as how many active patients you have, how many new patients you see annually, how many procedures performed per patient visit, how many statements are mailed monthly. You'll also need to estimate your projected growth as accurately as possible. For example, at the present time there are three physicians in your group but you plan to have four physicians within 2 years and five physicians within 5 years. The practice characteristics would change accordingly and the statistical data must be projected for the increased growth.

To help ensure that you'll be getting a system that can grow with the practice, you'll need to project the computer applications that you'll be adding to the system. Your current needs may be only for the accounts receivable software, but within a 5-year period you may expect to add general ledger, accounts payable, payroll, and word processing. Let your expectations be known.

The vendor will determine the system you need based on the information you provide. Consequently, there are no shortcuts for selecting the right computer for your practice. It takes work on your part. It requires a culmination of knowledge about your practice and the patients you serve.

SELECTING APPROPRIATE SOFTWARE

Selecting an office computer is not an easy task. Cost is by no means the only consideration. No computer system is completely satisfactory for everyone, nor will it fulfill every dream.

Begin the selection process by viewing computers in action. It's essential to see computer demonstrations and the actual operation in other physicians' offices. Ask questions! How does the system work? You have analyzed your needs and the needs of your office—now make sure that the computer will work for you.

Know what's different about your practice. For example, as a surgeon, it would probably be necessary to have a computer-generated census listing of patients and surgical procedures performed. If you have a group practice and some patients are treated in your ambulatory surgery facility and others at one of three hospitals, you may need the report to be generated by physician—by treatment location, but with the capability of generating a report for "all physicians—all locations" for the physician who is on-call for the group. Don't assume that the computer can do it without costly program changes. Be specific about your requirements.

Know what's not different about your practice. For instance, your specialty should indicate the length of time a patient must stay in the data base. (Your requirements, however, could be different.) The needs of all specialists are not the same. This is why it's necessary to evaluate computer systems.

Your accounting, claim processing, and billing needs should be similar. However, if 90% of your practice represents minors, your requirements may be different.

Recognizing similarities between practices should reduce the time you spend investigating systems. The complexities of practicing medicine also should indicate the need to deal with a vendor who has expertise in the health care field.

There are three basic areas of software: operating systems, language translators, and application programs. A computer will come with a built-in operating system. The operation software is a communication network between the computer programs and the hardware. Some variety of machine language is inherent to every computer. The use of higher-level languages has led to computer systems that are more user-friendly (easier for the user to use). Application software are the programs you select, such as the accounts receivable program, for your office.

To evaluate application software properly, you need to know exactly what your requirements are. You will need to choose between batch and on-line processing, between customized and prepackaged programs. Other factors to consider would include user-friendly, reliability, flexibility, security.

Most often prepackaged software programs have options available that will allow them to be customized to your needs, eliminating the need to have a customized program written for your practice. However, it's essential to know not only the needs of your practice, but also the minimal acceptable features that would be necessary in a system for your practice. Your objective is to select software that will do your present procedures better—faster, more cheaply, more accurately—than you're doing them now.

When you look at computers in action, you no doubt will note that a patient's account can be retrieved almost instantaneously with just a few key strokes. Amazing? Yes! No time is lost compared with manually flipping through ledger cards. Don't assume, however, that all computers have the same capability for account inquiry. Can a search be accomplished by patient's name, guarantor's name, and account number or is the search restricted to account number only? Will the system allow for a search by entering the first two alpha characters of the patient's last name? For example, can you enter CA and have the system display all patients whose last names start with CA? If so, does the demographic information displayed on the screen provide you with sufficient information to aid you in selecting the proper account? (Helpful information may include an address, date of birth, social security number.) When doing an inquiry, can the operator see the detailed transactions, as well as all the demographic information? Do you see how easy it might be to select a system based on assumption without ever evaluating the "nuts and bolts" that will make the software more efficient for you?

The need to evaluate each function and each feature of a software program should become more apparent as you evaluate your choices. Don't expect the vendors to tell you what their programs won't do. It's up to you to analyze the differences between the programs.

Suppose the program allows for insurance claim processing. Can you assume the program will handle all your needs? Definitely not! Do you sign off on many disability claims? Does the program even allow you to enter disability dates for processing disability claims? Does the program allow you to file for secondary insurance coverage? Will it automatically invert the primary and secondary insurance coverage demographic information?

Does the software program allow for multiprocessing? That's allowing for two or more functions being performed at the same time. For instance, an employee checking account inquiry, another employee posting charges, and another employee doing a demand statement—a statement given to a patient at the time the service is rendered. A program that restricts you to performing only one function at a time can decrease office efficiency.

Are you beginning to see how important it is for you to know what the program can do for you? Do you see how easy it might be to select a program that doesn't satisfy your requirements?

A thorough evaluation of software applications is essential for determining what the computer can and cannot do for you. A computer can do just about anything you want it to do—but there is a price tag associated with it. During the investigation process, you'll probably find vendors who have different software modules available for the system to grow with you, such as a module for accounts receivable, another for accounts payable, another for word processing, etc. On the other hand, you may see a demonstration in which many features are combined in one package. Your analysis should provide the data for selecting the best possible system for your office.

Your staff also can be a valuable resource for helping you select the best system. Use your key people—those who best understand your office procedures—and allow them to try some of the available systems and voice their opinions. They, no doubt, can help you choose a computer that will enhance your business operations.

SELECTING APPROPRIATE HARDWARE

Your vendor's software has probably been tailored to run on one major brand of hardware. The quality of state-of-the art hardware is fairly even from manufacturer to manufacturer. If you don't buy your computer and all its peripheral components from the same company, however, repair service could be a problem.

Most vendors will probably offer a turnkey system, that is, a complete computer system for which a single vendor assumes total responsibility for hardware and software construction, installation, and testing. However you still need to understand a sales pitch. You also need to be assured that the system has sufficient power and memory for running your software application programs.

The storage disk is equivalent to file space; it's where the information you feed the computer goes. The main unit is called the central processing unit (CPU) and it is composed of three parts: the control unit, the arithmetic unit, and the storage unit. Each unit performs specific functions.

Core memory manages the disk. It's important to have sufficient core memory, as well as disk storage. Can you add additional core memory and disk storage to accommodate your projected future growth?

Can the CPU support your demands? How many CRT terminals can it handle? Will it allow all of them to be used at once? Does the computer have the capability of multi-programming—executing two or more programs during the same time period? Can you add another printer? If the printer breaks down, does the entire system shut down?

The vendor should determine how much disk storage you'll need, based on how much detail you want to keep on your accounts and for how long. Thus, the accuracy of the information you provide is vital for figuring disk storage space.

Drawing up a "request for proposal" (RFP) will force you to take a careful look at how your office functions. It should include a detailed analysis of the record keeping performed in your office, as well as list special requirements and your objectives. It can be given to the vendors to respond to your needs and it will make it easier for you to compare their offerings.

If you're planning to purchase an inexpensive personal computer, you don't need a RFP; but for a more sophisticated system, a RFP should enable you to evaluate systems better. For example, suppose you want to start with three terminals. Terminals come in many styles and the price can vary significantly. In all probability you don't need the most sophisticated, complex terminal on the market, nor would you want the cheapest one made. You will need one that will work for you. A keyboard full of hieroglyphics would be asking for trouble—remember, your staff will be using it.

As you compare vendors' bids, the quoted price may trigger the need for additional investigation. If one vendor quotes you $1000 for three terminals and another vendor quotes $2000, you need to know why. If the quotes were about equal but the maintenance agreement costs were significantly higher on the one bid, find out why. It could be that maintenance costs are higher because they offer a full-color screen. Do you want or need this additional expense?

When you first look at a computer system, everything looks good. But if you take the time to evaluate each piece of equipment and each feature, you'll find there are differences and the learning process can be extremely beneficial. For instance, if you purchase three terminals but do not select a system that offers multiprocessing, you'll defeat your purpose because only one job can be performed at any given time. Why would you need three terminals? On the other hand, if you have the advantage of multiprocessing and you only have one terminal, you simply cannot use this most important function. An extra terminal would be a small extra expense, but it would allow you to operate the system to your advantage.

Printers are classified by speed, ranging from 30 characters per second to 1200 lines per minute (LPM) or more. A printer is an electromechanical device and, therefore, more prone to breakdowns and failures, compared with all-electronic devices. Faster printers generally have higher maintenance costs.

Most offices don't need a high-speed printer; in fact, some consultants will recommend two or three medium-speed printers, rather than one 1200 LPM, for large clinics. Some microcomputers also cannot handle extremely fast printers.

Discuss printers in detail with the vendors. A cheap,

off-brand printer could be a maintenance nightmare. You need a printer that is fast enough to get your work done; otherwise, the printer could hinder the efficiency of your business operations.

A dot-matrix printer may be sufficient for all your needs, or the size of your practice could be large enough to justify more than one printer. A letter-quality printer would be necessary for a stand-alone word processing program, whereas if the system only allows for some basic word processing, you may only want to consider near-letter-quality printing.

Seeking information on the warranty period for hardware and the cost for a maintenance service contract is essential and could influence your preference for one supplier over another. The warranty period may be as short as one month or as long as one year. When the warranty period expires, it's usually necessary to obtain a service contract to help ensure that when the system is down, service will be provided.

Down-time is a period of time during which a computer system is not functioning. There are times when the system is not available, not because it has failed, but because preventive hardware maintenance is being done or it's performing functions, such as backup. This is classified as scheduled down-time. Unscheduled down-time is unexpected system failure. When this occurs, you need to get the system back in operation as quickly as possible. If you don't have a maintenance service contract, you may stay down for a much longer period of time while you wait for a service representative to come to your rescue. At that time, should you need a special part, there may be another delay in getting it.

PURCHASING MECHANISMS

The final price tag of even a basic microcomputer system may be more than you had anticipated—and this is common. If you have received bids from your RFP, the quotation has a limited period of validity. But while it is valid, the supplier is committed to supplying the system at the prices given. For most computer systems, you'll probably be given only a purchase or lease option, since the availability of a rental arrangement is unusual when small systems are involved.

It's almost always cheaper to buy than to acquire equipment in any other way; however, you simply may not have the money sitting around or you may not want to commit to a single purchase.

The loan-for-purchase depends on many factors—loan rates, lease rates, prevailing stock-, bond-, and money-market rates, depreciation schedules, etc. It is more expensive to borrow than pay cash. Of course, you must have enough credit to qualify for a loan.

Many physicians want obsolescence protection and that's a big reason for leasing. They're afraid new technology might make their system obsolete.

A lease is basically an agreement that allows you to borrow money for the system. It will typically run for at least 5 years. When the lease expires, you usually have three options—you can extend the lease at a greatly reduced monthly rate; you can purchase the equipment outright for a lump sum; or you can return the equipment to the lessor. The arrangements usually demand that you buy a maintenance service contract. The lease also may allow for an escape clause. If you give several months notice, you may "opt out" the old equipment to bring in new equipment. The escape clause, however, may require you to pay a penalty and/or a higher monthly rate. A leasing company also may be willing to structure the lease to fit your budget and cash flow best. For example, you pay less during the first year because of your previous financial commitments and then pay more heavily during the later years of the contract—when you know you'll be better able to afford the payments. With leasing, it is important for you to know about all hidden costs. Find out what you're responsible for.

In a rental agreement, you pay nothing toward ownership and therefore the monthly charge is often substantially lower than in a lease. It also usually includes maintenance. When the term of the rental agreement expires, you may return the equipment or renegotiate the contract. The contract also may contain an "opt out" clause with a financial penalty for prematurely terminating the contract.

There are alternatives to procuring your own in-house system. If the cost is excessive in proportion to your projected use of the machine, you may want to consider a service bureau.

Before you make your final decision, meet with your accountant or tax advisor. Their expertise may save you from making a costly mistake.

In all probability your system will be obsolete by the time you are through with it. Consequently, don't count on recouping anything from it. There are companies, however, specializing in the sale of used computers and they might be helpful to you. There are times when even bargains can be found.

MANAGING YOUR DATA-PROCESSING PROCEDURES AND SAFEGUARDING YOUR DATA

Management and control of a computer system are not built into it but must come from other resources. Entering data into the computer is the easy part. Developing controls for the system to ensure maximum benefits from it takes thoughtful planning.

To utilize any system fully, work must be well planned. If you only have one terminal, one printer, and one operator, it's still essential to make the computer work for you through management and control of the system.

Evaluate the forms used in your office. Will the computer accommodate the information you require for a new patient registration? Will you continue to use this source document, or will you register patients directly into the computer at the time of arrival? What method will you use for obtaining signatures for release of information and assignment of benefits for filing insurance claims? Many new patients also may come from hospital consultations. How will the required information be obtained and how will it be entered into the system? If you practice at more than one location, do you have a check and balance system to assure entry of all patients into the computer?

Exercising management and control of data is essential for the success of any information system. It's not efficient to interview some patients and process the data directly into the computer, and then have other patients complete a form. You need to be consistent. If you need more demographic information for collection purposes than what the computer allows for input, a form definitely should be completed and kept as part of the permanent record.

Switching back and forth among computer tasks can decrease efficiency, as can constantly moving different kinds of paper and forms in and out of a printer. Personnel should be assigned tasks not only according to good accounting principles but also for maximizing office efficiency.

The computer may generate a prenumbered fee slip or charge slip for recording transactions to be posted into the system, or you may desire to continue to use your current form or redesign it. It may be necessary to use two different forms; one for office patients and the other for hospital patients, particularly if surgery is being performed. Would it be feasible to list all procedures you do on one form?

The fee slip must be completed with accurate information; an incorrect diagnosis or procedure code could create serious problems for you. Does someone in your office do your coding or do you check the proper diagnosis and procedure codes from the listing on your fee slip? Periodically auditing codes will result in better control.

Accuracy must be maintained for posting transactions (charges and payment) into the computer. For example, run an adding machine tape total on the fee slips to be posted and compare this total to the computer total after posting the fee slips. If they don't equal, the error needs to be found and corrected. The same is true for posting payments or adjustments. A check and balance procedure done on a daily basis is the best way to detect mistakes because they minimize the number of transactions reviewed per audit, and discrepancies can be found early. If daily audits and controls are adequate, audits at longer intervals should merely substantiate the accuracy of your computer data.

A step-by-step approach for examining each function performed on the computer should be instituted. Your computer administrator or office manager should implement the necessary management and control to help ensure that all data are accurate and that the work flow has been planned to maximize office efficiency.

Computer-generated insurance claim processing and billing should increase cash flow and decrease the accounts receivable, but it won't just happen. It requires good management and control. Insurance forms may need to be processed on a daily basis and you may need to cycle bills, if you are to accomplish your objective.

Many reports will be computer-generated. If data are not accurate, reports can be misleading. If the reports are not used, how can they enhance your business operations? Are you beginning to understand why the lack of management and control is a common reason cited for computer failure?

Your staff also will be an integral part of the overall success or failure of a computer system. Orientation sessions and training time should be provided for those who are directly involved in the operation. Human elements play an important part in implementing change and you need to create positive action for greater achievements.

Security for computer systems holding private information includes not only controlled access to terminals and information, but also physical measures, such as limited access to the facility or a lock on the computer room door. There also must be fire protection, as well as a halon fire extinguisher installed in the computer area.

As far as insurance protection is concerned, consult with your insurance agent. You may need a separate policy for your computer system or you may need to add the equipment to your current policy.

You can enhance security by controlling the functions operators can perform, as well as the terminals they can use for performing their tasks. Each operator may be given a special password to enter the system, but you should have the flexibility to change passwords at any time. Some systems may only allow for one password to be used by all operators. Consequently, the security of the system would be poor.

Don't overlook that codes for diagnosis and procedures represent confidential information (these codes can be interpreted) and the utmost caution should be used when handling these data. Place terminals away from the patients' view. The video screen holds a wealth of information.

The backup media you use for safeguarding your data should be safely secured. Remember, your backup is a complete copy of your business operations. Backup of your system should be done on a daily basis to avoid losing data or having to repeat entering data into the system.

THE FUTURE OF COMPUTERIZATION IN THE MEDICAL OFFICE

The ultimate impact of computer technology in medicine will, no doubt, be determined by how it is used. Once you have your system in full operation, you can begin to incorporate other programs that may be beneficial for you. Just as you cost-justified your original purchase, you should also justify the purchase of any additional hardware and software. It's also essential to go through the same type of evaluation process; analyze your needs and state your objectives.

There are many business application programs on the market that can enhance administrative procedures, such as appointment scheduling, general ledger, accounts payable, payroll, inventory, etc. There are also clinical applications. In addition, clinical software is easily accessible by telephone from a national data base.

Don't overlook that support and maintenance are vital to the success of the programs. Your computer operators also must be trained for each new program you acquire. To help ensure the continued success of the system, there should be an established office organizational pattern that will enable the data to flow smoothly and regularly to the personnel responsible for computer input. Specific duties to be performed must be categorized and assigned. The system must be managed and controlled.

Automation is playing—and will continue to play—a substantial and beneficial role in medicine. The trend in computer hardware is toward miniaturization. The microprocessor has already changed the design and cost of hardware. Software development, no doubt, will continue to keep pace with hardware technology. Just think—today patients can go to the supermarket to have their blood pressure checked by a machine. Is this bad for medicine? Not necessarily! These machines cause many patients to see physicians who probably would never go to a doctor otherwise.

The future of computerization in the medical office will be determined by how it is used. It's a tool that should increase office efficiency and help you make better decisions. The success of the system will be limited—or helped—by the quality of the management.

CONCLUSION

An overview as brief as this cannot prepare physicians for office computerization but it does begin the educational process. The success or failure of any computer system depends on many factors. Certainly, bad business practices will defeat all the advantages that a computerized system has to offer.

As you increase your knowledge of computer systems by reading, attending seminars, and talking with your colleagues who have already computerized their operations, you'll begin to recognize some potential pitfalls that you'll want to avoid, and you'll strive to experience all of the potential benefits computerization has to offer. The improvements in office efficiency that can result from a properly designed, implemented, and operated system is a big dividend you can earn from the investment of your time and money.

9 Space Planning Your Medical Facility and Negotiating an Office Lease*

RUSSELL D. RICHARDSON

DEVELOPING YOUR MEDICAL OFFICE FACILITY

Two out of three private practice physicians rent their office space, according to a 1985 survey by *Medical Economics*. The remainder own their own new or remodeled medical building or office condominium.

Advice on whether to rent or buy, however, is *not* what this chapter is all about. That decision is something each physician must make for himself after weighing the pros and cons of renting and buying.

Suffice it to say that those who opt to buy are sufficiently established to obtain financing, see real estate as a good investment, like the freedom (and do not mind the headaches) of property ownership, and can benefit from the tax deductions for mortgage payment interest, real estate taxes, insurance, maintenance, and depreciation. They are not overly concerned that medical buildings are specialty buildings, not easily converted to other uses, and therefore difficult to sell if the need arises.

Physicians who opt to rent are not necessarily without the means to buy. They simply may prefer other forms of investment, enjoy the freedom to move elsewhere when the lease ends, or dislike property management responsibilities. They cannot claim the same tax deductions as property owners, but since rent itself is a legitimate business expense, they may deduct that.

Whether you choose to lease or buy office space will not alter certain basic facts about what is a good site, a well-constructed building, and an efficient office design. In fact, these three topics—explored from the vantage point of both renters and buyers—are the subject of this chapter. (If you plan to lease, see later for a detailed analysis of what is negotiable in each section of a typical medical office building lease.)

SITE SELECTION FACTORS

With a dozen or more factors contributing to a successful practice site, the task of finding and comparing several sites can be daunting. Actually, with the right tools, it's easy. As many facial plastic surgeons have learned, a city map and a dozen boxes of colored pins are all you need. Assign one color of pin to each of the factors listed below; then stick the properly colored pin in the map at each point you identify the presence of the corresponding site factor. Before long, the pins will converge on the sites with the most potential.

Growth Area

It's a proven fact that most successful medical practices are located close to successful commercial areas. A corollary: If the commercial area near your practice continues to grow, so will your practice. Locating in a growth area assures you of a site convenient to a large number of potential patients. To pinpoint growth areas, visit the local chamber of commerce.

Prestigious Area

The chamber of commerce or local realtors also can tell you which growth areas have a prestigious reputation. The type of medical practice you endeavor to develop dictates that you locate in the vicinity of well-established, well-recognized medical colleagues. Surrounding yourself with success is always important; it's critical when starting your practice. If you choose an office in a medical building that is identified with excellent medical services, your very location will generate new patient inquiries as people tend to go to well-known professional buildings for new medical needs (Table 9-1).

---

*Many physicians developing surgical facilities choose to lease space in a new or existing building. This section is adapted from American Academy of Facioplastic and Reconstructive Surgery Monograph; *Developing a Practice in Facioplastic Surgery*, William H. Beeson, M.D., Editor. The Education and Research Foundation for the American Academy of Facioplastic and Reconstructive Surgery, 1101 Vermont Avenue, NW, Suite 404, Washington, DC 20005, 1986. The author provides valuable tips on negotiating a lease and on space planning. Copyright 1986 by The Educational and Research Foundation for The American Academy of Facial Plastic and Reconstructive Surgery. All rights reserved. Reprinted by permission.

116 Developing a Practice in Ambulatory Surgery

Table 9-1. More Tips for Medical Office Developers

Topography. If you are looking for land on which to build, consider the fact that more level ground costs less to develop. It also is more approachable from access roads than is a steeper incline.

  Lot size. To determine the minimum lot size required, first figure how many square feet the building must be. A solo practitioner typically requires a minimum of 1000 square feet of usable space. Multiply that by the number of physicians you plan to accommodate. Then figure that the product is equal to only 80% of the total space you need, since most building plans achieve an 80% efficiency in layout. For instance, for four doctors, a building would have to be 4 × 1000 square feet divided by 80%, or 5000 square feet.

  Now apply the formula 1-1-4. The first "1" equals the building size; the second "1" tells you how many square feet are desirable for landscaping; the "4" tells you how many square feet are desirable for parking and future expansion. Thus, from the above example for four doctors, a 5000 square foot building needs another 5000 square feet for landscaping and 20,000 square feet for parking and expansion, for a total lot size of 30,000 square feet.

  Zoning. Local government agencies control how land in their jurisdiction may be used, targeting some land for residential development and others for agricultural or commercial purposes. These zoning codes vary from region to region, but everywhere it is a costly and lengthy procedure to petition authorities to rezone land designated for some other use than the one you plan. Results may not be favorable. Before plans progress too far, you should consult the landowner or his real estate agent about zoning on property you are considering.

  Building orientation. If winds in your area sweep down from the northwest, you can cut utility costs by placing most windows and doors on the southeast side of your building. Likewise, keeping drives and parking lots clear of snow and ice is easier if the building shields them from the wind. The cost of bringing utilities to the building also can be reduced by orienting the building favorably in relation to existing power, water, and sewage lines.

Physician Mix

Where do competing and referring physicians practice? The telephone directory's Yellow Pages have the information. If two sites are very close in all other factors, the one that suggests the greatest potential for referrals should sway your decision. Some physicians use one color of pin for each specialty.

The map pins you use to chart these first three factors should tell you which prestigious, high growth areas are understaffed by doctors in your specialty.

Proximity to Hospitals, Ancillary Facilities

For the convenience of patients and to save time for yourself, the best site will be near the hospitals where you will perform surgery, and near medical laboratories and other facilities whose services you may employ.

Proximity to Restaurants, Shopping

The availability of restaurants, shops, banks, and other support facilities is key to your ability to attract and retain good office staff. An employee's ability to enjoy lunch or make productive use of break-time for personal errands can greatly affect her willingness to work hard on your behalf and continue employment in the environment you have created. For yourself, too, the availability of neighborhood restaurants and services—to entertain referring physicians or run personal errands—should not be underestimated.

Visibility

If your office building is visible from major highways or shopping centers, it silently will advertise your services to passersby.

Proximity to Major Roads, Public Transportation

The closer you locate to major highways, the easier it will be for patients to find your office and the less trauma they will experience on their first visit. Ease of access will be a time saver, too, for you and your employees.

Your Travel Time

Your time is, in fact, one of your most valuable assets, and the amount of time you could spend in transit should weigh heavily in selecting a practice site. The trend today, of course, is to practice in a medical office structure adjacent to or within walking distance of a hospital. If you plan to limit your practice to one hospital, the measurement of travel time will be simple. However, if you will perform facial plastic surgery in more than one hospital, you must measure time from office to hospital, hospital to hospital, and hospital back to office. On top of that, add your travel time from your residence. If your time is worth $200 per hour and a certain location saves 15 minutes per day, then you may save $12,000 per year, based on a five-day work week and a 48-week work year.

Parking

Which office buildings (or building sites) offer enough parking space for patients, your employees, and yourself? In fact, how many parking spaces do you need? Careful planning for parking is especially critical in urban areas, where there's more often a shortage than a surplus of nearby spaces. Medical office building planners typically advise a solo physician to reserve 10 to 12 parking spaces, six to eight for patients and four for staff. Often, a rental or condominium agreement will include one parking space for every 100 to 200 square feet of office space. Beyond that, parking must be paid for, either by staff and patients or by the physician as an amenity. Other features to check out on parking include: indoor spaces, night lighting (if you plan to keep evening office hours), covered areas for patient drop off and pick up, covered areas for office deliveries.

Room for Expansion

Which sites have room for expansion if your practice should grow, or you take on a partner, or you decide to add a surgical suite to your office? If you are a small tenant in a large building, beware that you may be asked to move out of your space at the end of your lease to accommodate a larger tenant's expansion.

"Curb Appeal"

This real estate term refers to the emotional appeal a building has, from the outside, before a person ever steps foot inside. Curb appeal is completely subjective, but it's worth thinking about what type of building you instinctively will be comfortable in and will be happy to call home for a number of years. New patients and staff will form their first impressions of you from the curb, as well.

BUILDING CONSTRUCTION FACTORS

A little knowledge of the physical characteristics of office buildings will help you when it comes time to talk with building landlords, builders, or space planners about the office features that are important to you. Here are the chief characteristics:

Building Shell

Its shell is to a building what the skeleton is to the human body. It is all those components that support and give shape to the rest of the building—the foundation, plus the beam and girder system. The beams and girders can be made of wood, steel, or precast concrete, with the size of the building usually dictating the appropriate material.

Exterior Skin

As the name implies, the exterior skin is what covers the outside of the shell. Glass, brick, wood, concrete, or architectural panels are a few of the skin materials available. Choice may be dictated by what is regionally available, within your budget, allowed by local ordinances, helpful in reducing insurance rates, conserving of energy, low in maintenance, and acceptable to your personal taste. Remember that the exterior skin sets the tone ("curb appeal") for the entire building.

Interior Improvements

This term covers everything done to complete the building interior, from laying down subflooring to partitioning off common areas and individual offices to installing adequate soundproofing. Choice of materials here can affect total building or rental costs more than any other single item. In the long run, buying or renting high quality interior improvements pays off. The initial costs may be higher, but installation may go more smoothly, maintenance costs will drop off, soundproofing will be assured, building codes will be adhered to, and the building will have the appropriate professional and aesthetic appeal. (For a comparison of ceiling, flooring, and interior wall materials by initial cost, maintenance cost, ease of installation, etc., see *Planning Guide for Physicians' Medical Facilities*, published by the American Medical Association.)

Tenant Improvements

The improvements in your office, both those provided by the landlord and those paid for by you, are the tenant improvements. (See later for a list of standard improvements provided by landlords.)

Core Area

Every feature that supports all building tenants is part of the core area—elevator shafts, restrooms, mechanical rooms, stairwells, public corridors, and lobbies. Some of these terms warrant additional definition.

HVAC

The heating, ventilating, and air conditioning systems (HVAC) is perhaps the one office feature most important to the comfort of yourself, staff, and patients. An office that is too hot or too cold not only is a discomfort to all, but also has a definite adverse effect on office productivity.

The wide variety in HVAC systems available makes it a challenging task to find the one best for a facial plastic surgery office. One building may have a central plant—a central cooling tower and heat source—that provides your office with a "variable air volume." Other buildings have "split systems" that have several rooftop units to supply forced air to individual offices. A third type popular for individual comfort and control is the electrohydronic system, which works much like a heat pump in today's new home construction.

Building codes usually specify the number of zones or thermostats a building must have. Generally, there will be one thermostat for every 700 to 1,200 square feet of area, depending on the system design. It's possible the control will be in your office, but it may be in the neighboring tenant's suite—not the ideal situation if his practice demands different temperatures from yours. Try to keep control of the thermostat.

To educate yourself about HVACs in general, talk to builders, building managers, and heating contractors. Learn the methods by which each system operates, its ability to give you air conditioning year-round, its availability 24 hours per day and on weekends, its link to an efficient exhaust system, and its operating costs (you will be paying the bill whether the landlord includes it in your rent or you are separately metered).

Plumbing Stacks or Loops

Although the plumbing requirements for each doctor's office vary, there is one characteristic common to all: expense. Most buildings will have plumbing in the core area, as well as in plumbing "stacks" located next to building support columns. Some buildings also have "loops" that go around the entire floor for ease of access and cheaper installation. The closer your office is to a stack or loop, the lower your costs are going to be for plumbing installation.

Since most medical offices require more plumbing than other kinds of office facilities (at least two lavatories for staff and patients and for yourself, plus laboratory and examining room sinks), locating your office near main plumbing conduits can save considerable cost.

Elevators

A rule of thumb is that builders will install one elevator for every 25,000 to 30,000 square feet of gross floor area. Too few elevators waste time and guarantee that you, your staff, and patients all will be frustrated by the time your office is reached.

Slow elevators will do the same. Electric-geared elevators generally are the fastest; hydraulic elevators the slowest.

Oversized, "hospital" elevators are a must because of their depth and ability to accommodate wheelchairs and stretchers. They also are more likely to be able to accommodate the equipment and furniture you will have to move into your office.

A final item to inspect is an elevator's safety features. Does it have, for instance, a telephone for contacting the building management in the event the elevator sticks between floors?

Floor Load

How much weight can a floor accommodate? A typical building's floor load is 70 to 100 pounds per square foot. Any building constructed with less than a 70-pound floor load may not support heavy medical equipment or even filing cabinets.

Ceiling Heights

Most ceilings will be 8' to 8'6"; however, you may find 7' to 9' ceiling in some buildings. Stay within this range, as anything higher may make small examining rooms look and feel smaller, and anything shorter may give you a closed-in feeling. The 9' ceiling will give you additional storage area (Table 9-2).

Life Safety and Security Systems

Typically the most overlooked of a building's features, the life safety and security systems are the occupant's most important protection from hazards and physical harm. They include everything from clearly marked emergency exits and properly posted emergency procedures to guard service after hours. Physical features may include:

Emergency power sources. Smaller buildings usually have battery packs located in the common areas or perhaps installed within each office. Larger buildings may have an emergency generator capable of powering elevators in the event of power failure. For physicians with office surgeries, control of an emergency power source may be critical.

Fire alarms. Fire alarms are activated manually to alert occupants to a fire. Newer buildings may have a visual strobe for hearing-disabled occupants, as well as the traditional audio alarm. Alarms may be connected to a central control system (see later) or may go directly to the fire department.

Sprinkler systems. When the temperature reaches a certain degree, automatic sprinklers turn on and pump water into the building. Sprinklers generally are used only

Table 9-2. "Building Standard" Construction

New buildings give tenants an allowance to complete their office interior, just as an allowance in older buildings is provided to remodel. Either way, the sum is the minimum amount required to bring the space up to "building standard." If the tenant wants more, his improvements are called "non-standard" and he pays for them.

As you are comparing building standard allowances, here are some points to consider in the six major areas on which allowances usually are given.

Walls. Will walls be constructed of drywall, plaster, or a module wall system? Will they be insulated for sound control? Do plans call for walls to go to the ceiling, just above the ceiling, or to the deck of the floor above? (Walls that go at least above the ceiling lines are imperative for sound control.) What type of wall covering is provided—vinyl or paint?

Ceilings. Are the ceilings drywall (its concealed spline system provides good sound control) or acoustical pads (its exposed grid system is less expensive, but has less ability to control sound).

Floors. Is the building standard carpet or tiles? Are colors and quality available through the owner appealing and durable?

Window coverings. Some buildings do not provide an allowance for this costly item, and yet require you to seek approval for your choice because it affects the building's exterior appearance.

Electrical allowance. How many electrical outlets and telephone outlets are provided? Is the number sufficient? Is the voltage/amperage sufficient for your equipment?

Plumbing allowance. If a plumbing allowance is offered, is it adequate for your practice? Will it allow for sinks in every exam room?

Who pays for maintenance of all improvements?

---

in buildings more than three stories tall; however, they are an excellent safety feature for any building. Most sprinkler systems also are set off when fire alarms are activated.

Smoke detectors. When smoke or fumes activate the sensor, an alarm is sounded for the occupants. Depending on the system, the alarm may also ring at a central control station.

Automatic elevator system. In the event of a fire, this system causes the elevators to go immediately to the first floor and release passengers. Since elevator shafts act just as the flue in a fireplace, providing draft to the fire, this safety feature is an important one.

Emergency stairs. Most buildings have two or more emergency stair exits, one located at least one-half the distance of the diagonal of the building from the other. Most modern high-rise buildings will provide pressurized stair towers for smoke control. Most walls in the stair towers are "2-4 hour rated," meaning they will withstand fire from two to four hours before burning through.

Fire fighter control panel. This panel, located on the first floor, indicates where in the building an alarm has been set off. Also, because communication jacks placed throughout the building are connected to this panel, it provides a means for firemen to contact one another, no matter where they are.

Security alarms. An alarm can be installed that will alert security if someone intrudes in your office after hours.

Central control. Larger buildings may have a central control area where security guards can provide electronic surveillance of all life safety systems, including fire alarms, sprinklers, and elevator location indicators. Control areas often have a loudspeaker paging system for emergency contact with all occupants.

OFFICE DESIGN FACTORS

A solo practitioner's office can have as many as 10 types of rooms—plus an office surgery. No matter what your taste or practice methods, no matter whether you are evaluating an existing office for rental purposes or constructing a new one, you can recognize a good office layout by certain design features. Obviously, if you lease space, you will not be able easily to change such features as room size or flow, but familiarity with design principles at least may steer you clear of problem office spaces (Table 9-3).

The following guidelines are written for an individual practice; however the basic ideas are applicable to partnerships or groups. Most office buildings employ a space planner who can help you apply these guidelines, or you may elect to hire an independent planner to help you with decorating as well as design (Table 9-4).

Layout Efficiency

The building with the highest rental rate per square foot is not necessarily the most expensive. If the layout of office space in building "A" is so efficient that only 1,000 square feet are required to give you every kind of room you need in just the size you need, it may cost you less than an office in building "B" where the rent is lower but an inefficient layout consumes 1,100 square feet. For instance, if building "A" rents for $10 per square foot, your annual rent will be $10,000, whereas 1,100 square feet in building "B" at $9.50 per square foot will cost you $10,450.

The figure of 1,000 square feet is the approximate amount of space a solo practitioner requires for his practice, including most or all of the rooms described

Table 9-3. More Tips for Tenants

Owner's reputation. Ask who the owner is and investigate his philosophy toward the building. If the owner regards the building only as a tax write-off or is looking for a quick return, he may not care about long-term commitments, resulting in high tenant turnover and poor service. Conversely, an owner with a reputation for long-term investments probably knows how to build long-term satisfaction among tenants.
   Management's reputation. Talk to the other tenants about the management of the building. Perhaps a management company handles this operation for the owners. Determine the management company's response time to various problems. Is the exterior of the building well maintained? Are grass and shrubbery trimmed? Is there rubbish around the building? Check the condition of the parking lots. Examine the mechanical rooms of the building; if they are well maintained, the entire building is probably maintained in that manner. Visit the management company's office. Its physical condition and the way its staff present themselves may be an indication of their management philosophy.
   Space planning service. Today, most landlords or leasing agents provide preliminary space plans for your office layout. Check to see if this service is available to you, and who does it. An experienced space planner can save you time and money. Only if the plans are not adequate—or if you want total design control—should you need to hire your own designer.
   Cleaning service. Talk to other tenants about the quality of cleaning services and examine common areas for cleanliness. If the service is part of your rent, ask the owner for a copy of the cleaning specifications that are part of his contract with the cleaning agency. How often is the service performed and at what hours? Who supplies paper towels, toilet tissue, and cleaning supplies for your restrooms? Who shampoos your carpets or waxes your floors?
   Building size. If you are a tenant of 1000 square feet in a 100,000 square foot building, you represent 1% of the occupied space. Your ability to negotiate with the owners will be far less than if you rent 2000 square feet in a 25,000 square foot building.

below, plus corridors sufficiently wide (5 feet) for two people to pass comfortably.

Reception/Waiting Room

No patient enjoys waiting for the doctor, but the anxiety of the wait can be dispelled in a reception area that heeds design rules about size, physical arrangement of furniture, and decor. A well-designed waiting room serves a second function for the facial plastic surgeon: It can be a showcase of the physician's own sense of detail and artistry, two personal traits of great importance to the patient awaiting facial plastic surgery. In the waiting room, the patient forms a strong impression of the doctor to whom he soon will entrust the face he shows the world.

Size

To determine how large your waiting room should be, first multiply the number of patients you see each hour by two. That will give you the minimum number of chairs you need. For each chair, allow 12 square feet. Some space planners suggest that beginning physicians increase these minimum numbers by 15% to accommodate the growth of their practice. Not allowing for growth is a common—and costly—mistake, they warn.

Arrangement

Not just the number, but the type and arrangement of chairs and other furnishings will affect the final dimen-

Table 9-4. Ergonomics: Factoring Human Comfort into Office Designs

Could this scene occur in any medical office building you know?
   Already nervous, a new patient wanders down an ill-lit corridor searching for the doctor's office. When finally a nameplate announces the doctor's presence within, the patient opens the door onto a dark and cheerless room. The only window, a frosted glass pane that separates the waiting room from the business office, abruptly opens; a hand thrusts out a form; a voice instructs, "You have to fill this out before the doctor will see you."
   Ergonomics, also called human engineering, is the applied science concerned with making sure that scenes like this never occur. Its basic goal is to find a way to design and arrange the things that people use so that the people and things can interact most comfortably and productively.
   For facial plastic surgeons, ergonomics may be only a new name for something they do already when they create waiting rooms with an ambience that calms patients and quietly reflects the physician's professionalism. Nevertheless, perhaps some of the facts ergonomics researchers have turned up may be new.
   • Patients are less anxious in offices where no door separates the waiting room from the corridor leading to examination rooms.
   • People do 12% more work under natural lighting, which derives its energy equally from all parts of the spectrum, than from indoor lighting, which derives its light from just one color band (yellow).
   • If sinks and desk are too low, every time you bend forward to work, you put nearly 300 pounds of pressure on your back.

sions of the waiting room. Again, a space planner can help, drawing a diagram showing the placement of each piece of furniture. Some important rules of thumb: Chairs are better than couches, as patients like a sense of privacy; for the same reason, avoid arranging chairs so that lines of patients stare across the room at one another; a small writing desk, for privacy and ease in filling out forms, is a bonus. The soft lighting of occasional lamps instead of flourescent overhead fixtures, good ventilation, coat racks, current magazines, accessible toilets, and music are nice finishing touches. So are wall hangings or some focal point of interest such as plants, an aquarium or an unusual outside view. Carpeting promotes quiet, costs less to maintain, and can be attractive.

Decor

Comfort and attractiveness are two important attributes of waiting room decor. Utility is another. Office furnishings come in five different grades. Insist on the more costly, industrial grade. Modern materials and styles can be combined in ways that avoid institutional drabness, giving you furniture that blends function and beauty and is reinforced and sturdy enough that you will not have to replace it in 2 or 3 years. High quality furnishings also give the appearance of an established, successful practice.

Business Office

Most medical offices today place the receptionist not in the waiting room (as once was the practice) but in a separate business office, set off from the waiting area with a sliding glass window. The window affords a view of patient arrivals at the same time that it blocks telephone noise from the waiting room and creates privacy for the confidential matters that will be discussed in the business office.

Several factors will affect how much space you need for business functions and, once you have considered them all, add more space for future staff additions, computer hardware, and other office equipment (Table 9-5).

To start, space planners advise that you allot 125 square feet for the first office worker, then add 75 more feet for each additional person. Even if you only have one worker now, allow for more work stations in the future. In laying out work stations, the rule is to allow five feet between two people who will work around one another. Work space should include plenty of counter space at desk height (30 inches) for writing and billing and at typewriter stand height (28 inches). Do not neglect storage for office forms and paper supplies (Table 9-6).

To ensure ample room for equipment, give the space planner one list of equipment essential to opening your practice and another of equipment you hope to purchase in the next few years. Adequate room for files to house all patient histories must be planned, and advice on the best file system for your needs should be obtained from an office furniture specialist.

The business office need not be plush, but your employees' work habits will be affected positively by your provision of work space that is pleasant and roomy. An outside window, if possible, is a great plus, as is carpeting for sound control.

Table 9-5. Equipment: Lease or Buy?

Sophisticated medical equipment—unarguably essential to the delivery of modern health care services—is undeniably expensive. Yet there are ways to acquire equipment without its consuming substantial amounts of working capital. Instead of buying outright, physicians can buy equipment on installment, or lease it. Here are the pros and cons of each method:

Leasing. Some lease agreements allow you to upgrade equipment as new developments appear on the market. If technology is rapidly changing the equipment you need, such agreements not only keep your equipment current but also guarantee that you will not be troubled with the outright ownership of obsolete equipment. Any equipment whose life is no longer than the period it would take to buy it on installment probably should be leased. When the life of the lease equals the life of the equipment, the lease is called a "true" or "pure" lease, and this is the only type of lease on which many third-party payors will reimburse, including Medicare.

Some leases include handling, delivery, and installation, as well as maintenance. Some do not, charging extra for every administrative detail and requiring a substantial deposit, too. The true cost of a lease is the sum of these extras, if any, and the installment payment.

Whatever equipment your lease provides at whatever cost, you know—because you are leasing—that your management of the equipment will be confined to the length of the lease. If you like the arrangement you can renew.

A last advantage: Sometimes leasing is the only way to fund new equipment. Any means of getting some equipment is justified if the revenue it will produce will exceed the cost of the lease.

Installment buying. When interest rates are low, buying on installment can result in lower monthly payments than a leasing agreement would. Ownership gives you certain tax benefits (depreciation) that leasing does not. If the life of the equipment is longer than the period of the installment loan (as is the case for much medical equipment), there is some salvage or residual value which you, as owner, can realize through sale of the equipment. Another financial benefit to ownership: Whereas lease companies used to be able to claim that leases did not tie up your line of credit like loans do, bankers today add up the total lease obligations and treat it just like a loan commitment when calculating your net worth.

Two other pointers, helpful whether you lease or buy on installment: (1) Either method puts less strain on your cash flow than buying equipment outright—cash that you may be able to use more effectively elsewhere. (2) Whatever company you go with, check its reputation with other customers first; make sure it provides service promptly, and is financially sound enough to provide service over the life of the equipment or lease.

Table 9-6. Office Building Comparison Form

Item	Bldg. A	Bldg. B	Bldg. C
Site factors			
Growing area	_____	_____	_____
Prestigious area	_____	_____	_____
Physician mix	_____	_____	_____
Proximity to hospitals, ancillary services	_____	_____	_____
Proximity to shopping, restaurants	_____	_____	_____
Visibility	_____	_____	_____
Proximity to roads, transportation	_____	_____	_____
Your travel time	_____	_____	_____
Parking	_____	_____	_____
Room for expansion	_____	_____	_____
Curb appeal	_____	_____	_____
Construction quality			
Building shell	_____	_____	_____
Exterior skin	_____	_____	_____
Interior improvements	_____	_____	_____
Tenant improvements	_____	_____	_____
Core area	_____	_____	_____
HVAC	_____	_____	_____
Plumbing stacks	_____	_____	_____
Elevators	_____	_____	_____
Floor load	_____	_____	_____
Ceiling heights	_____	_____	_____
Life safety and security features	_____	_____	_____
Office design			
Layout efficiency	_____	_____	_____
Waiting room	_____	_____	_____
Business office	_____	_____	_____
Examination rooms	_____	_____	_____
Consultation room	_____	_____	_____
Storage	_____	_____	_____
Toilets	_____	_____	_____
Utility space	_____	_____	_____
Laboratory	_____	_____	_____
Employee lounge	_____	_____	_____
Private office	_____	_____	_____
Miscellaneous			
Owner's reputation	_____	_____	_____
Manager's reputation	_____	_____	_____
Space planning service	_____	_____	_____
Cleaning service	_____	_____	_____
Building size	_____	_____	_____
Rental rate data			
Method of measurement			
—Usable square feet	_____	_____	_____
—Rentable square feet	_____	_____	_____
Full service	_____	_____	_____

Examination Rooms

The center of office activity, examination rooms should be designed for maximum physician efficiency and patient comfort. They also must be of sufficient size and number to accommodate a growing facial plastic surgery practice.

Efficiency Factors

Space planners have computed that 20 to 30 minutes can be saved each day by physicians who practice in examination rooms that have been designed for maximum efficiency. Personal fatigue also is reduced when design eliminates unnecessary footsteps. Key to a good design are these elements: identical layouts in each room, rooms stocked with identical supplies, equipment set up off the floor where it easily can be reached, writing areas at standing height, dictation systems in each room, everything within reach from examination tables (including light switches), chart racks on doors, and a visual system that signals to all staff when a room is in use.

Comfort Factors

Patients appreciate every detail that reduces anxiety—doors that open in a way that blocks a direct view of the patient from the hallway; dressing facilities that include a mirror, clothes hooks, and chair or bench; such aids to waiting as good lighting and current magazines, perhaps music; and soundproofing. Doorways wide enough to allow wheelchairs and stretchers to pass through may be important.

Size and Number

Examination rooms should be small enough to eliminate unnecessary steps, but large enough to accommodate the movements of you and your assistants. Space planners have determined that rooms 6'x9' allow space for the physician to work on one side of an examination table only; 7'x9' allows for work on both sides; and 8'x10' allows work on both sides, plus room for some equipment.

One rule of thumb for setting up an adequate number of examination rooms is to divide the number of patients seen in 1 hour by two. Another says that every physician needs somewhere between one and three rooms, the smaller number perhaps being adequate if another room is available for postexamination consultation (see later). Another reminds physicians that they should have a sufficient number of rooms to accommodate the staff's preparation of patients prior to the physician's examination.

Consultation Room

Some physicians believe examining rooms are too impersonal for postexamination consultations. They prefer a separate consultation room. Others use their private office for this purpose. Whatever your personal preference, it is important that some room be set aside for your discussions of procedures with patients, your staff's discussions of financial arrangements with patients, and perhaps patients' private discussions with their families. Properly equipped, such a room also can serve as a staff and patient library, or as a conference room for pharmaceutical representatives.

Even multipurpose consultation rooms need not be overly large. Most measure from 10'x10' to 12'x15', and use light colors to enhance the size. Other features are: audiovisual equipment, occasional lamps, comfortable furniture, bookcases, patient/staff pamphlets and other reading material, carpeting, good ventilation.

Storage, Toilets, Utility Space

It's easy, but shortsighted, to trim capital expenditures by trimming space not directly related to medical or business functions, space planners advise. Here's what they say about three such spaces.

Storage

Some supplies will be stored in each examining room, in the business office, and elsewhere, right in the areas where they ultimately will be used. Still needed, however, is an area for bulk storage of supplies from patient wraps and paper towels to medicinal supplies and old patient files. A central storage area, contiguous to the business office, should provide ample space so that supplies do not spill over into the business office itself. Adequate numbers of built-in cabinets, racks, shelves, and counters can be computed by space planners.

Toilets

Since most office buildings provide men's and women's restrooms on each floor, which your patients can use when arriving or leaving your office, your own office will probably need only one or two toilets. Plan 4'x5' areas for each. Some physicians plan one toilet for patients and staff to share, and a private one for themselves. Others plan a separate toilet for patients and share one with staff. If space and budget permit, you might consider a shower in your private toilet area.

Some tips from space planners: Install wall-hung tanks and wash basins, as they facilitate cleaning; assign staff to keep patient toilets clean; plan for one toilet to accommodate handicapped patients.

Utility Space

In one-story buildings, you may have to accommodate your own heating and cooling system, and hot water heater, right in your office. A janitor's supply closet —with sink—may also be essential. In multistory buildings, utility space may be shared with other tenants.

Laboratory

Before deciding that you want your own lab right in your office, check whether other lab facilities exist in or near your office building. If they do, can you provide the same services at less cost to your patients? Maybe you will want a small galley-shaped lab that can double as a nurses' workroom, storeroom, or spare examining room. A lab may be more essential if you plan an office surgery unit.

Space planners usually allot about 150 square feet per technician. They place labs adjacent to examination rooms, the operating room, or toilets. Minimally, a lab should have enough counter space (at 36" to 42" height) for a sink, sterilizer, and other equipment, as well as cabinets for supplies. Countertops should be constructed of the most durable material available and have splashboards at right angles to the wall. A small refrigerator, with ice maker, frequently is installed under the counter.

Employee Lounge

You may want to plan for an employee lounge "at the back of the house," away from the waiting and exam areas. A small table to seat two to four people will give your employees an area to relax away from the telephones and paperwork. An added benefit: Stock the refrigerator with fresh fruit, soft drinks, and salads. The thoughtfulness can return twice the investment in appreciation and productivity.

Private Office

Since you probably will spend more of your waking hours in your office than you will at home, provide yourself with a room that is appealing, comfortable, and relaxing, as well as functional. A music system, portable television, library, and communications equipment will be well worth the investment. Decorate with high grade carpet, fabric, or paneling on the walls, and selective lighting fixtures. Select your favorite desk, chairs, couches, bookcases, tables, and credenza. Coordinate paintings, pictures, certificates, and other wall hangings.

NEGOTIATING AN OFFICE LEASE

A lease is a binding, legal document, something from which no one can extricate you should its terms suddenly appear unfavorable to you. If you have agreed to pay $2,000 per month for 5 years no matter what, you will owe it whether you become disabled or of necessity must move to another city. If you move in and find that the previous tenant took the luxurious drapes you had counted on to adorn your office, chances are you missed the fine print about which fixtures stay. If you have agreed that the lease will automatically renew unless you notify the landlord by a certain date, so be it, even if the omission was merely an oversight and you have already signed a second lease on a new space.

It pays to know what you are signing. It also pays to negotiate the terms of any lease you are considering. Any lease is negotiable, and 99% of all leases have been amended at least once. There is no such thing as a standard lease, although landlords can buy preprinted leases. Convenient for the landlord, a preprinted lease also favors him. Nevertheless, landlords usually will negotiate— especially with doctors, who are considered desirable tenants.

Negotiating a lease is not something to attempt without the counsel of a good real estate lawyer, one knowledgeable in *local* leasing laws. As management consultant Michael Wiley writes in *Medical Economics* (September 23, 1985), "Only a lawyer from New York would know that if you nail something to a wall there, it belongs to the landlord; if you screw it to a wall, you can take it with you."

This section contains an analysis of a typical office lease. As you negotiate your own lease, do not be satisfied with verbal agreements. *Everything* should be in writing. That will eliminate misunderstandings with your present landlord and protect you in the event that ownership of the building passes to a third party.

OFFICE LEASE AGREEMENT

The lead statement in an office lease simply identifies who is the landlord and who is the tenant:

_____ ("Lessor") and _____ ("Lessee") hereby enter into the following office lease agreement.

The Leased Premises

The next section describes the actual space you will rent, as well as the common areas of the building to which your lease entitles you to use. It typically will include a reference to one exhibit that is a diagram of the lease space (see Fig. 9-1) and to another that provides a legal description of the real estate on which the office building is located (see Fig. 9-2). Any restrictions on the use of the common areas will be listed here, and if your lease entitles you to parking spaces, that too will be mentioned.

> Lessor hereby leases and demises to the lessee and the lessee agrees to lease from the lessor a portion of a certain medical office building located in (*city, state*), the street address of which is _____, which office building is referred to herein as the "office building." The portion of the office building hereby leased to lessee is identified on the floor plan attached hereto and marked Exhibit A ("The leased premises"). The rentable area of the office building shall be deemed to be _____ square feet and the rentable area of the leased premises shall be deemed to be _____ square feet.
>
> The lessor also grants to lessee, together with and subject to the same rights granted from time to time by lessor to other lessees and occupants of the office building the right to use the lobbies, and common areas within the office building and the common parking and any other public facilities located on the real estate described on Exhibit B attached hereto ("The associated common areas").

Term and Commencement Date

Leases typically run from 3 to 5 years. A longer term lease may be available if you want to make the commitment. A shorter term lease obviously gives you an opportunity to relocate at the expiration of the lease. The shorter term also enables the landlord to increase your rent at the expiration of the lease term.

Perhaps the most advantageous terms for you would be a term of 5 years with the option to renew at the existing rate or a prenegotiated rate. The commencement date of a lease is the date on which you agree to start paying rent. This date typically is the date on which you take possession or your first day of business. You may want to make explicit that the landlord's improvements or renovations must be completed by this date, or you have the right to cancel the lease. If you need a period of time in which to set up your office, you may wish to ask for an appropriate number of days in which to do so.

Some leases have an automatic renewal date; if so, you will want to keep that date firmly in mind, especially if you have plans to move.

> The term of this lease shall be for a period of _____ years (the "lease term"), commencing on _____ (the "commencement date").

SAMPLE LEASE EXHIBIT A — LEASED PREMISES
This diagram outlines the area of the office building that defines the premises covered by the "office lease agreement."

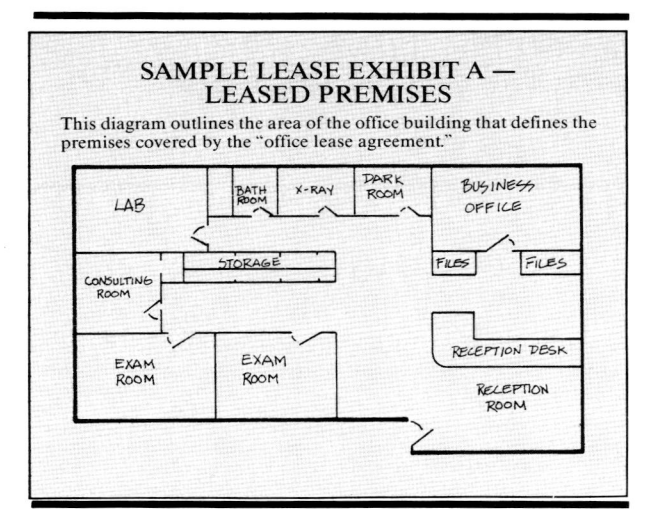

Figure 9-1.

Construction of Improvements

The obligation of the landlord to provide you with the construction or the remodeling of your office space is detailed in this section. Make sure all understandings pertaining to improvements are covered in writing. You may want to ask for the right to inspect work in progress.

The construction of the improvements may be covered by reference to an exhibit entitled "work letter agreement" (see Table 9-7) or may be agreed on by attaching as an exhibit plans and specifications for the office. If a method of payment and the terms of that payment are not outlined, you should make this part of your improvement exhibit.

Note the phrase that binds you to accepting the premises "as is." If, during your inspection, you fail to notice that plumbing does not work, keys are missing, and windows are broken, you must pay for those repairs unless they are included in the written work letter agreement.

> Lessee has personally inspected the lease premises and accepts the same "as is" without representation or warranty by lessor of any kind and with the understanding that lessor shall have no responsibility with respect thereto except to construct the improvements described in *Exhibit C* ("The work letter agreement"), so that the leased premises will be

SAMPLE LEASE EXHIBIT B — LEGAL DESCRIPTION OF REAL ESTATE
Part of the west half of the northwest quarter of section 21, township 17 north, range 3 east in _____, more particularly described as follows:
    Commencing at the northeast corner of said half quarter section; thence south 0 degrees 06 minutes 51 seconds west (assumed bearing) 603.98 feet along east line of said half quarter section to the point of beginning; thence continue south 0 degrees 06 minutes 51 seconds west 522.72 feet to the south line of the owner's land; thence south 89 degrees 14 minutes 29 seconds west 425.01 feet along said south line; thence north 0 degrees 06 minutes 51 seconds east 522.72 feet; thence north 89 degrees 14 minutes 29 seconds east 425.01 feet to the point of beginning and containing 5.100 acres, more or less.
    Subject to a 50.00 foot easement by parallel lines off the entire east side as described in a public street dedication for _____ Road in instrument number 24221.
    Subject also, to a 50.00 foot easement for pipeline in favor of _____ Utility Company.
    Subject also, to all other legal rights of way and easements of record.

Figure 9-2.

Table 9-7. Sample Lease Exhibit C—Work Letter Agreement

[This type of document outlines those construction items to be provided by the landlord at no additional expense to the tenant. This exhibit may be modified by indicating other improvements to be included and paid for by the landlord or other improvements to be included and paid for by the tenant. In lieu of the written work letter, you may elect to attach a full set of plans and specifications containing all of the construction work.]

In addition to the mutual covenants explained in the lease to which this *Exhibit C* is a part, landlord and tenant further mutually agree as follows:

1. PLANS AND SPECIFICATIONS FOR THE LEASED PREMISES

   (a) Tenant agrees to cooperate with landlord's architects and engineers, who shall prepare at landlord's expense detailed space plans for tenant finished improvements for the leased premises which shall include, but not be limited to, locations of doors, partitioning, reflected ceiling, electrical fixtures, outlets and switches, telephone outlets, plumbing fixtures, extraordinary floor loads and other special requirements; and tenant shall approve such space plans. Tenant may provide space plans by an architect selected by tenant at tenant's expense prior to the space plan approval date. Landlord shall be entitled, in all respects, to rely upon all plans, drawings and information so supplied. All working drawings shall be prepared by landlord's architect or engineer, which working drawings shall include architectural, mechanical, electrical and structural engineering drawings for building standard work as described in paragraph 2 hereof at landlord's expense.

   (b) Tenant may require work (hereinafter referred to as "building nonstandard work") different from or in addition to building standard work as described in paragraph 2 hereof. In such event, any architectural, mechanical, electrical and structural engineering drawings, plans and specifications required shall be prepared by landlord's architect or engineer at tenant's expense and shall be subject to the approval of landlord.

   (c) If tenant selects interior finish items such as wall paint and/or wall coverings, fixtures or carpeting from landlord's building standard work, tenant shall notify landlord of all such selections in writing within twenty (20) days following the space plan approval date. All interior decorating items and services selected by tenant in excess of building standard shall be provided by tenant at tenant's sole cost and expense.

   (d) All plans and specifications referred to in subparagraphs (a) and (b) of this paragraph are subject to landlord's approval, which approval shall not be unreasonably withheld.

   (e) Tenant's plans and specifications shall not be in conflict with building codes of the city of _____ or with applicable insurance regulations for a fire resistant building. All plans and specifications shall be in a form satisfactory for filing with appropriate governmental authorities for permits and licenses required for construction.

   (f) The extent to which any of tenant's requirements are building non-standard work or otherwise exceed building standard shall be determined by landlord's architect or engineer.

2. BUILDING STANDARD WORK AT LANDLORD'S COST AND EXPENSE

Landlord agrees, at its sole cost and expense, to furnish and install all of the following building standard work limited to the quantities specified by landlord and as indicated on tenant's final approved plans:

   (a) *Tenant entry door*. 3'0" × 7'0" tinted tempered glass door with anodized aluminum frame, closer and locking hardware.

   (b) *Interior tenant doors*. 3'0" × 7'0" solid core, selected oak finish with anodized aluminum frame, floor mounted doorstop and passage hardware—one door per 250 square feet of office area.

   (c) *Interior partitions*. Full height vinyl clad partition wall—4" vinyl covered baseboard, 10 linear feet per 100 square feet of office area.

   (d) *Ceiling*. Suspended acoustical ceiling 2' × 4' non-directional panels throughout.

   (e) *Carpeting*. All floor within the tenant's leased premises shall be carpeted. Tenant shall have the right to select carpeting for the leased premises from a group of samples furnished by landlord.

   (f) *Plumbing*. Two restrooms per office area—each restroom contains:

   Men's. One wall-hung lavatory with liquid soap dispenser; one paper towel dispenser, mirror and wall-mounted light fixture; one 20 amp duplex electrical outlet; one tank type water closet with toilet paper dispenser; one direct flush urinal and exhaust fan.

   Women's. One wall-hung lavatory with liquid soap dispenser, one paper towel dispenser, mirror and wall-mounted light fixture; one 20 amp duplex electrical outlet; one tank type water closet with toilet paper dispenser and exhaust fan.

   (g) *Electrical*.
   (1) One 20 amp duplex outlet per 100 square feet of office area.
   (2) One single pole switch per 200 square feet of office area.
   (3) One 2' × 4' four-tube recessed fluorescent lighting fixture per 75 square feet of office area.
   (4) One telephone outlet per 250 square feet of office area.
   (5) Emergency lighting, exit lights, fire alarm(s) as required by code.

   (h) *HVAC*. Year-round heating and air-conditioning system, including ducted supply and return distribution system above ceiling providing conditioned air to all tenant offices and rooms: System designed to maintain temperature in normal comfort zones based on a standard lighting and electrical load not to exceed four watts per square feet of rentable area and occupancy of one person per 100 square feet of rentable area.

   (i) *Window coverings*. All exterior windows within the tenant's leased premises.

3. BUILDING NON-STANDARD WORK AT TENANT'S COST AND EXPENSE

Provided tenant's space plans and specifications are approved or furnished not later than the time provided hereinabove in paragraph 1, landlord shall cause tenant's building nonstandard work to be installed by landlord's contractor, but at tenant's sole cost and expense. Prior to commencing any such building non-standard work, landlord shall submit to tenant a written estimate of the cost thereof. If tenant approves such estimate, it shall notify landlord in writing within seven (7) days and at the same time pay landlord in full the amount of such estimate; and landlord's contractor shall proceed with such work. If tenant shall fail to approve any such estimate in writing within seven (7) days after submission thereof, such failure shall be

Table 9-7. (Continued)

deemed a disapproval thereof; and landlord's contractor shall not proceed with such work or the building standard work affected thereby. It is understood that tenant shall thereupon be liable for the delay and increased cost, if any, in completing the affected building standard work. Tenant shall also be responsible for the design, function, and maintenance of such special improvements, whether or not installed by landlord at tenant's request.

Tenant agrees to pay landlord or its contractor, as set forth above, the cost of all such building non-standard work including contractor's overhead plus 10% for landlord's overhead and coordination of the work.

4. SUBSTITUTION AND CREDITS

Tenant may select different new materials (except exterior window draperies) in place of building standard materials which would otherwise be initially furnished and installed by landlord in the interior of the leased premises under the provisions of this *Exhibit C*, provided such selection is indicated on tenant's complete plans and specifications approved by landlord. If tenant shall make any such selection and if the cost of such different new materials of tenant's selection shall exceed landlord's cost of building standard materials thereby replaced, tenant shall pay to landlord, as hereinafter provided, the difference between the cost of such different new materials and the credit given by landlord for the materials thereby replaced plus a fee of 10% of the difference, if any, for landlord's additional costs resulting from such substitution.

No such different new materials shall be furnished and installed in replacement for any of building standard materials thereby replaced, tenant shall pay to landlord, as hereinafter increased cost thereof and landlord and tenant have agreed in writing on the increased costs of such different new materials and installation in excess of the cost of building standard. If tenant approves such estimate, it shall notify landlord in writing within seven (7) days and, at the same time, pay landlord in full the amount of such estimate; and landlord's contractor shall proceed with such work. If tenant shall fail to approve such estimate within seven (7) days after the submission thereof, such failure is to be deemed a disapproval thereof; and landlord's contractor shall proceed with the building standard work in lieu of the proposed substituted work. Tenant shall thereupon also be liable for the delay and increased cost, if any, in completing the affected building standard work.

All amounts payable by tenant to landlord pursuant to this paragraph 4 shall be paid by tenant promptly after the rendering of bills therefor by landlord or its contractor to tenant, it being understood that such bills may be rendered during the progress of the performance of the work and/or the furnishing and installation of the materials to which such bills relate. Any such different new materials shall be surrendered by tenant to landlord at the end of the initial or other expiration of the term of the lease. No credit shall be granted for the omission of materials where no replacement in kind is made. There shall be credits only for substitutions in kind, *e.g.*, a lighting fixture credit may be applied only against the cost of another type of lighting fixture.

5. COMPLETION AND RENTAL COMMENCEMENT DATE

The target commencement date of the lease as set forth in the basic lease provisions shall not be delayed by any of the following:

(a) Tenant's failure to approve or furnish space plans and specifications in accordance with date specified in paragraph 1 hereof;

(b) Tenant's request for materials, finishes or installations other than building standard;

(c) Tenant's changes in said plans and specifications after the approval or submission thereof to landlord in accordance with date specified in paragraph 1 hereof; or

(d) A delay in performance of building standard work as a result of tenant's failure to approve written estimates of the costs of building non-standard work or materials in accordance with paragraphs 3 and 4 hereof.

---

available for lessee's occupancy by the commencement date, unless prevented by causes beyond the control of lessor. Such improvements shall be in accordance with and at the expense of the party indicated in *Exhibit C*.

Minimum Rent

The minimum rent is that amount you agree to pay to the landlord for the term of the lease. In addition to this fixed rental, you also may be responsible for the increases in the operating expenses and real estate taxes of the building (see next section on "Operating Expenses").

> Lessee agrees to pay as minimum rent for the leased premises the sum of $_____ per year ("minimum annual rent") and $_____ per month ("minimum monthly rent") without relief from valuation or appraisement laws. The minimum monthly rent shall be paid in advance on the first day of each calendar month commencing on the commencement date. If the commencement date of this lease as provided above is on any day other than the first day of the calendar month, lessee shall pay a pro rata amount of the minimum monthly rent for the first and last partial calendar months of the lease term.

Operating Expenses

The landlord's ability to recover increases in the operating expenses and real estate taxes of a building are for the benefit of you and the landlord. If a landlord cannot do this, he will probably reduce or discontinue services. If you agree to the increases, there should be no legitimate reason for the landlord to cut back on services.

The lease should define operating expenses. Even if it does not list each and every one, you at least should insist on written details concerning the landlord's obligation for cleaning services, repairs, and maintenance.

There are several ways to establish your percentage of

the operating expenses. Common practice today is to establish a dollar amount that will be paid by the landlord. Any amount in excess of the established base will be paid by you. Your attorney or real estate agent should be able to advise you as to whether the landlord's established base rates are typical of the area, as well as to chart the escalation rate of base rates over the past few years. Usually, you will find a phrase that binds the landlord to operate the building "in accordance with sound management and generally accepted accounting principles and practices for medical office buildings."

Most leases give you and your accountant the opportunity to review the actual operating expenses and the annual rental adjustment. If your lease does not have this provision, ask for it.

> For the purposes of this lease, "operating expenses" shall mean the real property taxes and assessments and other taxes and assessments of any nature levied and assessed against the office building and associated common areas, or assessed against lessor as a result of the office building and associated common areas, all expenses incurred by the lessor in connection with the operation, maintenance and repair of the office building and associated common areas in accordance with sound management and generally accepted accounting principles and practices. Such maintenance, repair and operation shall include, without limitation, costs of resurfacing, repainting and restriping the parking areas, cleaning, sweeping, and other janitorial services, any policing or other security, purchase, construction, and maintenance of refuse receptacles, planting and relandscaping, directional signs and other markers, all utilities, improvements, machinery, and equipment used in connection with the office building and associated common areas, a reasonable management fee, premiums on public liability and fire and extended coverage insurance, including rental value insurance, and other costs necessary in lessor's judgment for the maintenance and operation of the office building and associated common areas, but maintenance and operation shall exclude depreciation for capital expenditures as determined in accordance with generally accepted accounting principles, and any costs not directly connected with the use, operation and upkeep of the office building and associated common areas.
>
> *Annual rent adjustment.* For the purposes of this lease, "annual rent adjustment" shall mean the amount of lessee's proportionate share of operating expenses (as hereinafter defined) for a particular calendar year.
>
> *Expense percentage.* For the purposes of this lease, "expense percentage" shall mean the percentage obtained by dividing the rentable area of the leased premises by the total rentable area of the office building. Which percentage shall for purposes of this lease be _____ .
>
> *Lessor's share of operating expenses.* For the purposes of this lease, "lessor's share of operating expenses" shall be an amount equal to three dollars ($3.00) times the rentable area of the leased premises. . . .
>
> *Lessee's proportionate share of operating expenses.* For purposes of this lease, "lessee's proportionate share of operating expenses" shall be an amount equal to the remainder of (1) the product of expense percentage times the operating expense less (2) lessor's share of operating expenses.
>
> *Payment obligation.* In addition to the minimum annual rent specified in this lease, lessee shall pay to lessor an additional rent for the leased premises, in each calendar year or partial calendar year during the term of this lease, an amount equal to lessee's proportionate share of operating expenses for such calendar year.
>
> *Payment of lessee's proportionate share of operating expenses.* The amount of lessee's proportionate share of operating expenses for each calendar year (herein referred to as the "annual rental adjustment") shall be estimated annually by lessor, and written notice thereof shall be given to lessee at least thirty (30) days prior to the beginning of each calendar year. In the case of the calendar year in which the lease term commences, written notice of the estimated operating expenses shall be given lessee prior to the commencement date. Lessee shall pay to lessor each month, at the same time the monthly rent is due, an amount equal to one-twelfth (1/12) of the estimated annual rental adjustment.
>
> *Increases in estimated annual rental adjustment.* If real estate taxes or the cost of utility or janitorial services increases the estimated annual rental adjustment during a calendar year, lessor may increase the estimated annual rental adjustment during such year by giving lessee written notice to that effect; and thereafter lessee shall pay to lessor, in each of the remaining months of such year, an amount equal to the amount of such increase in the estimated annual rental adjustment divided by the number of months remaining in such year.
>
> *Adjustment to actual annual rental adjustment.* Within ninety (90) days after the end of each calendar year, lessor shall prepare and deliver to lessee a statement showing

Table 9-8. Methods of Measuring Space and Calculating Rent

Building owners use several ways to measure rental space. To draw a true comparison among rental rates in several office buildings, you need to ask exactly what method is being used.

The two most common methods are to measure "rentable" space and "usable" or "net" space.

Rentable space typically is calculated by multiplying (a) the distance from the inside of the exterior wall (or glass line if more than 50 percent of the exterior wall is windows) to the inside of the public corridor wall by (b) the distance from halfway into the wall separating your office from another office to the same spot on the other side of your office space. Added to this figure is a pro-rata share of all the common areas.

For instance, if common areas account for 10% of the gross floor space in the building, your rentable area would be the usable area multiplied by 1.10. Put another way: A rental rate of $10 per rentable square foot equals a rental rate of $11 per usable square foot.

Quoting usable square feet is a bit more straightforward. Your usable office space is all that is being measured; no extra figure has been added for areas used in common with other tenants.

Annual rent and rental rate. The annual rent is calculated by multiplying the rental rate (quoted as so much per square foot) by the number of usable square feet. Some rates are "full-service," that is, they include utilities and cleaning services, another factor to consider when comparing buildings.

lessee's actual annual rental adjustment. Within thirty (30) days after recepit of the aforementioned statement, lessee shall pay to lessor, or lessor shall credit against the next minimum monthly rent payment or payments due from lessee, as the case may be, the difference between lessee's actual annual rental adjustment for the preceding calendar year and the estimated amount paid by lessee during such year. If this lease shall commence, expire or be terminated on any date other than the last day of a calendar year, then lessee's proportionate share of operating expenses for such partial calendar year shall be prorated on the basis of the number of days during the year this lease was in effect in relation to the total number of days in such year.

Lessee verification. Lessee or its accountants shall have the right to inspect, at reasonable times and in a reasonable manner during the ninety (90) day period following the delivery of lessor's statement of the actual amount of lessee's annual rental adjustment, such of lessor's books of account and records as pertain to and contain information concerning such costs and expenses in order to verify the amounts thereof.

Obligations of Lessor

The landlord's obligations to provide services during certain hours should be specified. A standard lease clause (like the one below) will say that the landlord has no liability for damages incurred or business lost if those services are not provided. Nor will you automatically get a reduced rent for the time services were not provided—unless you ask for it and get that provision in writing in your lease. Withholding rent, a practice common among residential renters, is not upheld by the courts for commercial renters, who must sue landlords who ask for rent even when business could not be conducted.

If you plan to have evening or weekend hours, be sure that this clause states that services will be provided during those hours.

Subject to the provisions for additional rent provided for under "operating expenses" above, the lessor agrees during the term of this lease at its cost and expense to furnish the following.

Services. Furnish for normal office use such heat, air conditioning, electricity and water and such elevator and janitorial service as in its judgment is reasonably necessary for the comfortable use and occupation of the leased premises during normal business hours on all generally recognized business days. Failure to furnish such utilities and other services shall not render lessor or its employees or agents liable for damages or injury to persons, business or property suffered by lessee, its employees, agents, licensees or invitees, nor be construed as an eviction of lessor or work an abatement or diminution of rent.

Repair. Maintain the exterior and structure of the office building, the associated common areas and the underlying land and improvements in a manner compatible with good quality office space.

Obligations of Lessee

This section is a fairly straightforward statement of your willingness to be a good tenant, plus a promise that you will use your office for a specific function only, in this case, the practice of medicine. If you are in a building designated for physicians' offices only, you may want to add a provision in this part of the lease stating that the landlord does not have the right to lease to a nonconforming tenant without the prior consent of the majority of the other tenants.

Table 9-9. Building Cost Comparison Form

Item	Bldg. A	Bldg. B	Bldg. C
Square feet			
Rent psf			
Annual rent			
Estimated rent increase			
—Base rent			
—Operating expenses			
Utilities (if extra)			
—HVAC			
—Other electric			
—Water			
—Cleaning services			
—Other			
Security deposit			
Parking costs			
Moving costs			
Cost of non-standard improvements			
Other			

The section also obligates you to care for the premises and make necessary repairs. It typically prohibits your making alterations without the landlord's consent—something you may want to change, asking for permission to improve the premises without consent so long as no structural changes are made.

A prohibition against your subletting the premises also is a usual provision of this section. Nonetheless, permission to sublet your offices to another physician may not be unreasonably withheld. This means the landlord may not refuse consent of your subtenant if your subtenant meets the use requirements and has the ability to perform under your lease.

> During the term of this lease, the lessee agrees as follows:
>
> *Use of premises.* Lessee shall use the leased premises solely as physicians' offices and for no other purpose without the prior written consent of lessor.
>
> *Compliance with law and regulations.* Lessee shall comply with all laws, regulations and orders of any governmental authority and with the rules and regulations, as reasonably adopted and modified from time to time by lessor (the "rules and regulations"). Lessee shall not do or permit anything to be done in or about the leased premises or the associated common areas that will in any way obstruct or interfere with the rights of other tenants or occupants of the office building or injure or annoy them, and shall not do or permit anything to be done that will increase the premiums of fire insurance on the office building. Lessor shall not be responsible to lessee for the nonobservance of the rules and regulations by any other tenant or occupant of the office building. Lessee shall not use the leased premises without any necessary approvals by an applicable medical licensing or health agencies.
>
> *Care of leased premises.* Lessee shall maintain and take good care of the leased premises, shall commit no waste therein or damage thereto and shall return the leased premises on the termination of the lease term in as good condition as they were at the beginning of lessee's occupancy or were placed in during the term of this lease, ordinary wear and tear and casualty excepted.
>
> *Compressed air.* Lessee, at its expense, shall furnish end facilities for compressed air or similar service for the normal use of the leased premises in the practice of medicine or dentistry. Only such facilities shall be installed only with lessor's prior written permission and under lessor's supervision.
>
> *Alterations.* Lessee shall make no alterations in or to the leased premises, unless and until the plans have been approved in advance by lessor in writing. As a condition of such approval, lessor may require lessee to remove the alterations and restore the leased premises upon termination of this lease. Nothing in this lease shall, however, be construed to constitute the consent by lessor to the creation of any lien, and no person shall be entitled to any lien on the office building, the leased premises or the underlying land and improvements. In the event, despite this provision, a lien is placed thereon, lessee shall cause such lien to be removed or shall, immediately upon request of lessor, provide a corporate surety bond satisfactory to lessor which shall save lessor harmless under such lien and from any interest, costs and attorneys' fees incurred by lessor in connection therewith.
>
> *Repair.* Lessee, at its sole cost and expense, shall repair any damage to the leased premises or the associated common areas caused by any act or neglect of lessee, its employees, agents, invitees or licensees, ordinary wear and tear and casualty excepted. If lessee shall fail to make such repairs within a reasonable time not exceeding thirty (30) days after receiving notice thereof from lessor, lessor may cause such repair to be made at lessee's expense, and lessee shall immediately reimburse lessor therefor.
>
> *Assignment and subletting.* Lessee shall not assign or sublet the leased premises or this lease, in whole or in part, without the prior written consent of lessor. Without in any way limiting lessor's right to refuse to give such consent for any other reason or reasons, lessor reserves the right to refuse to give such consent if in lessor's sole discretion and opinion the use of the leased premises or quality of operation is or may be in any way adversely affected or if the financial worth of the proposed new occupant is less than that of lessee. In the event of any assignment of subletting, lessee shall, nevertheless, remain primarily liable to perform the obligations imposed on lessee hereunder. Lessee further agrees to reimburse lessor for reasonable attorneys' fees incurred in conjunction with the processing and documentation of any requested transfer, assignment, subletting, change of ownership or hypothecation of this lease or lessee's interest in and to the leased premises.

Rights Reserved to Lessor

This section, too, is a straightforward statement, reserving to the landlord the right to inspect the leased premises, alter common areas at will, and approve window coverings because their visibility from the building's exterior affects the property's appearance.

The sample clause below also includes standard language stating that, under some circumstances, the ownership of improvements a tenant might make may well pass to the landlord when the lease expires. Many physicians do not realize that this may apply to expensive medical fixtures, but it does. Some physicians have successfully negotiated an amendment to allow them to take such items with them. To be effective, such statements should be specific and written.

> Lessor shall have the following rights:
>
> *Entrance.* To inspect the leased premises at all reasonable times, and to show them after lessee gives notice of intended vacation or within ninety (90) days of the expiration of the lease term, and to enter the leased premises at any reasonable time to make such repairs, additions or alterations as it may deem necessary for the safety, improvement or preservation thereof or of the office building.
>
> *Fixtures and improvements.* On termination of this lease, to retain any improvements to the leased premises, any equipment and cabinet work furnished by lessor, and to retain bookcases, special cabinet work and fixtures attached to the leased premises by either party, except fixtures attached by lessee that can be removed without material damage to the leased premises, provided lessee is not in default hereunder, and shall, upon removal, promptly repair any damage.
>
> *Common areas.* Lessor shall have the right at any time to change or otherwise alter the common areas of the office building and associated common areas.
>
> *Window coverings.* Lessor shall have the right to approve all window coverings and other materials that are visible from the outside of the office building prior to their installation. Lessee shall promptly remove any such materials not approved by lessor.

Rights of the Parties in the Event of Eminent Domain or Casualty

In this section, a lease states what happens to lease obligations if something destroys the building or the leased premises. Most casualty clauses (like the sample below) give the landlord 120 to 180 days in which to reconstruct the premises. Obviously, you cannot continue your practice without an office space for this period. Try to negotiate a shorter time frame for reconstruction and investigate your own insurance carrier's policy on temporary relocation expenses due to a casualty.

> *Eminent domain.* In the event the leased premises or any part thereof shall be acquired by the exercise of eminent domain by any public or quasi-public body in such a manner that the leased premises shall become unusable by the lessee for office purposes, this lease shall terminate as of the date that possession thereof is taken by the condemning authority. Lessee shall have no claim against lessor or the condemning authority on account of such taking for the value of the unexpired term of this lease remaining, and all damages awarded or compensation given as a result of such taking shall belong to and be the sole property of lessor, except lessee shall be entitled to any specific award or compensation allocated to the cost of removal of equipment or property of lessee or relocation by lessee.
>
> *Casualty.* In the event the leased premises are substantially damaged or destroyed by fire or other casualty and the same is not or cannot be repaired and restored within one hundred twenty (120) days from the date of such casualty, either lessor or lessee may cancel this lease by written notice to the other at any time within thirty (30) days thereafter. Rent shall abate proportionately during the period that the leased premises or any part thereof are unusable as a result of such casualty.

Security Deposit

In most cases, you should be able to have the landlord waive the security deposit. In the event you are unable to negotiate this provision and must have a security deposit, ask for interest to be computed on your deposit.

> Lessee hereby deposits with lessor the sum of $_____ as security for the performance of its obligations hereunder. Such deposit shall not be a trust fund but may be commingled with the general funds of lessor, and no interest shall be payable in respect thereof. In the event lessee shall default in performing its obligations hereunder, lessor shall have the right to apply such deposit against the rent and other amounts to which lessor shall be entitled hereunder, without thereby waiving any right or remedy hereunder. Lessee shall, upon notice from lessor, promptly restore such deposit to the extent it is so applied hereunder by lessor. The deposit of lessee shall be refunded to lessee upon termination of this lease unless applied by lessor in accordance with the terms of this paragraph.

Fire and Extended Coverage Insurance

The fire and extended coverage insurance provisions of most leases simply state that you as the tenant must be responsible for the destruction or loss of your property no matter what the cause, including the negligence of the landlord, the landlord's employees, or the landlord's agents. Conversely, you as a tenant are not required to insure the entire building and the landlord will obtain the fire and casualty insurance for the building as well as undertake the liability risks for the common areas and the parking lots. In addition, both landlord and tenant generally agree to waive the insurer's right of subrogation against the other party. This means that any rights that the landlord and tenant have waived against each other also binds their respective insurance companies to the extent of fire and extended covered insurance. In other words, you have agreed that your insurance company cannot file a claim against the landlord for loss of your property. Most insurance companies have agreed to this provision.

> During the term of this lease, lessor shall maintain fire and extended coverage insurance on the office building, but shall not protect the lessee's property in the event of damage however caused. Lessee shall be responsible for insuring its property located on the leased premises, in the office building or the associated common areas, and neither lessor nor any other tenant or occupant of the office building shall be liable to the lessee for damage to lessee's property however caused. All insurance policies maintained by the lessor or lessee as provided in this paragraph shall contain an agreement by the insurer waiving the insurer's right of subrogation against the other party to this lease or agreeing not to acquire any rights of recovery that the insured has expressly waived prior to loss. Lessor and lessee each hereby waives and releases any and all rights of recovery that either have against the other for any loss or damage, whether or not caused by any alleged negligence of the other party, its agents, licensees or invitees, to the extent that such loss or damage is or would be covered by any insurance required to be maintained under this lease.
>
> Lessee shall not use the leased premises in any manner or store anything in or upon the leased premises that would result in an increase in the premiums for the fire and extended coverage insurance.

Lessee's Indemnification of Lessor

The lessee's indemnification of lessor simply states that the landlord or owner may not be held responsible for any injury or death to persons due to the condition of the leased premises, the office building, or the associated common areas. However, if the injury or death is due to the sole negligence of the owner or landlord, then the landlord may be held accountable.

Depending on the landlord's mortgage commitment or, more importantly, the landlord's insurance commitments, this provision may be changed. It would be more appropriate for the tenant to be responsible for personal injury that occurs in the leased premises, and for the landlord to be responsible for same in the common areas and parking lot.

> Lessor shall not be liable to lessee or to any other person for damage to property or injury or death to persons due to the

condition of the leased premises, the office building or the associated common areas, to any occurrence or happening in or about the leased premises, the office building or the associated common areas or to any act or neglect of lessee or any other tenant or occupant of the office building or of any other person, unless such damage, injury or death is the direct result of the sole negligence of lessor. Lessee shall be responsible and liable to lessor for any damage of the leased premises, the office building or the associated common areas and for any act or neglect of lessee or any other person coming on the leased premises, the office building or the associated common areas by the license or invitation of lessee, express or implied, except where such damage is a result of a casualty loss covered by lessor's fire and extended coverage insurance provided for above. Lessee shall save lessor harmless from any and all liability to any person for any damage to property or for injury or death to any person resulting from use of the leased premises or the associated common areas. Lessee shall pay the premiums for a policy or policies of insurance in companies satisfactory to lessor and its mortgagee, and shall keep the same in force during the lease term and furnish a certificate thereof (or such other document or duplicate policy evidencing such insurance in a form satisfactory to lessor and its mortgagee) covering the following risks and protecting lessor, lessor's mortgagee and lessee:

Public liability and property damage insurance in standard form, with limits of bodily injury and death liability not less than five hundred thousand dollars ($500,000.00) for an accident affecting any one person, and one million dollars ($1,000,000.00) for an accident affecting more than one person, and providing property damage coverage of at least five hundred thousand dollars ($500,000.00) aggregate. If it becomes customary for other similar facilities in the area to carry higher limits of liability coverage, lessee shall, if requested by lessor, increase the above liability coverage to such customary limits.

Rental value insurance payable to lessor.

Such additional risks or greater coverage of the above risks as shall be required by lessor's mortgagee.

Defaults and Remedies

The default provisions of a lease generally focus on the rent and additional rent to be paid. Typically, the landlord puts the tenant in default if rent is not paid within 10 days after written notice is given by the landlord. This 10-day period can be extended; however, keep in mind that, if you and the other tenants do not pay your rent on a timely basis, the landlord will have a difficult time paying his mortgage commitment on a timely basis. Mortgage companies typically are less lenient than landlords.

Nonetheless, you may be able to negotiate a more lenient clause than the one in the sample below should the default result from your disability or death. Many landlords are willing to grant you and your heirs some amount of relief from this possible burden.

Defaults. Each of the following shall be deemed a default by lessee:
(1) Failure to pay the rent as herein provided when due;
(2) Failure to make additional payments provided for in this lease when due;
(3) Failure to perform any act to be performed by lessee hereunder or to comply with any condition or covenant contained herein; or
(4) The abandonment of the leased premises by lessee or its adjudication as a bankrupt; the making by lessee of a general assignment for the benefit of creditors by or against lessee; lessee's taking the benefit of any insolvency action or law; the appointment of a permanent receiver or trustee in bankruptcy for lessee or its assets; the appointment of a temporary receiver for the lessee or its assets if such temporary receiver has not been vacated or set aside within thirty (30) days from the date of such appointment; the initiation of an arrangement or similar proceedings for the benefit of creditors by or against lessee; termination of lessee's existence, whether by dissolution, agreement, death or otherwise, as the case may be.

Remedies. In the event of any default of lessee, and the continuance of default for a period of ten (10) days after written notice is given by lessor to lessee, this lease shall terminate at the option of lessor. In the event of termination of this lease, lessor may, in addition to its other rights and remedies at law and in equity, re-enter the leased premises, take possession of all or in part thereof and remove all property and persons therefrom and shall not be liable for any damage therefor or for trespass. No such re-entry shall be deemed an acceptance of the surrender of this lease or deemed satisfaction of lessee's obligation to pay rent as provided herein or of any other obligation of lessee hereunder.

Miscellaneous Provisions

About the sample miscellaneous provisions below, only two comments are necessary, both on the landlord's right to mortgage the office building. First, when the landlord applies for a mortgage, he may ask you to execute instruments indicating that your lease is indeed in full force and effect and to certify this to the lender. At this point, you will have the opportunity to list any modification to the lease or to state any obligations you feel the landlord is not performing. (This provision also is covered in the estoppel certificate provisions of the lease.)

Second, you want to make sure there is some protection for you if the landlord defaults on the mortgage, as there is in the sample below.

Right of quiet enjoyment. Lessor agrees that if lessee shall perform all the covenants and agreements herein provided to be performed by lessee, lessee shall, at all times during the lease term, have the peaceable and quiet enjoyment of possession of the leased premises, except as provided under the "defaults and remedies" provisions above and except for interference in such enjoyment caused by acts of lessee.

Lessor's right to mortgage. Lessee agrees at any time, and from time to time, upon request by lessor, or the holder of any mortgage or other instrument of security given by lessor, to execute, acknowledge and deliver to lessor or to the holder of such instrument, a statement in writing certifying that this lease has not been modified and is in full force and effect (or if there have been modifications, that the same are in full force and effect and state such modifications), that there are no defaults hereunder by lessor, if such is the fact; and the dates to which the fixed rents and other charges have been paid, it being intended that any such statement delivered pursuant to this paragraph may be relied upon by the holder of any such mortgage or other instrument of security or any authorized assignee of lessor.

Lessee's rights shall be subject to any bona fide first mortgage now existing upon or hereafter placed upon the leased premises by lessor; provided, however, that if the mortgagee shall take title to the leased premises through foreclosure or deed-in-lieu of foreclosure, lessee shall be allowed to continue in possession of the leased premises as provided for in this lease so long as lessee shall not be in default.

Rights of assigns. Except where specifically limited, the rights and liabilities of the parties hereto shall run for the benefit of and shall be binding upon the personal representatives, heirs, assigns and successors in interest of lessor and lessee.

Indemnification. Lessor and lessee shall be liable for and hereby agree to pay to the other party any and all costs and expenses, including reasonable attorneys' fees incurred by the nondefaulting party in connection with any default under the terms, covenants and conditions contained herein, without relief from valuation or appraisement laws.

Waiver. No waiver of any covenant or condition or the breach of any covenant or condition of this lease shall be taken to justify or authorize a nonobservance on any other occasion of such covenant or condition or any other covenant or condition or to constitute a waiver of any subsequent breach of such covenant or condition. Acceptance of rent by lessor at any time when lessee is in default of any covenant or condition hereof shall not be construed as a waiver of any such default or of lessor's right to terminate this lease on account of such default.

Notice. Any notice, consent or wavier required or permitted to be given or served by either party to this lease shall be in writing and either delivered personally to the other party or mailed by certified or registered mail, return receipt requested, addressed as follows:

Lessor: _____

Lessee: _____
_____
_____
_____

Either party may change its address for such purpose by serving notice on the other party.

Severability. If any provision of this lease or the application thereof to any person or circumstance is invalid, such invalidity shall not affect other provisions or applications of this lease that can be given effect without the invalid provision of application, and to this end the provisions of this lease are declared to be severable.

Signature Page

The signature page of the lease is for your execution. If possible, it would be to your benefit not to guarantee the lease personally. Discuss with your attorney alternate means of executing your lease as a medical corporation or other entity.

Executed in (*location*), this _____ day of _____, 19____
 By:_____
 Its:_____
  (Lessor)
 By:_____
  (Lessee)
ATTEST:
_____
_____

STATE OF
        SS:
COUNTY OF

Before me, as notary public in and for said county and state, personally appeared _____ and _____, by me known and by me known to be the _____ of _____, a (*state name*) corporation, who acknowledged the execution of the foregoing "office lease agreement" on behalf of said corporation.

WITNESS my hand and notarial seal this _____ day of _____, 19____ .

_____
Notary Public

_____
(Printed Signature)

My commission expires:
_____

My county of residence:
_____

STATE OF
        SS:
COUNTY OF

Before me, a notary public in and for said county and state, personally appeared _____ and _____, by me known and by me known to be the _____ and _____ respectively, of _____, who acknowledge the execution of the above and foregoing "office lease agreement" for and on behalf of said corporation.

WITNESS my hand and notarial seal this _____ day of _____, 19____ .

_____
Notary Public

_____
(Printed Signature)

My commission expires:
_____

My county of residence:
_____

10 Office Surgical Facility—How I Do It

Developing an office surgical facility is a complex process that takes considerable time and effort. Facilities can be developed in free-standing, independent facilities or in multistory medical office buildings. The authors have selected five office surgical facilities to serve as examples on how ambulatory surgical facilities can be adapted to a variety of practice styles and physical facilities. All five facilities are accredited by the Accreditation Association for Ambulatory Health Care. Each facility is unique in its physical structure. Dr. Tobin's facility is a free-standing office surgical facility occupied entirely by his surgical practice. Dr. Mangat's facility is also a free-standing structure. However, additional space is available in his facility that is leased to other physicians and dentists. Drs. Gilmore, Strahan, and Patseavouras have office surgical facilities in multiphysician medical office buildings.

The authors hope that the following floor plans and the pictorial review of these facilities will be helpful to readers in stimulating the design and characteristics of their personal facility.

**Facial Plastic and Cosmetic Surgical Center
Abilene, Texas
Howard Tobin, M.D.**

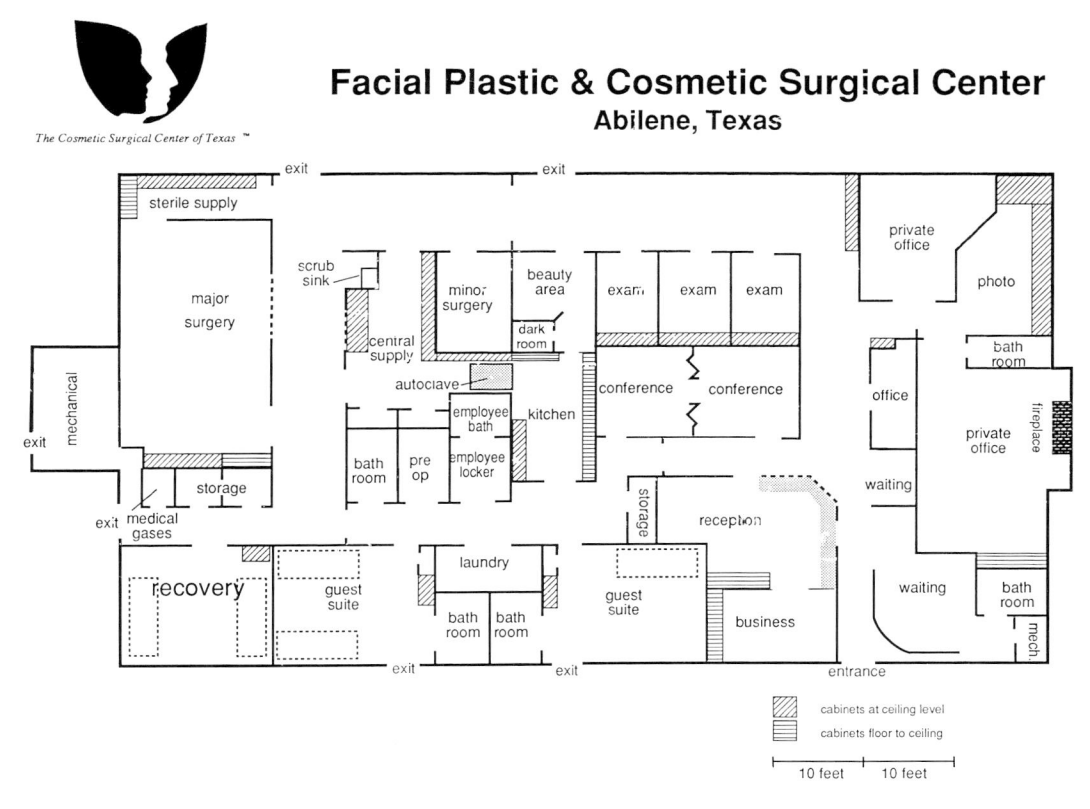

Figure 10-1. Blueprint of Howard Tobin's office and ambulatory surgery center

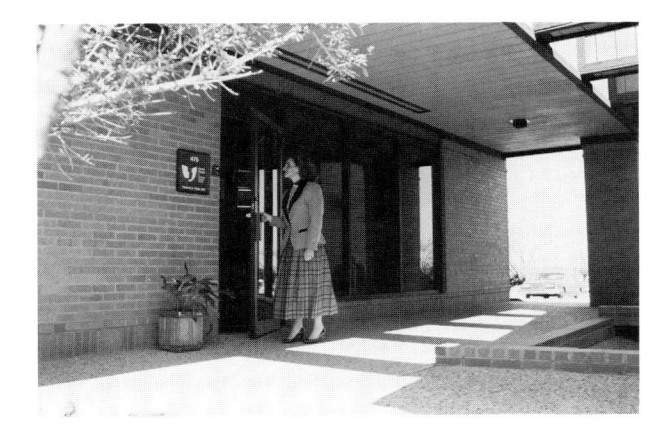

Figure 10-2. Exterior of building

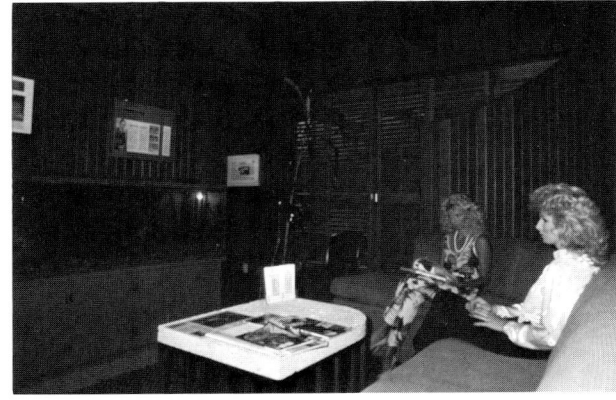

Figure 10-3. Waiting room

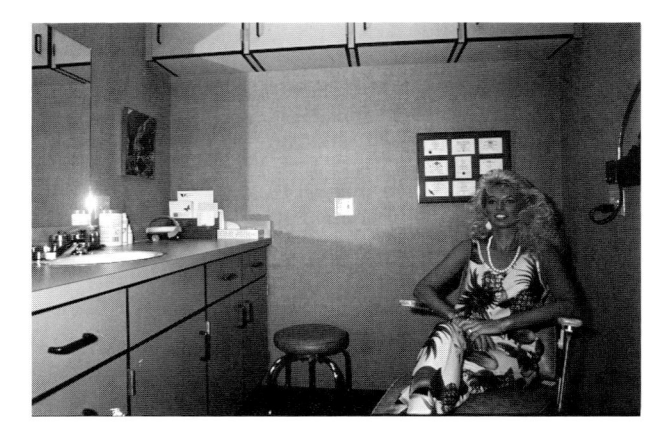

136 Developing a Practice in Ambulatory Surgery

Figure 10-4. Patient examination room

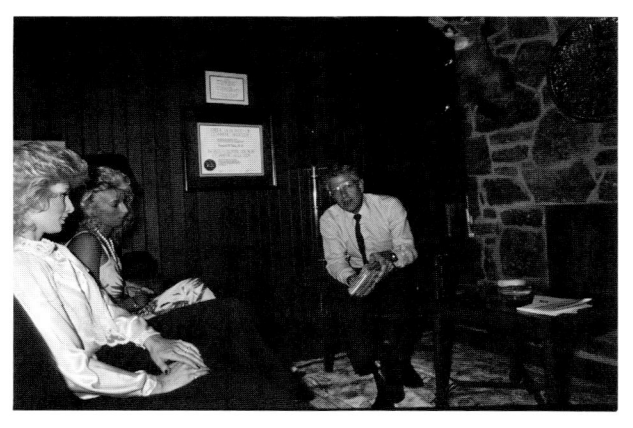

Figure 10-5. Private office and consultation room

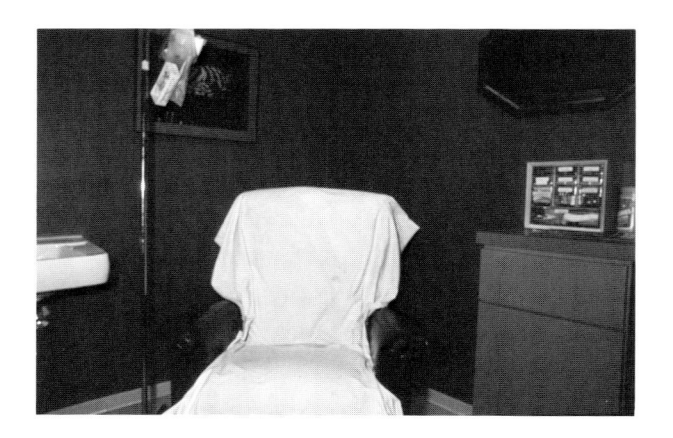

Figure 10-6. Pre-operative suite

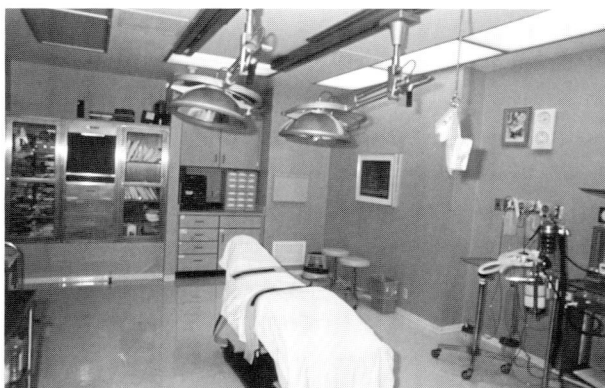

Figure 10-7. Operating room

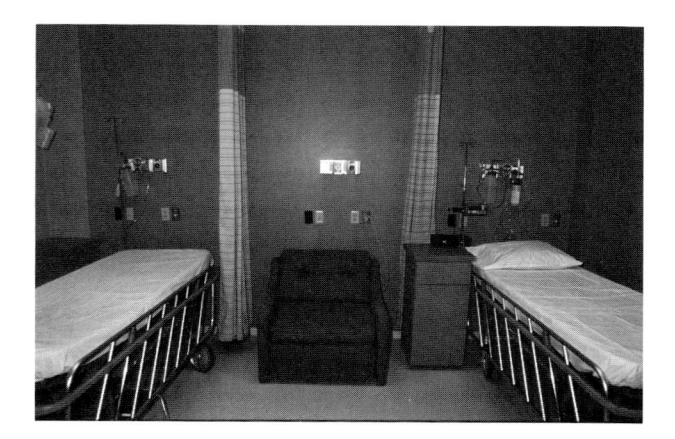

Figure 10-8. Recovery room

**Outpatient Surgical Center
Greensboro, North Carolina
Louie L. Patseavouras, M.D., F.A.C.S.**

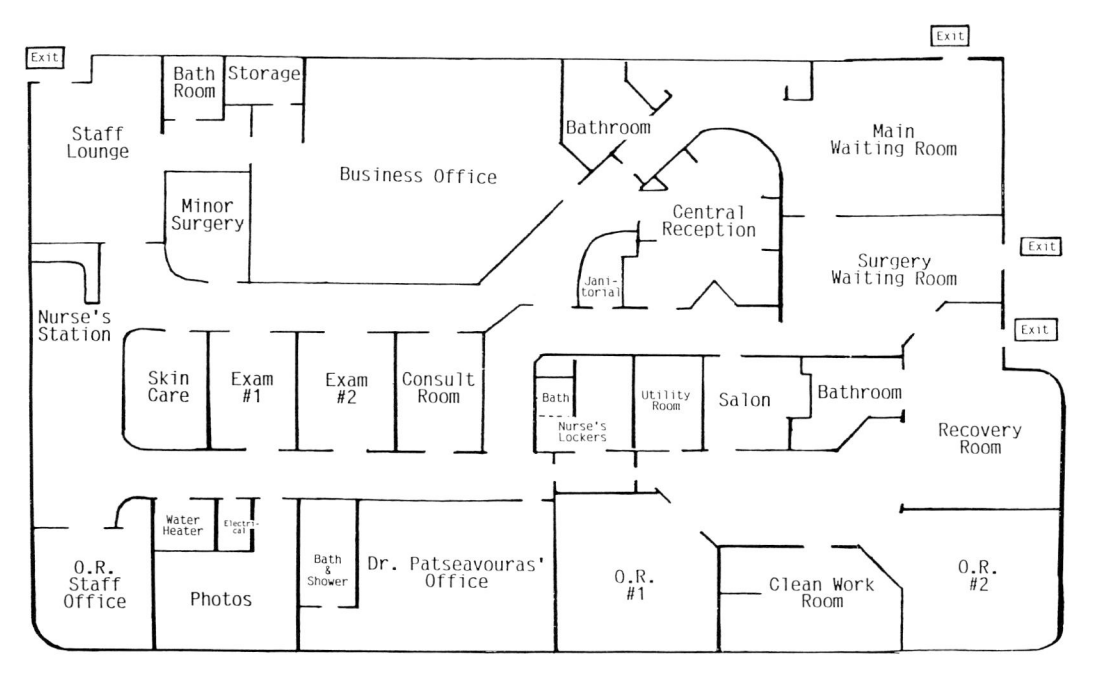

Figure 10-9. Blueprint of Dr. Patseavouras' office and ambulatory surgery center

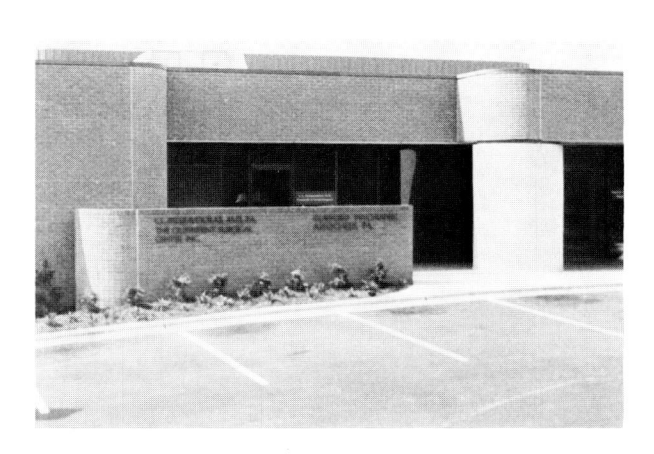

Figure 10-10. Exterior of building

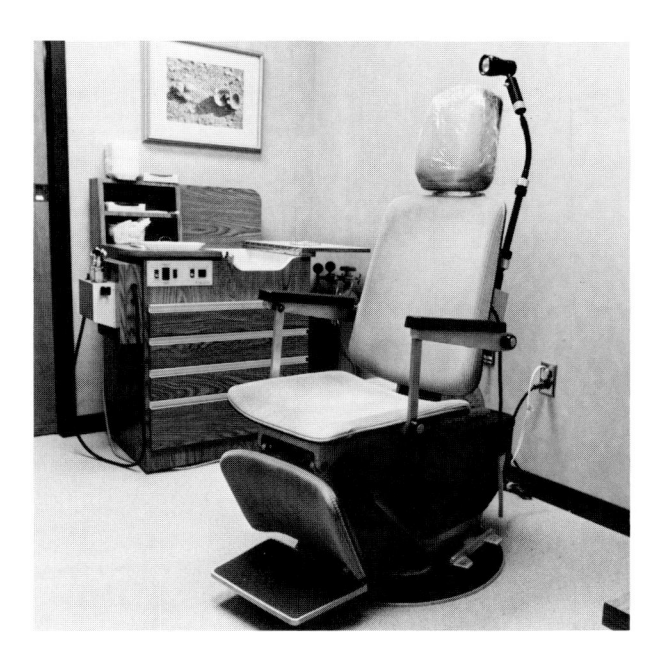

Figure 10-11. Patient examination room

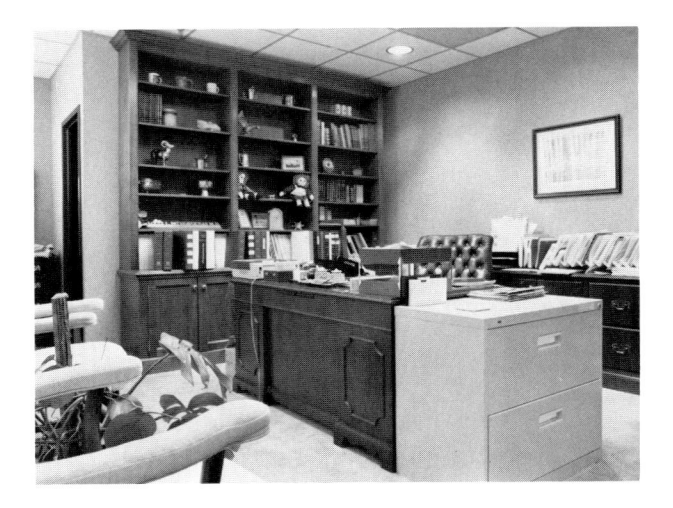

138 Developing a Practice in Ambulatory Surgery

Figure 10-12. Private office

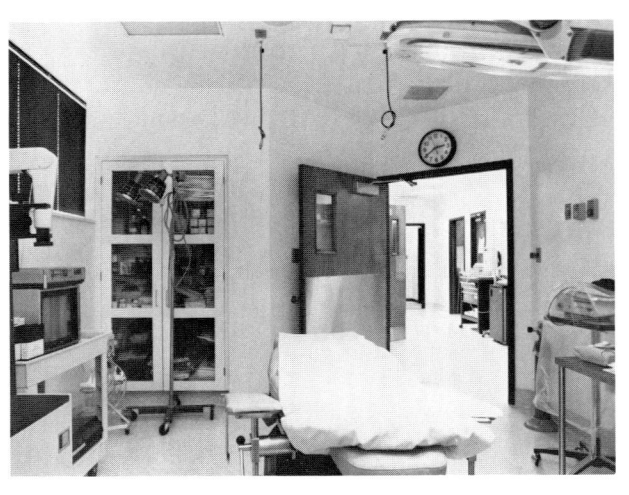

Figure 10-13a. Operating room

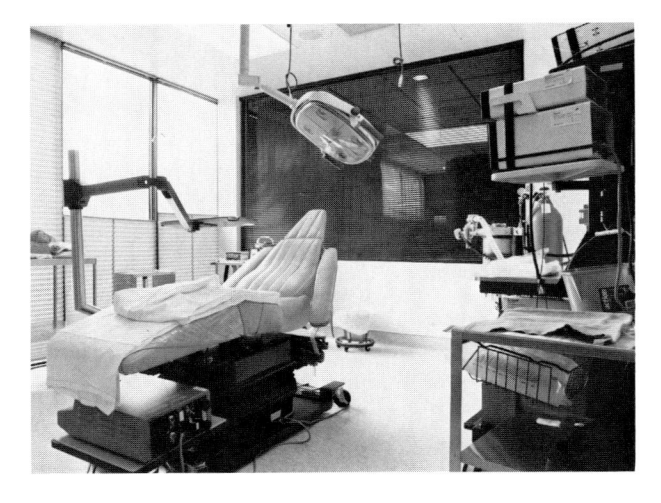

Figure 10-13b. Operating room

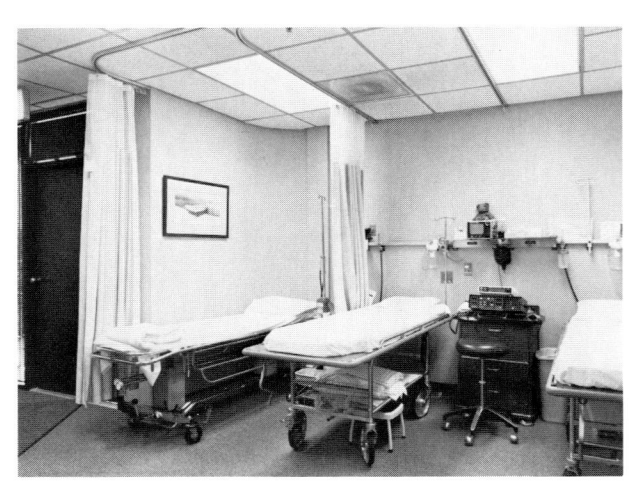

Figure 10-14. Recovery room

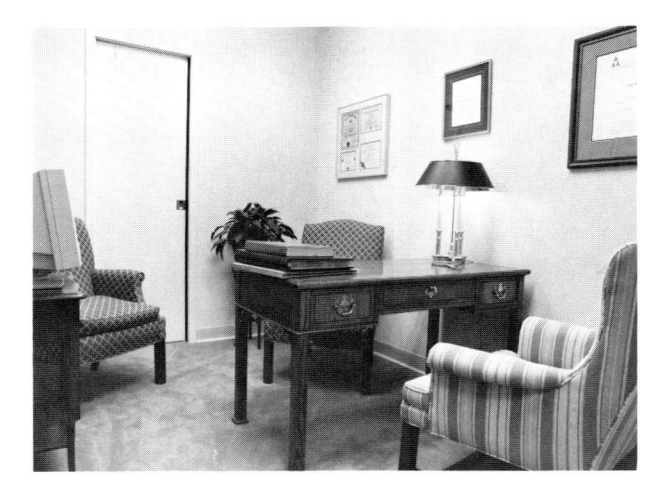

Figure 10-15. Consultation room

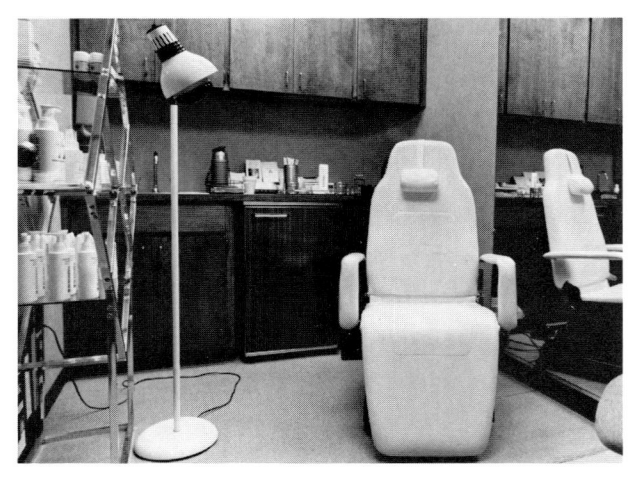

Figure 10-16. Skin care room

**Aesthetic Plastic Surgery
A Medical Corporation
Los Angeles, California
Ronald W. Strahan, M.D.**

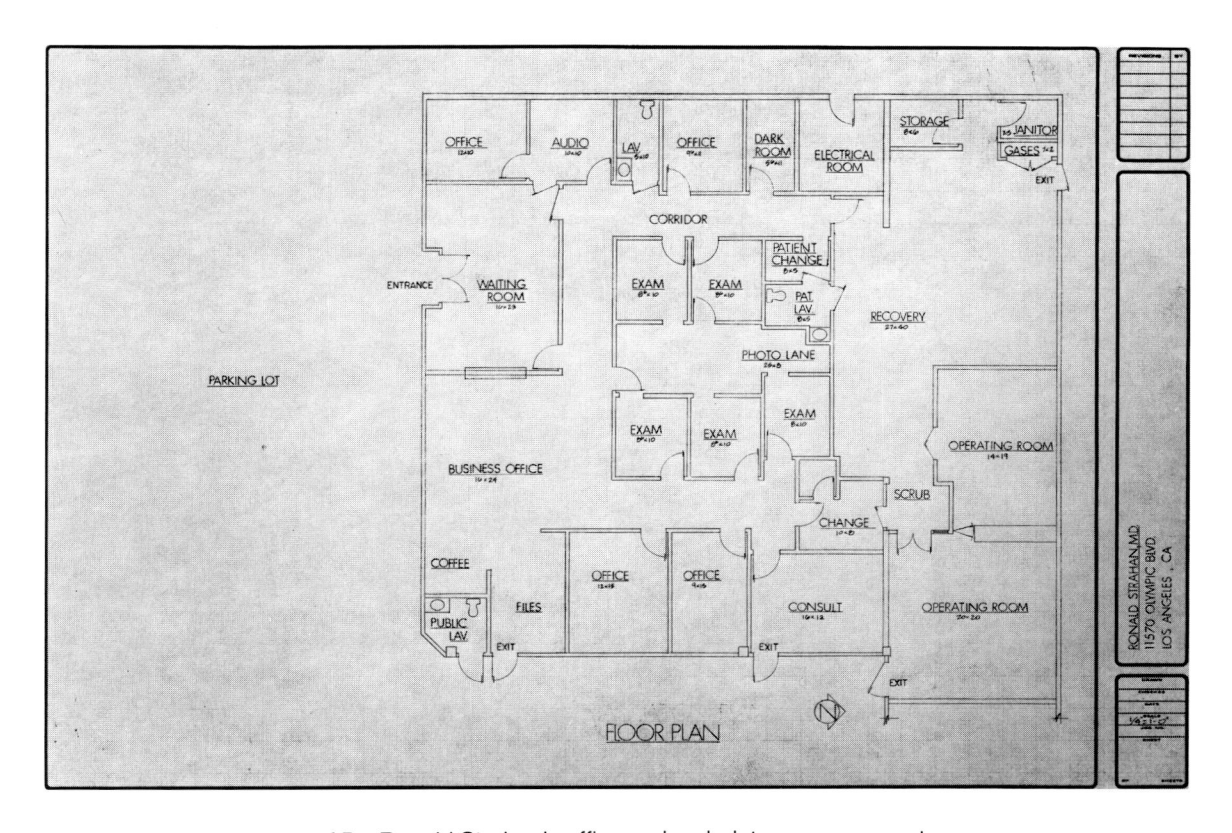

Figure 10-17. Blueprint of Dr. Ronald Strahan's office and ambulatory surgery center

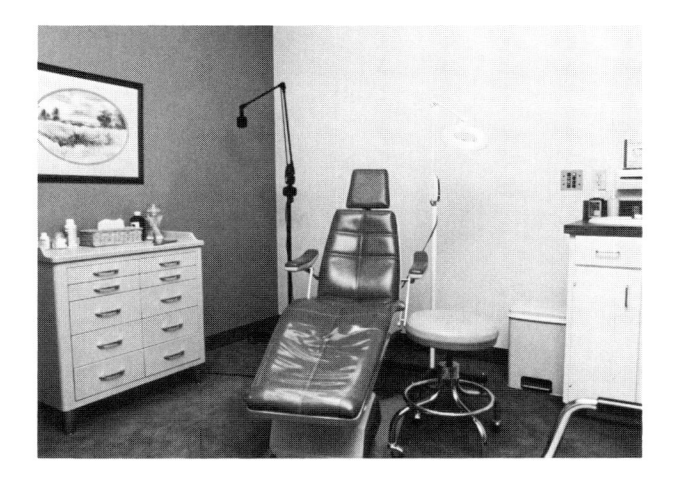

Figure 10-18. Patient examination room

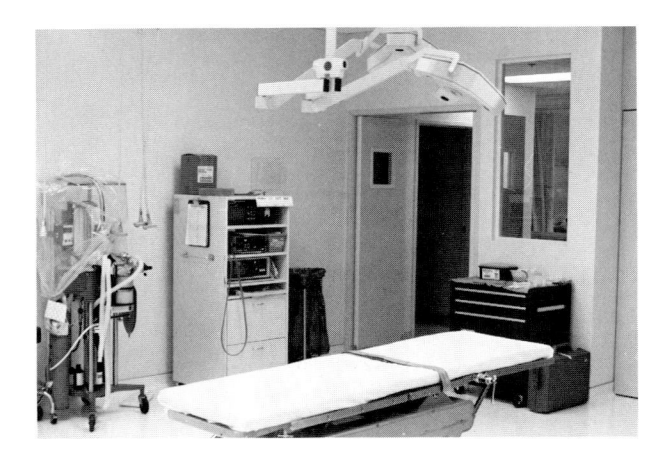

140 Developing a Practice in Ambulatory Surgery

Figure 10-19. Operating room

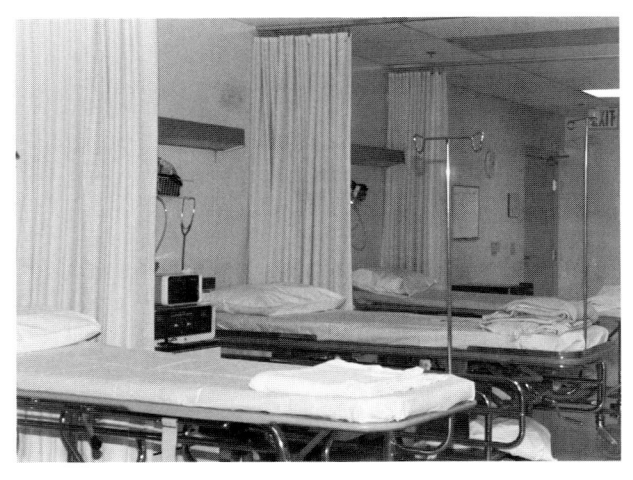

Figure 10-20. Recovery room

Office Surgical Facility—How I Do It 141

**Jim Gilmore, M.D., Associated
Facial Plastic and Cosmetic Surgery
Dallas, TX
Jim Gilmore, M.D.**

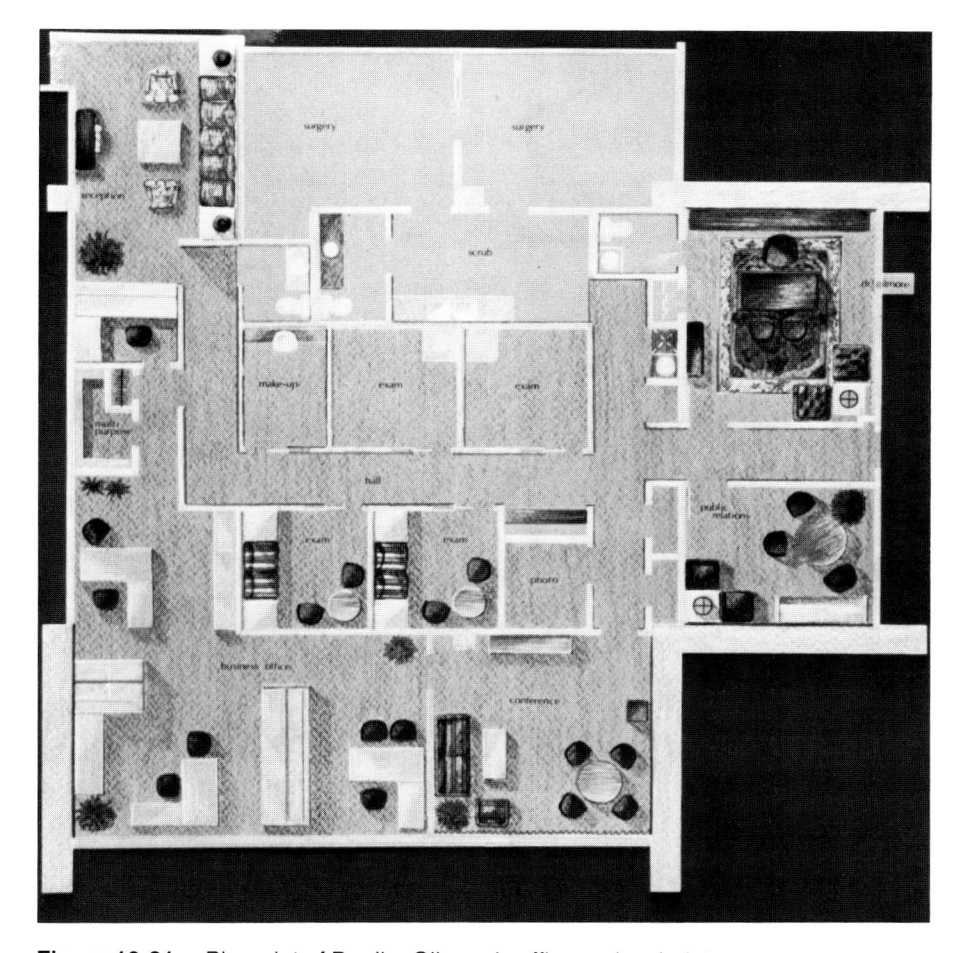

Figure 10-21. Blueprint of Dr. Jim Gilmore's office and ambulatory surgery center

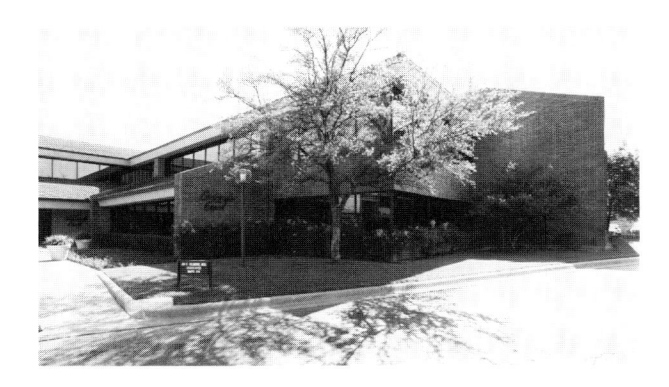

Figure 10-22a. Exterior of building

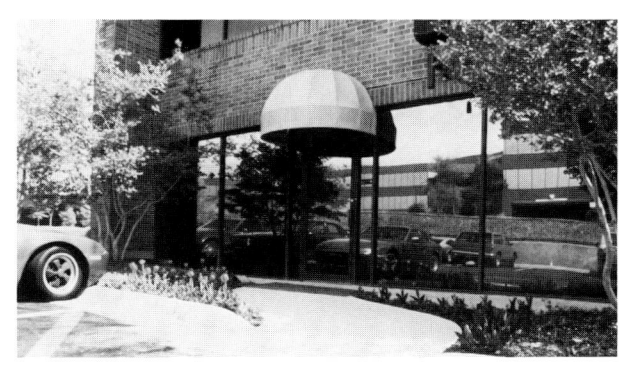

Figure 10-22b. Private entrance

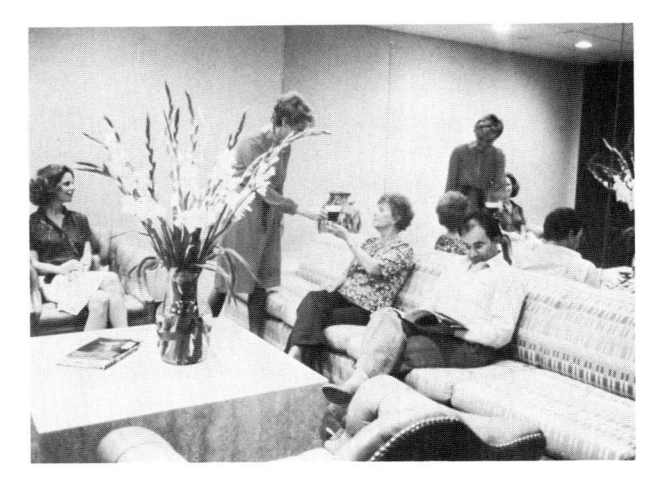

142 Developing a Practice in Ambulatory Surgery

Figure 10-23. Waiting room

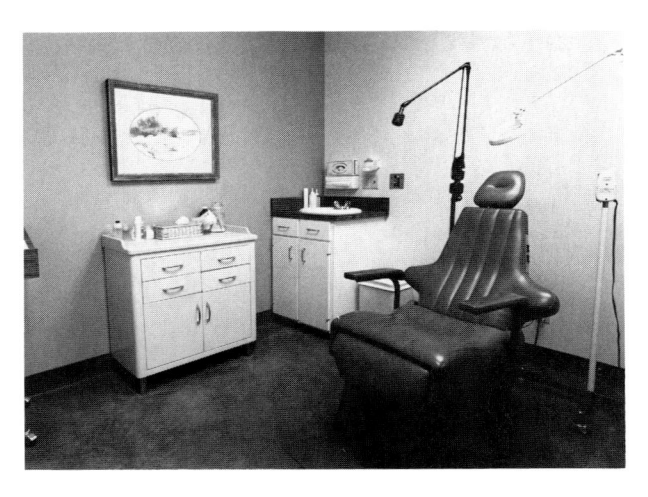

Figure 10-24. Private examination room

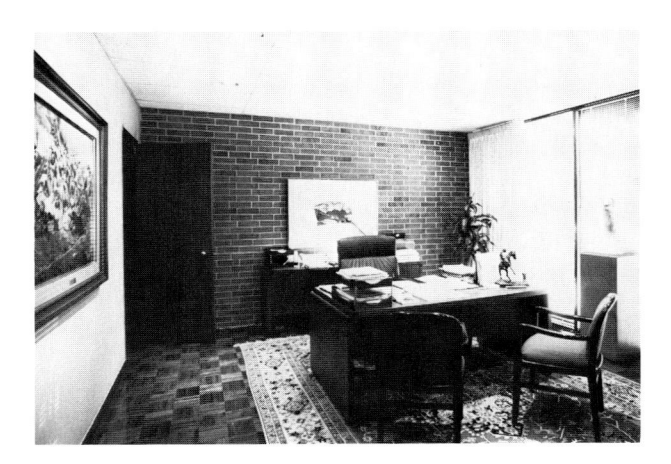

Figure 10-25. Private office

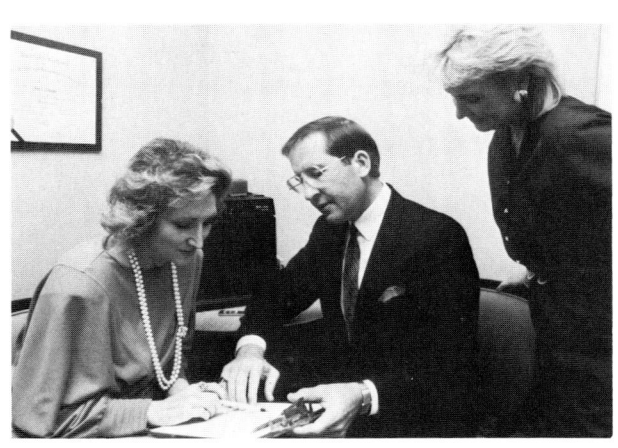

Figure 10-26. Consultation room

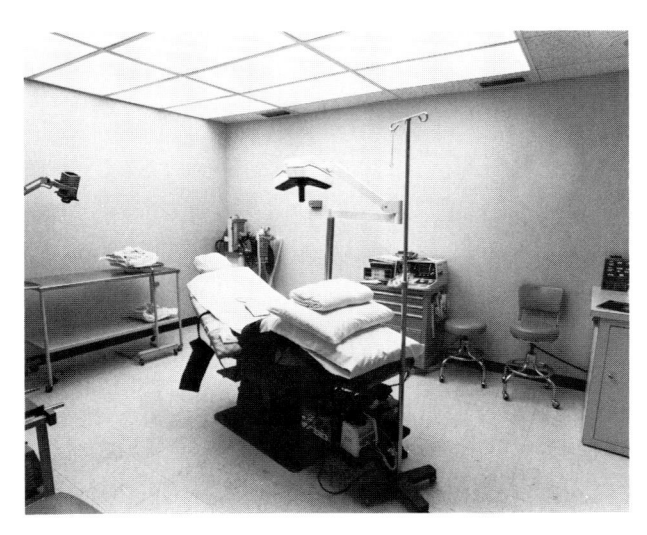

Figure 10-27. Operating room

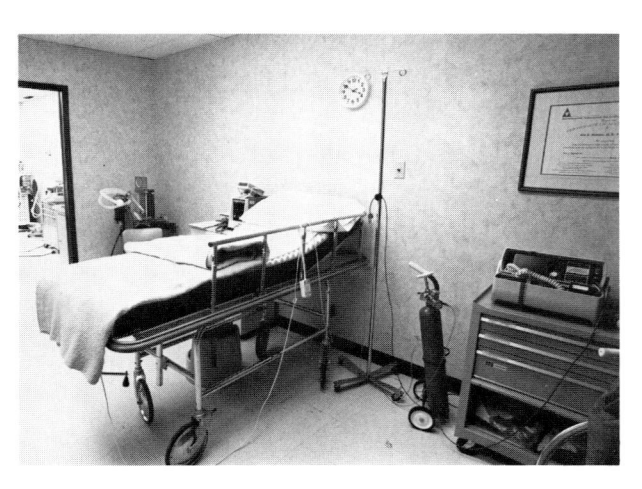

Figure 10-28. Recovery room

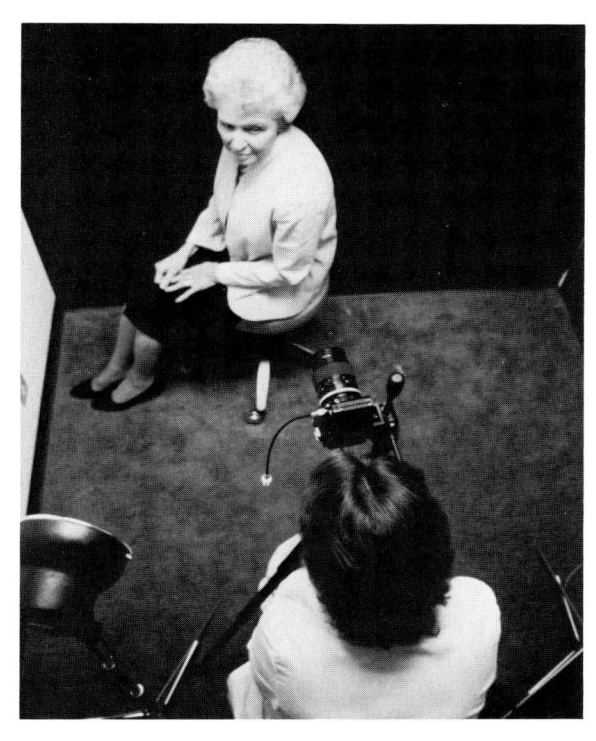

Figure 10-29. Photography room

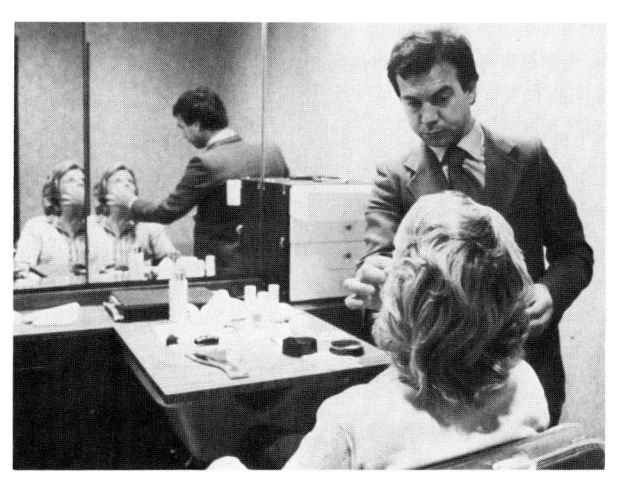

Figure 10-30. Make-up room

144 Developing a Practice in Ambulatory Surgery

**The Facial Plastic and Cosmetic
Surgery Center
Edgewood, Kentucky
Devinder S. Mangat, M.D.**

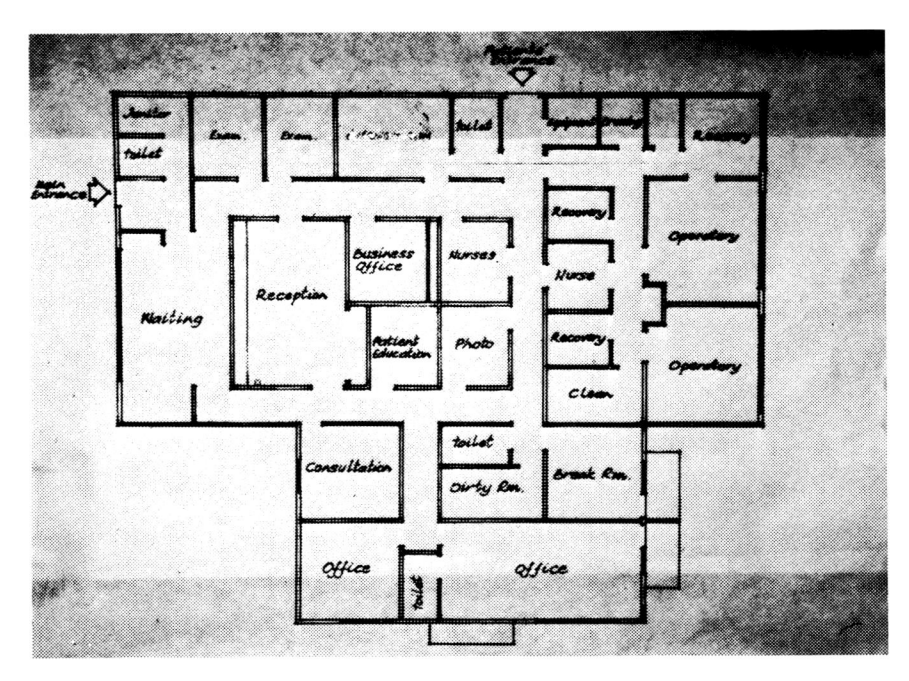

Figure 10-31. Blueprint of Dr. Devinder Mangat's office and ambulatory surgery center

Figure 10-32. Exterior of building

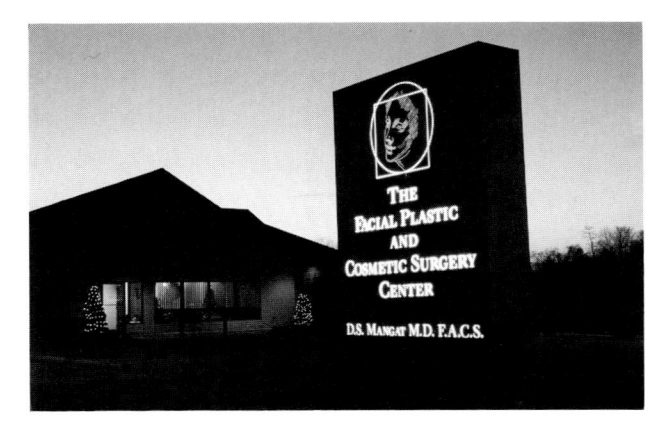

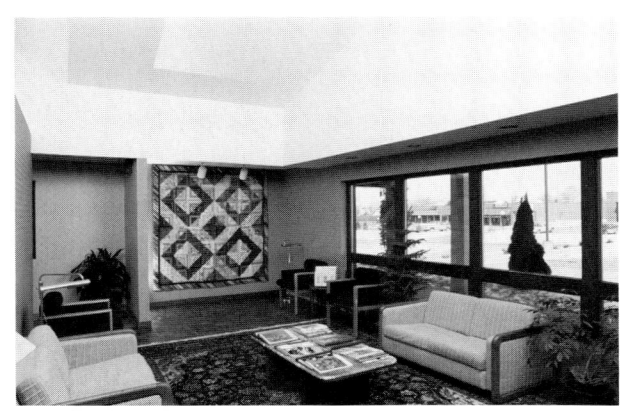

Figure 10-33. Waiting room

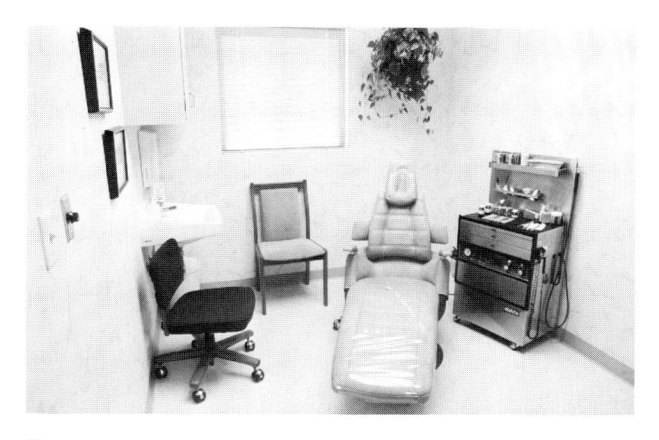

Figure 10-34. Patient examination room

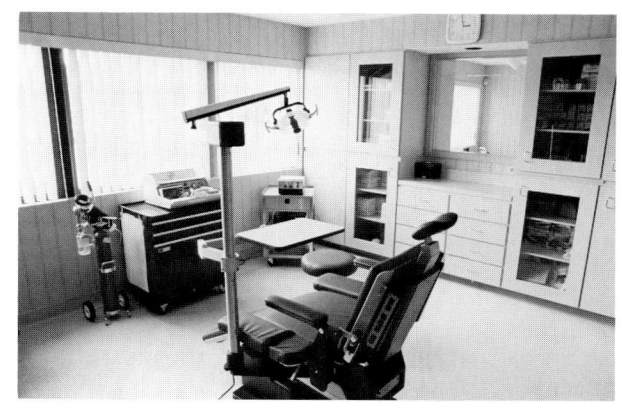

Figure 10-35. Operating room

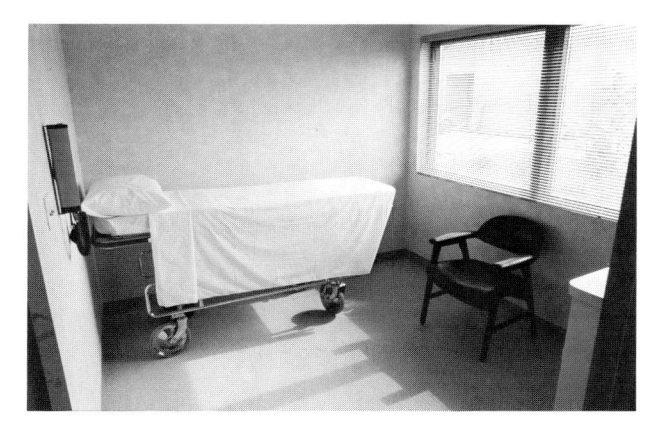

Figure 10-36. Recovery room

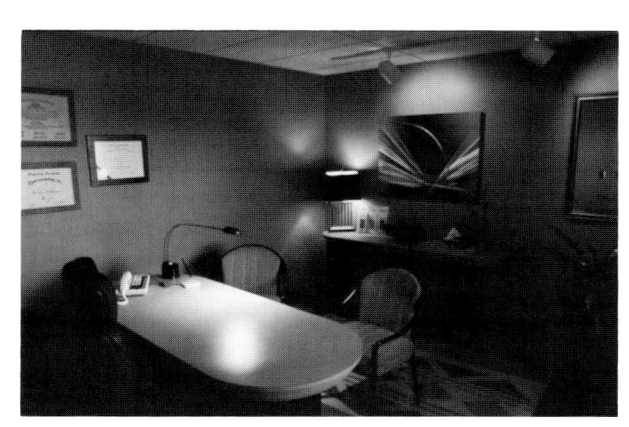

Figure 10-37. Consultation room

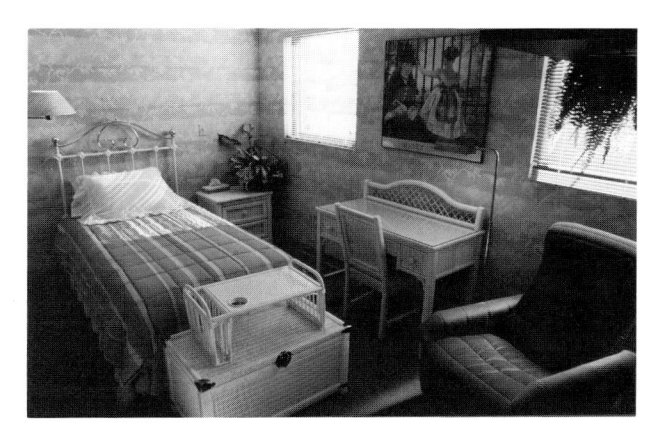

Figure 10-38. Overnight patient suite

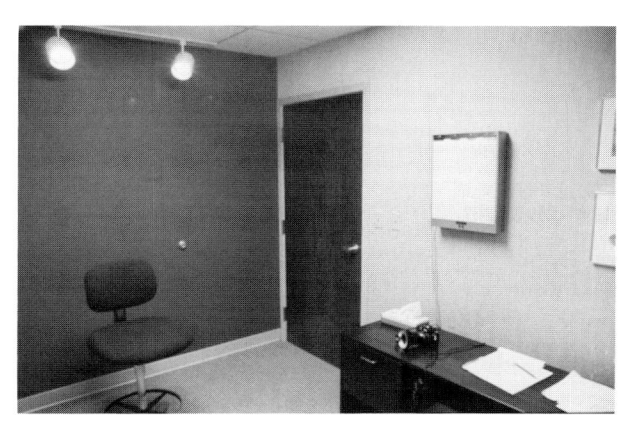

Figure 10-39. Photography room

Appendixes

FORMS, PROTOCOLS, AND GUIDELINES

The following are examples of forms, protocols, and guidelines utilized by the authors. The authors provide these as information only and do not offer a direct or implied guarantee of any sort. It is recommended that individuals review the enclosed material and utilize it as a starting point for development of their own personalized forms, protocols, and guidelines. When doing such, it is obviously recommended that information from a multitude of sources be obtained. The following should serve as only one of those sources.

In addition, the Association of Operating Room Nurses (AORN) has authorized the reproduction of their "Recommended Practices." We appreciate the inclusion of this valuable information.

Publishers Note: The following forms, protocols, and guidelines are offered as examples only and each individual should develop his or her own guidelines to suit individual needs. The recommendations set forth herein are those of the authors and in no way reflect the opinions of the publisher or the American Academy of Facial Plastic and Reconstructive Surgery.

Appendix 1: Anesthesia

SURGICAL CARE PROTOCOL

Selection of Cases:

1. Only local infiltration anesthesia or supplemented IV sedation will be utilized in Beeson Facial Surgery. No general anesthesia will be utilized.
2. Only patients of Class I or Class II American Society of Anesthesia Risk Classification will be performed in its facility. Only patients age 18 or older will undergo IV sedation unless specifically authorized by Dr. Beeson.

PREOPERATIVE GUIDELINES

**MINOR PROCEDURES
(shave excisions, cyst excisions, small scar revisions, perioral or periorbital peels)**

1. Physical exam by doctor prior to surgery [recorded on short form—operative record sheet].
2. Vital signs and surgical consent will be obtained prior to surgery.
3. Preoperative laboratory evaluation will be obtained at discretion of doctor.

**MAJOR PROCEDURES
(those requiring IV sedation)**

1. Pre-operative physical exam by doctor prior to surgery.
2. Contact with patient's personal physician will be made by doctor prior to surgery.
3. Ophthalmologic evaluation prior to blepharoplasty—we will submit our guideline letter to the patient's doctor.
4. EKG on patients over 40 [performed within 12 months of surgery]
5. Laboratory evaluation to include: CBC, PTTU/A, CHEM-12, VDRL, BETA SUB [on female patients age 13 to 45 of possible childbearing status]. [Labs performed within 12 months of surgery].
6. Provide patient with post-operative instruction booklet, prescription, medications, and instruction sheets prior to surgery.
7. Patients informed prior to surgery about the need to have responsible adult accompany them to the office on the day of surgery and to stay with them the night of surgery.
8. Consent signed at pre-operative evaluation.
9. Pre-operative photographs obtained—both prints and slides.*

DAY OF SURGERY

1. Verify that responsible adult will be staying with patient and review post-operative instructions with patient and responsible adult. Patient valuables should be sent with responsible adult and not left with patient.
2. Obtain vital signs, perform brief physical exam, observing for any changes from preoperative physical exam. Question patients as to any recent changes in their health. Review labs and physical exam on chart. Inquire as to time food or beverage was last ingested. In females, inquire as to time of last menstrual period.
3. Patient evaluated by doctor.
4. Patient washes face and is provided with "welcome pack." Pack provides gown, slippers, and bags for clothing and other personal items.
5. Patient sedated in pre-operative room. [Patient given call button or bell].
6. Patient transferred [gowned] into surgery.

Surgery

1. Laminar Flow Unit turned on 30 minutes prior to surgery.
2. Patient monitoring. All patients will be monitored with blood pressure, EKG, and pulse oximeter.
3. IV sedation—intravenous sedation will be performed by Dr. Beeson or by nursing staff under the direct supervision of Dr. Beeson. Patients will receive no sedation until Dr. Beeson is present in the operating room.
4. Personnel. A scrub nurse, surgical assistant, and circulating nurse will be present for all cases.

---

*Pre-operative exams should be scheduled approximately two weeks prior to surgery. Patients undergoing facelift, blepharoplasty, nasal surgery, or the first stage of hair transplantation surgery will usually be required to convalesce the first night in the facility adjacent to St. Vincent Hospital [Sheridan Martin House]. Patients must have a responsible adult staying with them the night of surgery. Nursing services can be arranged for patients who so desire such. Patient's charts will be reviewed at the weekly nurse's administrative meeting one week prior to surgery. Nursing staff will contact patients the night prior to surgery to review schedule of events and to answer any questions.

Circulating nurse must be present in room at all times during case.

At the discretion of the doctor, a surgical assistant on a specific case may not be necessary. Under such circumstances, a scrub nurse and circulator will be present in the operating room at all times.

Recovery

A 2-stage recovery system will be utilized. Stage 1 Recovery will be the operating room and Stage 2 Recovery will be the preop sedation area.

Stage 1 Recovery

Patients will be continually monitored with blood pressure, EKG and pulse oximeter for a minimum of 20 minutes following the end of their surgical procedure or until vital signs are stable and patient is ambulatory. Evaluation guidelines are as follows:

   a. Vital signs within 20% of pre-operative values
   b. No respiratory problems
   c. Patient handling secretions normally without difficulty in swallowing
   d. Patient moving all extremities and responding appropriately to verbal commands
   e. Patient verbalizing to commands
   f. Patient ambulatory with assistance*

---

*Patient will be transferred to Stage 2 Recovery only after evaluation and approval by doctor.

Stage 2 Recovery

Patients will remain in Stage 2 Recovery under direct supervision of nursing staff until the following discharge criteria are met:

   a. Vital signs continue to be within 20% of pre-operative value
   b. No nausea and vomiting
   c. Patient taking fluids well
   d. Patient able to dress self and ambulate with minimal assistance

Discharge Procedure

1. Patient will be released only to responsible adult. If patient is convalescing first night in extended care facility adjacent to hospital, they will be transported by nursing staff in the facility van to the patient's motel room where they will be released to the care of a responsible adult.
2. Post-operative care instructions will be reviewed with responsible adult caring for patients by nursing staff. Written instruction booklets will be again provided if they are not in the possession of the adult caring for the patient.
3. A return appointment time will be given to patient.
4. Emergency call number will be given to patient with instructions to call if there are any questions.
5. If patient is convalescing in the extended care facility, they will be evaluated following surgery by the doctor.†

---

†Doctor will remain in facility until patient is discharged.

THE FACIAL PLASTIC AND COSMETIC SURGERY CENTER

DATE	SURGEON	

PROPOSED PROCEDURE

HISTORY: AGE:_____ SEX:_____   MEDICATIONS: (steroids, eye drops, ASA, over-the-counter)

ALLERGIES:

HEAD/NECK: ☐CVA ☐GLAUCOMA ☐BLEEDING DISORDER ☐THYROID DISEASE   **PULMONARY:** ☐TB ☐COUGH ☐BRONCHITIS
☐SEIZURES ☐DIABETES ☐FACIAL FRACTURES ☐CONTACT LENS   ☐SOB ☐ASTHMA ☐PNEUMONIA
☐SYNCOPE ☐SICKLE CELL   ☐URI ☐SPUTUM

CARDIAC: ACTIVITY TOLERANCE _____ NY CLASS: (circle) I II III IV
☐CHF ☐RHD ☐HPT ☐PALPITATIONS
MI: _____ ☐ANGINA ☐EDEMA ☐MURMURS ☐ARRHYTHMIAS

ABDOMEN: ☐JUANDICE ☐HEPATITIS ☐RENAL DISEASE ☐N&V ☐HIATAL HERNIA   **PREGNANCY:** ☐YES ☐NO
☐BACK PROBLEMS/ARTHRITIS

OTHER ILLNESSES: _____

PREVIOUS ANESTHETICS/OPERATIONS: _____

PROBLEMS/COMPLICATIONS: _____

FAMILY ANESTHETIC DIFFICULTIES: _____

TOBACCO: _____ppd _____yrs   ETOH: AMOUNT _____   DRUG ABUSE: _____

HT: _____   B/P: _____   PULSE: _____   TEETH: ☐DENTURES ☐CAPS ☐BRIDGEWORK

WT: _____   TEMP: _____   ☐OTHER: _____

AIRWAY: HEART: OTHER: (Renal, GI, CNS)

NECK: (Bruits, ROM)   LUNG:

LABS: CXR   LYTES   H/H   U/A

EKG   CHEM   PLATS

NPO STATUS: _____

ASA PHYSICAL STATUS: (circle)
I II III IV V E   ANESTHESIA PLAN: ☐M.A.C.   ☐G.A.   ☐REGIONAL: _____

POSTANESTHESIA PAIN RELIEF: _____

SPECIAL MONITORING: _____

The anesthesia plan was explained to the patient and the patient understands and agrees.

_____   _____
CRNA SIGNATURE   ANESTHESIOLOGIST SIGNATURE

DISCHARGE NOTES FROM RECOVERY ROOM

Date: _____/_____/_____   Time: _____ AM/PM

COMMENTS:

_____
_____
_____
_____
_____
_____
_____
_____
_____

_____
SIGNATURE - ANESTHESIOLOGIST

POST ANESTHESIA NOTES

Date: _____/_____/_____   Time: _____ AM/PM

COMMENTS:

_____
_____
_____
_____
_____
_____
_____
_____
_____

_____
SIGNATURE - ANESTHESIOLOGIST

The Facial Plastic and Cosmetic Surgery Center

Patient Name: _____

Age _____ Date of Birth _____

Address _____

Physical Status ASA _____ Date _____

Surgeon _____ Anesthetist _____

Pre-Operative Diagnosis _____

Operative Procedure _____
_____

Pre-Anesthetic Medication _____

Pre-Medication Effect: Satisfactory _____ Apprehensive _____ Depressed _____

Anesthetic Techique: Inhalation _____ Intravenous _____ Spinal _____ Epidural _____

Block (Specify) _____ Local _____ Other _____

Anesthetic Agent: Primary _____ Supplement _____

	0	15	30	45	1 hr.	15	30	45	2 hr.	15	30	45	3 hr.	Total Drugs Used
O_2														
N_2O														

IV Fluids

B.P. ∨∧
P (•)
R (○)

180, 160, 140, 120, 100, 80, 60, 40, 20, 0

EBL | Urinary Output

Monitors:
 EKG
 Temperature: Esoph/Rectal
 Steth: Esoph/Precordial
 Line: CVP/Arterial
 Other _____

Intubation:
 Oral
 Nasal
 Cuff
 Other _____

Anesthetic Begun _____ A.M./P.M.   Ended _____ A.M./P.M.
Operation Begun _____ A.M./P.M.   Ended _____ A.M./P.M.

Remarks _____
_____
_____
_____
_____

Position:
 Supine Prone
 Trendelenburg/Reverse
 Lithotomy
 Jacknife
 Sitting
 Foot Down
 Kidneyrest (up)
 Lateral R L (up)
 Gas Machine and
 Equipment Checked ☐

_____
Anesthetist

Preoperative Notes

Date: _____ Signed _____ M.D.

Operative Comments

Postoperative Notes

Date: _____ Signed _____ M.D.

Appendix 1: Anesthesia 153

PREOPERATIVE RECORD

	CHART #
NAME_____ AGE____ WT _____ DATE _____	SURGICAL CHECK LIST
ARRIVAL TIME_____ NPO STATUS_____	ALLERGIES
PERSON PICKING UP PT._____ RELATION_____	History/Physical done
PT. STAYING AT_____ WITH _____ PH#_____	Consent Signed
PRESENT MEDS._____ LAST DOSE/TIME____ DATE___	Lab work in chart
ASA_____ BP_____ PULSE_____ TIME_____	Opthamology report
PREOP MEDS. VALIUM____mg. DRAMAMINE____mg. GIVEN @	Contact Lens Removed
WBC____ RBC____ HGB____ HCT____ K____ UA____	Voided Pre-OP
PT____ PTT____ PLATELETS____ EKG____ CHEST FILM___	BP, Pulse taken Pre-OP
PREGNANCY TEST_____	ID band in place
	Permit checked with scheduled surgery
	Pictures checked
	Called Pre-op

OPERATIVE RECORD

PERSONNEL	SPECIMENS & IMPLANTS	TIMES
OPER. RM._____	PATHOLOGY_____	INJECTION TIME_____
SURGEON_____	OTHER_____	STARTING TIME_____
ASSISTANT_____	IMPLANT_____	ENDING TIME_____
ANESTHES._____	MANUFACTURER_____	ANES. START_____
TYPE ANES._____	LOT_____ BATCH_____	ANES. END_____

PRE-OPERATIVE DIAGNOSIS: _____

POST-OPERATIVE DIAGNOSIS: _____

OPERATION PERFORMED: _____

COUNT   CORR.___ INCORR.___
NEEDLES_____
BLADES_____
WOUND CLASS   I   II   III

RECOVERY RECORD

EVALUATION — SCORE									
PULSE VOLUME	Strong	2							
	Weak	1							
RHYTHM	Regular	2							
	Irregular	1							
COLOR	Pink	2							
	Pale, mottled	1							
	Cyanotic	0							
VENTILATION	Exchanging well	2							
	Diminished	1							
AIRWAY	Clear	2							
	Obstructed	1							
CONSCIOUSNESS	Fully awake	2							
	Arousable	1							
	Unresponsive	0							
MOVEMENT	Purposeful	2							
	Involuntary	1							
	Not moving	0							

DISCHARGE

TIME_____ DCG. BY_____
DCG. TO: _____
Rx: _____
INSTRUCTION BOOK: _____
SURGICAL SITE/DCG. _____
RETURN VISIT: _____
ADDITIONAL INFO: _____
_____
_____
_____

Date

TIME	T	P	R	B/P	INTRAVENOUS FLUIDS MEDICATIONS	ORAL AMT. TAKEN	PARENTERAL FLUID INTAKE		OUTPUT		TREATMENTS		NOTATIONS
							Total Reading In Bottle	Absorbed	IV Checked	Urine	Ice Compress	Change Nasal Dressing	

BEESON FACIAL SURGERY
PRE-OPERATIVE RECORD

Name_____ Age_____ Date_____ Allergy_____ Chart_____

PRE-OPERATIVE CHECK LIST:

__Fee Paid	__EKG on Chart	__Washed Hair	__Has Instruction Books	Wt._____
__Opth. Eval.	__Has Sitter	__Washed Face	__Knows Post-Op Instr.	B/P_____
__Visual Acuity	__Has Resp. Adult	__Mascara Removed	__Gowned	Pulse_____
__Consent	__Has Medication	__Hose Removed	__LMP	Resp._____
__Neg Preg Test	__Up-dated Photos	__Contacts Removed	__Bathroom	Temp._____
__Labs	__NPO Since___AM/PM	__Dentures	__Jewelry sent with family_____	
			(name)	

NURSE:_____

PHYSICAL EXAM:

	Normal	Abnormal	Remarks
Head	_____	_____	
Eyes	_____	_____	
Ears	_____	_____	
Nose	_____	_____	
Mouth	_____	_____	
Skin	_____	_____	
Neck	_____	_____	
Chest	_____	_____	
Cardiac	_____	_____	
Abdomen	_____	_____	
Neuro	_____	_____	

_____Hx and PE essentially without change from prior exam
_____Primary care doctor notified of surgery_____(Name)
_____Ophthalmologic clearance_____(Name)
Nurse:_____ Doctor:_____

PRE-OPERATIVE MEDICATIONS:

TIME	MEDICATION	NURSE
____	___mg. Valium p.o.	____
____	___mg. Dramamine p.o.	____
____	___mg. Prednisone p.o.	____
____	___mg. Scopolamine p.o.	____
____	_____	____
____	_____	____
____	_____	____

INTRA-OPERATIVE RECORD:

SURGERY:

Pre-Operative DX:_____

Post-Operative DX:_____

Procedure:_____

Surgeon:_____

TIMES:
____Enter O.R.   ____Start Surgery   ____End Surgery   ____Length of Procedure

VITAL SIGNS UPON ENTERING O.R.:
____BP   ____Pulse   ____Resp.   ____O2 Sat   ____EKG Strip Obtained/Labled

MONITORS UTILIZED:
____EKG   ____Dynamometer   ____Pulse Oximeter

IV FLUIDS:
TIME:_____   LOCATION OF LINE:

FLUID:
____R/L   _____cc   ____R Anticubital
____D5W   _____cc   ____L Anticubital
____D5 N/S   _____cc   ____Other
____Other   _____cc   ____Good blood return noted on check

INTRA-OPERATIVE MEDICATIONS:

Time Valium	Time Dilaudid	Time Dramamine	Time Decadron	Time Xylocaine	Time Other
__ ____	__ ____	__ ____	__ ____	__ ____	____
__ ____	__ ____	__ ____	__ ____	__ ____	____
__ ____	__ ____	__ ____	__ ____	__ ____	____
__ ____	__ ____	__ ____	__ ____	__ ____	____
__ ____	__ ____	__ ____	__ ____	__ ____	____
__ ____	__ ____	__ ____	__ ____	__ ____	____
__ ____	__ ____	__ ____	__ ____	__ ____	____

TOTALS _____

COMMENTS _____

Condition at the End of Procedure: COMMENTS:_____
____Satisfactory
____Vision Normal   Complications_____
____Facial Nerve Normal
____EOM Normal   Specimen sent to Pathology_____
____No Hematomas or Bleeding
____Vital Signs Stable ____B/P ____Pulse ____Resp. ____O2 Sat.
____Release to Stage I Recovery
     Time_____AM/PM   PHYSICIAN:_____

NURSING CHECK LIST:
____Charting Completed
____EKG Strip Attached /Labeled
____B/P Record Attached/Labeled
____Specimens Labled and Pathology Forms Completed
____Eyelid Tissue Banked

NURSE:_____

Beeson Facial Surgery
Post-Op Recovery Record

Name _____   Date _____ Chart # _____

Procedure:

FL	H.T.	Otoplasty
Bleph	Scalp R.	Mentoplasty
D.B.	NSR	Other _____
Peel	SML	_____

BLOOD PRESSURE / PULSE / RESPIRATION chart (240–20), time intervals 15/30/45

Time	Nurse's notes	Nurse sign.

Stage I Recovery:
Start at:	Condition:
Discharge:	Condition:

Stage II Recovery:
Arrived at:	Condition:
Discharge:	Condition:
Assessment Scale:	Min. in R.A.

	in	15	30	45	60	90
Moving all extremities:						
Taking Fluids						
Ambulating						
Dressed self						
Fully awake						
BP + 20/-20 of Pre-OPBP						
Bp + 20-50 or -50-50 of Pre-op						
Arouses easily on calling						
Pink color						
Able to deep breath and cough						

Medication in R.R.:

Time:	Drugs	Dosage	Nurse Sig.

_____ Tylenol #4   _____ Erythromycin
_____ Percocet   _____ Keflex
_____ Tigan Supp   _____ Novafed
_____ Darvocet   _____ Zovirax Pill
_____ Ampicillin   _____ Zovirax Ointment
_____ Tetracycline

Others _____

Released to: _____
Hotel _____ Home _____
_____ Post-Op instructions given
_____ Has Post-Op Booklets
_____ Has Post-Op meds.
_____ Tylenol #4   _____ Novafed
_____ Percocet   _____ Zovirax Pill
_____ Tigan Supp   _____ Zovirax Oint.
_____ Darvocet   _____ Ampicillin
_____ Tetracylcline   _____ Erythromycin
_____ Keflex   _____ Other

Return in a.m. at _____
May release:

_____ Nurse
_____ M.D.

PRE-ANESTHESIA QUESTIONNAIRE

SIGNATURE _____ AGE _____

DATE _____ TIME _____ WEIGHT _____ HEIGHT _____

	Yes	No
Have you had any operations or anesthesia?	( )	( )
If so, what type and in what year? _____		
Have you ever had trouble with anesthesia?	( )	( )
If so, what happened _____		
Has any member of your family had trouble with anesthesia?	( )	( )
If so, what? _____		
Have you ever had or do you now have:		
Seizures or fits?	( )	( )
If so, are you on medication? Give name. _____		
Does any member of your family have seizure or fits?	( )	( )
Do you have:		
Fainting spells?	( )	( )
Paralysis?	( )	( )
Loose teeth?	( )	( )
Dental plate, bridge, or false teeth? Which?	( )	( )
Difficulty opening your mouth?	( )	( )
Thyroid trouble?	( )	( )
Yellow jaundice, hepatitis, or liver disease?	( )	( )
If so, when? _____		
Kidney disease?	( )	( )
Stiffness or blood clots?	( )	( )
Varicose veins?	( )	( )
Heart attack or coronary?	( )	( )
High blood pressure?	( )	( )
Swelling of ankles?	( )	( )
Strokes?	( )	( )
A persistent cough?	( )	( )
Any lung disease?	( )	( )
If so, what? _____		
Shortness of breath after climbing stairs?	( )	( )
Shortness of breath after physical exercise?	( )	( )
Shortness of breath at any other time?	( )	( )
Any chest injury?	( )	( )
Any reaction to adhesive tape?	( )	( )
Any reaction to iodine, mercury, merthiolate?	( )	( )
Have you ever received or taken cortisone or steroids? If so, for what? _____	( )	( )
Have you ever had a blood transfusion?	( )	( )
How many cigarettes do you smoke a day? _____		
How much alcohol do you consume a day? _____		
A week? _____		
Motion sickness?	( )	( )
Medications now taking: _____		
Is there a possibility that you are pregnant at this time?	( )	( )

ANN COAN   Record Reviewed by _____
Certified Registered Nurse Anesthetist

Date:_____

Name_____ Date of birth_____ Age_____

<u>This is Part of Your Medical Record and is Kept Absolutely Confidential</u>

Reason for Consultation_____

Allergies:_____

Drug Allergies:_____

Medications Taken Regularly: _____

_____

Are you taking aspirin or any aspirin containing medications?_____

Are you taking Vitamin E?_____

Have you had any reaction to injections of a local anesthetic?_____

Date of last physical:_____Physician:_____

List previous surgeries you have had, dates and attending Physician:____

_____

Have you had any type of implants?_____What type?_____When?_____

Have you had an electrocardiogram in the past year?_____Normal?_____

General Health problems and have you been, or are you now, under treatment for any major medical condition:

Cancer	Yes ( ) No ( )	Eye Problems	Yes ( ) No ( )
Diabetes	Yes ( ) No ( )	Psychiatric Disorders	Yes ( ) No ( )
High Blood Pressure	Yes ( ) No ( )	Neurological Disorders	Yes ( ) No ( )
Heart Disease	Yes ( ) No ( )	Ulcers	Yes ( ) No ( )
Anemia	Yes ( ) No ( )	Rheumatic Fever	Yes ( ) No ( )
Lung Problems	Yes ( ) No ( )	Do you get nauseated	
Do you smoke?	Yes ( ) No ( )	easily?	Yes ( ) No ( )

_____
_____
_____
_____
_____
_____

Appendix 2: Employee Training

DAILY DUTIES

1. Assist Dr. Beeson with early morning rounds at the hospital p.r.n. to discharge and/or clean up post-operative patients from the previous day.
2. Staff meeting each morning:
   a. Go over post-operative patients coming in that day. What type of surgery they had and when. Discuss if they are coming in for regular post-op check or if they have problem.
   b. Surgery patients of the day. Make sure they have H&P, lab work, fee paid, etc.
3. Assist Dr. Beeson with post-op patients each morning. Stay one step ahead of them answering questions, taking photographs, etc. Route Dr. to next patient to be seen. Keep patient flow moving. Prepare consultation room for new consults as needed.
4. Meet surgery patients for the day and their families or care person. Get them prepared for surgery. Answer any questions they may have. Check that Dr. Beeson has seen them that morning, check for allergies, check for lab work, have patient wash surgical site. Medicate patient after vital signs have been checked and post-op arrangements have been made with family. Give family member or care person time to check into the Martin House. If no family or friend staying with patient, double check to make sure sitter has been arranged.
5. Assist with anesthesia and sedation pre-operatively.
6. Assist with surgery and dressing following case.
7. Note on surgery check list all medicines given during surgery and pre-op and times given. Attach blood pressure read-out and monitor strips to check list. Complete sheet prior to discharge.
8. Chart any medication given to patients at end of day and total. List name of patient, date given, and amount given.
9. Make sure crash cart is locked and safe is locked after returning medicines.
10. Instruments are to be milked following each 5 cases.
11. Charts and pictures are pulled daily for patients coming in the next day, and checked for appropriate information.
12. Record any injections and chemical peels done in record book.
13. Sterilize equipment for the next day and pull supplies for cases.
14. Check surgery charts for the next day for any abnormal lab results or need for any special supplies.
15. O-Syl disinfect floors in surgery room and clean with foam cleaner in between cases.
16. Master log surgeries daily (date, patient's name, age, chart number, procedure, doctor, and assistants).
17. Soak suction tips, speculums, and other instruments after each use in sporicide or cidex.
18. Be sure exam rooms and nurse's station are clean and in neat order.
19. Record biopsies taken or reports received in biopsy record book.

WEEKLY DUTIES

1. Check supplies and drugs and reorder p.r.n.
2. Check the next weeks surgeries and prepare for any different supplies or instruments (i.e. chin implants).
3. Check supply of chin implants, nose splints, x-ray splints, and petri dishes.
4. Check supply of chemical peel solution, make new solution p.r.n.
5. Check oxygen tank, emergency equipment, drugs and document.
6. Stock supplies in patient exam rooms.
7. Have nasal spray available in nose room and reorder p.r.n.
8. Check camera film supply, batteries, and flash supply and reorder p.r.n.
9. Check biopsy book and call for delayed reports.
10. Clean ultrasonic cleaner and change solution.
11. Culture chemiclave and log into 3-M monitor log.
12. a. Change sonic washer solution.
    b. Clean ultra sonic.

NURSE'S DAILY DUTY CHECK SHEET

Date _____   Done   Intl.

1. Assist Dr. Beeson with A.M. rounds
2. Attend staff meeting
3. Assist with post-op patients
4. Prepare patient for surgery
5. Prepare operating room for surgery
6. Pre-op preparation of patient
7. Move patient to O.R. suite and prepare for surgery
8. Assist with surgery
9. Clean O.R. suite after each surgery
10. Check on pre-op pts and recovery pts & discharge
11. Oxygen turned off
12. Crash cart locked
13. Care for surgical instruments
14. Clean & reorganize nurse's station
15. Document information in record book
    —Biopsies
    —Medications
    —Surgery procedures
    —Chemical peels
    —K 20's
16. Prepare patient charts for next day
17. Lock medicine cabinet
18. Charts in order before turning in
19. Pull instruments and supplies for next day
20. Prepare rooms for next day
21. Call Surgery patients for next day
22. Call consults for next day
23. Call post-op patients
    —Pam
    —Lynn
    —Kelly
    —Amy
24. Stock patient rooms and consult room
25. Check with hospital to confirm any surgeries for the preceding day
26. Schedule patients for
    —Surgery
    —Admitting
    —Sitting Service
    —Hotel
    —Flowers
27. File cabinets locked
28. Answering service turned on and checked
29. Patient room numbers at Martin House or Hospital
    _____
30. Person to make rounds with doctor in A.M. if hospital patient
    _____
31. Labs and voucher sheets ready for Med Path pick-up
32. Procedure charge list turned in to secretary or placed on daily ledger

Other

WEEKLY DUTIES

Week Ending _____   Done   Intl.

1. Check supplies and drugs
2. Plan for unusual supplies needed for next week
3. Check supply of nasal splints
4. Check supply of cartilage
5. Check supply of x-ray
6. Check supply of chin implants
7. Check supply of petri dishes
8. Check supply of chemical peel solution
9. Check crash cart, defibrillator, & oxygen tank
10. Check nasal spray supply
11. Culture autoclave
12. Call for delayed biopsy reports
13. Clean ultrasonic cleaner
14. Drug counts

Appendix 3: Quality Assurance

QUALITY ASSURANCE PLAN

OBJECTIVES:

1. To assure that the patient care being provided is maintained at an optimally achievable level of quality and is delivered in a safe, efficient, cost-effective manner.
2. To identify opportunities to improve care.
3. To provide administration and the medical staff with valid, reliable data about strengths and weaknesses in the clinical care being provided.
4. To protect the fiscal resources of the organization.

DESIGN:

To accomplish its objectives, the program is designed to:

1. Monitor and evaluate the quality of care being provided.
2. Determine that the care given is at the appropriate level.
3. Identify the causes of problems or deficiencies in care.
4. Implement appropriate corrective action.
5. Ensure that problem resolution endures over time.
6. Demonstrate, at least annually, that the program is effective.

Methodologies and Activities:

Quality Assurance Activities encompassed by the program include:

1. Credentialing and privileging of medical and nonmedical health care personnel and performance evaluation of staff.
   This activity will be performed by Dr. Beeson and will include review of past education, licenses and certifications, contact with personal references, etc. After an individual is accepted for employment, his past performance, continuing medical education, and licenses and certificates will be reviewed by Dr. Beeson and discussed with the employee in an attempt to maintain the highest standard of quality care. If situations exist as relate to poor patient care, such cases may be discussed with the Physician Peer Review Group, at the discretion of Dr. Beeson. Copies of annual employee reviews will be kept in the employee personnel file.
2. Medical records review—surgical case review, including indications for diagnostic and therapeutic procedures:
   A group of physicians will be selected one to two times a year to randomly review approximately 50 charts of surgical patients. Among other things, these physicians will review the indications for discrepancies and recommendations in this regard will be placed in writing by the Peer Review Group, discussed with Dr. Beeson and with other members of the Peer Review Group. The results of these discussions will be placed in the Quality Assurance file for documentation purposes.
3. Drug use monitoring:
   Detailed records of narcotics used, wasted, and currently in stock will be kept by nurses. These will be reviewed on a monthly basis and reviewed by Dr. Beeson and the Peer Physician Group on their review.
4. Patient Questionnaires:
   Patient questionnaires will be reviewed by Dr. Beeson and discussed with staff when appropriate. All patient questionnaires will be filed and will be available for review by the Peer Review Group.
5. Anesthesia Services Review:
   At least yearly a comprehensive review will be made of any case which incurred an adverse anesthetic reaction. The anesthetic regimen used will be reviewed as well as the appropriateness of preoperative laboratory regimens, etc. The aforementioned review may include consultation with an anesthesiologist or pharmacologist.
6. Postsurgical Infections:
   At least yearly a comprehensive review of all postsurgical infections will be made. A log of all such infections will be kept and report forms completed on each case by the nursing staff and Dr. Beeson. In addition, a computer review of the medical literature regarding infections associated with facial cosmetic surgery and prophylactic antibiotic use and head and neck surgery will be made. Consultation with an infectious disease specialist or other physicians may be made.
7. Analysis of injuries allegedly sustained at the facility.
8. Surveillance over the equipment maintenance program.
9. Continuing medical education for Dr. Beeson and nursing staff:
   All nursing personnel will be required to be certified in Advanced Cardiac Life Support. All office personnel must be certified in Basic Cardiac Life Support. Copies of these certificates will be kept in the Quality Assurance—Continuing Medical Education file. The medical staff will be required

to read selected journals and articles on a monthly basis. In-servicing training lectures will be given periodically and recorded in office Minutes. The medical staff will also attend selected medical meetings and the office staff selected office and business meetings. Pertinent information obtained at these meetings will be discussed with the entire staff at morning meetings. Records of such meetings will be made in the office Meeting Minutes. A list of CME courses attended will be kept in the Quality Assurance—Continuing Medical Education file.

10. Disaster drills:
Disaster drills will be held at least twice yearly and results will be filed.

11. Confidentiality:
All documents, reports, minutes, findings, conclusions and recommendations that are generated for the Quality Assurance Program are confidential for use in the Peer Review process. The material is protected from discovery under the laws of the State of Indiana. Records are stored in a manner ensuring strict confidentiality.

12. Reappraisal:
The structure and function of the Quality Assurance Program will be reappraised at least annually by Dr. Beeson. Revisions will be made to ensure that the program is achieving its objectives.

QUALITY ASSURANCE PROGRAM EVALUATION FORM

1. Review of routine patient flow and management protocol.
   Comments: _____
   _____

2. Review of sterilization protocol.
   A. Surgical procedures
   B. Instrument sterilization
   C. Sterilization report log
   D. Infection control log
   Comments: _____
   _____

3. Review of emergency equipment and emergency protocol.
   Comments: _____
   _____

4. Review of narcotics records.
   Comments: _____
   _____

5. Review of patient questionnaires.
   Comments: _____
   _____

6. Random review of patient charts: (20)

Problem	# Occurrences	Recommended Corrective Measures

7. Summary Comments:
   _____
   _____
   _____
   _____
   _____

   Signature of reviewers: _____

   Date: _____

Q A TRACKING SHEET

Special monitors (Nursing)

Problem	Plan	Action	Evaluation	Re-Evaluation

Q A TRACKING SHEET

Routine Duties (Nursing)

Task	Jan.	Feb.	Mar.	Apr.	May	Jun.	Jul.	Aug.	Sep.	Oct.	Nov.	Dec.

✓ = satis.,   0 = unsatis.   — = incompl.

AAAHC Medical Record Worksheet

Organization: _____

Site/Location: _____

Instructions: Check all items that appear in chart with "X" or "+". If *no* documentation is present, mark "O" or "−" in the appropriate box.

(Indicate Medical Record Numbers below)

Record legible to clinical personnel	1.
History and physical adequate	2.
Diagnosis or assessment appropriate	3.
Diagnostic procedures adequate	4.
Treatment consistent with diagnosis	5.
Consultation and referral adequate	6.
Follow-up adequate	7.
Diagnostic summary or problem list present	8.
Diagnostic summary/problem list used appropriately	9.
Allergies recorded	10.

Were any serious diagnostic or therapeutic problems (which place a patient at significant risk) noted during review of records? If so, indicate problem(s) and medical record number(s) on reverse side of this form.

Overall comments about quality of care (please use reverse side of this form).

Appendix 4: Risk Management

RISK MANAGEMENT PROGRAM

In order to develop a risk management program which will continue to be upgraded and updated, it is felt that a multi-tiered process is needed. The risk management team will consist of all nurses and physicians. We will attempt to utilize the administrative staff meetings as the main-stay functioning aspect of the risk management team, but will also utilize all additional clerical and medical personnel as well as our peer review group of physicians and our attorney. To this end, it is anticipated that risk management will be reviewed on a weekly basis and with periodic activities being initiated annually.

Risk Management Activities to be Conducted at Weekly Administrative Meetings:

1. Review of infection control log and discuss any infections noted during the preceding week.
2. Review of biopsy log to be sure appropriate logging and review of biopsies is being conducted.
3. Review of narcotics logs and records.
4. Review of any incident reports for the week.
5. Review of any pertinent items identified in patient questionnaires which have been received during the preceding week.

Additional Risk Management Activities:

1. At unannounced times during the year have narcotics officers from the State Police or City Police Dept. come in to the office to review narcotics records and procedures—we have already had our office thoroughly evaluated in this regard by the head of security for one of the Indiana University Medical Center Hospitals. We have also previously contacted the prosecutor's office and the DEA Office in Indianapolis and have asked that they have field representatives and investigators review the office at unannounced times during the year. They have previously stated they would do this when their investigators were in the area and had free time.
2. Incident Reports—Incident reports have been devised and will be completed whenever an act or omission occurs which might in any way affect patient safety or quality of care. These will be given to the doctor immediately and will be discussed at the weekly administrative meeting.
3. Conduct fire drills quarterly—Encourage the fire department ambulance crew to come to the office on an annual basis to fully review the office and the protocols we are using for our disaster plans and emergency patient evacuations.
4. Arrange for an attorney to review charts on two occasions during the year to assess our documentation process and to identify "weaknesses" in our recording and documentation systems. In addition, our attorney will discuss risk management and medical legal items with office personnel on those occasions.
5. On a yearly basis review our anesthesia protocols. Keep a list of any cases where there is any anesthetic problem or reaction of significance and review this with anesthesiologists on a yearly basis. Also review hospital cases to see how our office patients compare to those who have been hospitalized for procedures performed in that environment.
6. Infection control—On a yearly basis do a Medline search for all articles dealing with infections following facial cosmetic surgery or in the use of prophylactic antibiotics. Also review any infections we have had during the year and possibly consult with an infection disease specialist regarding these issues.
7. Patient questionnaire forms should be given to patients at three months postoperatively to be returned and reviewed.
8. Peer Review—Encourage peer review physicians to make suggestions and review our risk management protocols.

MONTHLY DUTIES

1. Check crash cart drugs for expiration dates and replace p.r.n.
2. Check fire extinguisher and emergency lighting.
3. Change sporicide or cidex solution.
4. Clean autoclave.
5. Check dates on sterilized equipment.

SEMIANNUAL DUTIES

1. Fire drill and disaster drill.
2. Emergency equipment (defib. and BP monitor) checked.

YEARLY DUTIES

1. Recertification of CPR once a year.
2. ACLS recertification every two years.
3. Obtain lab work and TB skin tests for all employees.

INCIDENT REPORT

Patient: _____   Visitor: _____   Employee: _____   Other: _____

Date of incident: _____ Date of report: _____

Location of incident: _____

Description of incident: _____

_____

Signature: _____

Physician Examination

Date: _____ Result: _____

_____

Signature: _____

Treatment

Date: _____ Type of treatment: _____

_____

Signature: _____

Follow up

Date: _____ Type of follow up: _____

_____

Signature: _____

Was this avoidable? _____ Measures taken to prevent recurrences: _____

_____

INFECTION CONTROL REPORT

Patient _____ Age _____ Chart # _____
Procedure _____ Date of procedure _____
Site of infection _____ Date Dx _____
Specimen source _____
Medications patient on _____ _____ _____
prior to infection   _____ _____ _____
Medications RX today _____ _____ _____
                                          Nurse: _____

Culture Report: Organisms   Sensitive to   Resistant to
Date _____
                                      Nurse: _____

Physician Review: Significant PMH   Hx of prior infections

Clinical follow-up:
  (Date)

Recommendations:

                                      Physician: _____

Appendix 5: Handling of Infectious or Hazardous Medical Waste

FACILITIES AND ENVIRONMENT

Included are protocols for:

1. Sterilization
2. Instrument Care
3. Handling of Specimens
4. Contamination Precautions
5. Sterilization of Operating Room
6. Instrument Care—Decontamination—Sterilization
7. Gas Sterilization—Gas Sterilization For Known Contaminated Cases
8. Use of Biological Test Indicators
9. Surgical Scrub Technique
10. Care and Disposal of Surgical Specimen
11. Steam and Gas Sterilization Guidelines

STERILIZATION PROTOCOL— OPERATING ROOM

Any discussion of cleanup methods must be based on acceptance of the concept that every surgical procedure deserves the same care as every other. That is, every patient merits the same degree of safety and precaution. Additionally, personnel working in surgery must be protected.

Therefore, every case should be treated as potentially contaminated. Cleanup techniques must be set up to contain and confine organisms so as to prevent contamination of the entire operating suite.

Definition

Any chemical or physical process which results in the destruction or removal of infectious agents outside the body.

Considerations

1. Blood and tissue fluids from any patient may contain organisms that are pathogenic to other persons.
2. Operating room practices have been developed which provide complete isolation for each patient.
3. Isolation procedures established by the office should be put into effect for the patient who, in addition to a surgical wound, has a known communicable disease.

Purpose

To prevent an infectious organism from being transmitted from one area to another on the same patient and/or from one patient to another.

Procedure

Precautions:

1. Excess furniture and equipment need not be removed from the room. Place as far from contamination as possible.
2. The only contaminated articles in the room are the furniture and equipment in direct contact with the operative field.
3. Use as much disposable linen as possible.
4. All personnel wear shoe covers—change before leaving room.
5. Scrub nurse should have sufficient water in her basin to submerge the open instruments.

Preoperative Preparations

1. All personnel entering even an empty OR must be properly garmented and wearing a cap and mask.
2. Using an alcohol soaked cloth, wipe down all flat surfaces of tables, equipment, and overhead lights at least one hour before scheduled incision time.
3. At the same time, the tops and rims of autoclaves and countertops in substerile rooms should also be damp dusted with an alcohol soaked cloth.
4. Place plastic bag inside trash container for disposables.

Operative Period

1. Areas contaminated by organic debris—blood and sputum—during the operation should be sprayed with germicidal and wiped up immediately.
2. Sponges should be discarded into plastic-lined kick-buckets.
3. Use glove or sponge stick to count sponges. Place counted sponges directly into plastic bag and tie. Do not place sponges on any item on the floor.
4. Once patient is in the room and operation has started, supplies and equipment should not leave the room.

5. Traffic in and out of room must be kept at a minimum to curtail dust turbulence created by the activity.
6. Circulating nurse should anticipate needs to avoid having to leave and return frequently.
7. Circulating nurse keeps floor and room neat and clear of debris.

Interim Cleaning

As soon as operation is completed and the patient is taken from the room, cleanup is initiated to ready the room for the next patient.

1. Be sure surgeon removes his gown first and then his gloves.
2. All personnel should change shoe covers as they leave the OR, if bloody.
3. Scrub nurse places all linen and disposable drapes in appropriate hampers, then clears back table of all disposable items and places in garbage bag. Needle book is disposed of in designated box. All sponges in or out of plastic bags are placed in appropriate containers by the scrub nurse.
4. Scrub nurse assembles unused instruments and places in tray.
5. Removes gown but leaves her gloves on.
6. Takes tray of instruments and basin of dirty instruments to sink area for cleaning. After cleaning, flashes instruments for next case or covers tray with plastic bag and carries to instrument processing area.
7. Circulator or scrub nurse removes back table cover by folding toward center to prevent spreading of airborne contaminants.

Interim Housekeeping

1. Horizontal surfaces of tables and equipment involved in the surgical procedure should be cleansed with detergent germicide.
2. Wet-mop floors using a fresh mop and bucket of detergent germicide.
3. Saline from back table may be disposed of in sink.
4. Room is made up for next case.

INSTRUMENT STERILIZATION—CHEMICLAVE

Purpose:

1. To sterilize all equipment supplies needed for operating room.
2. To assure the safety of the patient.
3. To protect against cross-contamination.
4. To provide a means by which all forms of microbial life is killed.

Procedure:

1. All equipment is brought into the nurse's area (left of sink) to be prepared for sterilization following protocol of Instrument Processing—Decontamination guidelines.
2. After decontamination has been accomplished, instruments are checked for breakage and placed on the counter opposite the sink area.
3. If instruments are to Chemiclaved in an unwrapped state, this may be done in 10 minutes.
4. Wrapping of equipment
   A. Disposable wrappers should be double thickness and indicators should be placed in the middle of the package. Tape with autoclave tape.
   B. Steri-peel packages should be taped so that all folded edges of package are sealed. Indicators should be placed inside package regardless of outside indicators.
5. Mark each package with contents and date of expiration.
   A. Disposable wrapped packages are dated to expire in one month.
   B. Double wrapped steri-peel packages may be dated to expire six months after sterilization.
6. All wrapped packages are to be Chemiclaved for 20 minutes.
7. All outdated materials should be washed, rewrapped and resterilized.

PROCEDURE FOR USE OF CIDEX

This method should be used when Steam Sterilization will destroy or damage instruments.

1. Use a sterile stainless steel soak basin with lid.
2. Use a similar pan and lid for sterile water to rinse instruments.
3. Always wash items thoroughly to remove blood, pus, oil, etc.
4. Rinse under tap water, dry and submerge in Cidex for the required time.
5. Rinse thoroughly in sterile water, changing as often as possible.

Note: All cidex basins should be changed daily. All cidex basins should be covered with lid when not in use.

INSTRUMENT PROCESSING—DECONTAMINATION

Purpose

The chief objective of the decontamination procedure is to render the environment microbiologically safe for the patient and for the personnel who come into contact with patient used items.

Procedure

1. Instruments should be kept as free as possible from blood and other gross contaminants by wiping with wet sponge during case.
2. At end of case, scrub nurse places opened dirty instruments in basin of water on back table, replaces unused instruments in instrument trays. Remove dirty gown. Take all instruments to the nurse's area, left of sink.
3. The gloved scrub nurse removes gross contaminants from dirty instruments using brush and running water in the sink.
4. Once every day, when the sink is used, wipe down sink and countertop with germicidal. (O Syl or Dow Germicidal Foam)
5. Instruments are then placed in ultrasonic cleaner. Place one ounce of Caviclean in sonic cleaner and set for 5 minutes. If there are many instruments this may need to be done in two loads.
6. Upon completion of sonic cleaning, the instruments must be thoroughly rinsed in cold running water to remove any residue of sonic solution or soap.
7. Instruments should then be placed in instrument milk for 30–45 seconds. Allow to drain. Rinsing or drying is not necessary.
8. Instruments are then placed in their assigned spaces in instrument trays. They may then be wrapped for sterilization.
9. IF INSTRUMENTS ARE TO BE USED FOR ANOTHER CASE TO FOLLOW: In this case, milking of instruments is not necessary and towel drying of instruments is preferred before they are placed into the Chemiclave.

INSTRUMENT STERILIZATION— GAS

Procedure

1. All equipment and supplies to be gas sterilized are taken to Methodist Hospital 4th floor surgery Instrument Room.
2. They should be given to the person in charge of the workroom on that shift. That person should record the name of the item and that it belongs to Dr. Beeson. They will wrap items.
3. The length of time required for sterilization varies upon the item. Items for general surgical use will be ready for pick-up or use the next day as they require 12 hours for aeration.
4. Any item to be used for implantation (chin implants) require 72 hours for aeration. BE SURE TO PLAN AHEAD!

STERILIZATION PROTOCOL— KNOWN CONTAMINATED CASE

It is not anticipated that a known contaminated case will ever knowingly be scheduled in the office surgical area. However, in the event that such a case does occur, this protocol has been established.

Purpose

To establish a procedure and controls which will further reduce the possibility of cross-infection of the surgical patient following a "septic" case. (Defined as a Class IV.)

Equipment

1. Housekeeping cart, which includes:
   A. Germicidal solution
   B. Color-coded plastic bags for contaminated articles
   C. Cloth towels
   D. Disposable gloves
   E. Shoe covers

Procedure

Thoroughly anticipate need for the entire case. Unless absolutely necessary, do not handle items in the room with hands that have handled items coming into contact with patient fluids. *Wear gown and gloves.*

1. Bring patient to the operating room in the usual manner.
2. All linen is placed in a color-coded plastic bag. Hand out to a clean person at end of case to be received in a hamper bag at the door.
3. All trash is placed in a color-coded plastic bag in the O.R.; received into a second color-coded plastic bag at the door.
4. Sharps are placed on the needle mat, folded and placed in the room trash.
5. Soiled instruments:
   A. Put germicidal in instrument water to wash instruments *after* the patient leaves the room.
   B. Wash dirty instruments and brush and assemble tray. All instruments are taken to autoclave for decontamination.
   C. Place germicidal in all containers holding water or saline and suck into suction containers. Seal and place in trash bag.
   D. Wipe down with germicidal all room furniture, both sides of table pads, pillows, etc. Tourniquet cuffs and blood pressure cuffs are wiped with germicidal and placed in a color-coded plastic bag and sent for *gas sterilization*.
   E. Power equipment, cords and hoses should be wiped with germicidal and sterilized for ten (10) minutes. Fiberoptic cords should be wiped, bagged, and sent for gas sterilization.
   F. Housekeeping will then clean the entire O.R., including the floor.

Points to Remember

1. Contain contamination to as small an area as possible.
2. Restrict traffic to an absolute minimum. Post "Contaminated Case" signs on doors.
3. Circulator should wear gown and gloves when coming into direct contact with a known septic case.
4. Reduce amount of contaminated goods by removing water and saline bottles before patient comes into room.

Beginning of Case

1. Set up hampers with color-coded plastic bags and place kick buckets on chux.
2. Have spray bottle of germicidal available.
3. Remove all unnecessary furniture.

During Case

1. Bag all sponges as soon as countable units occur.
2. Have extra needed supplies brought to you by a clean person. If necessary to leave room, change gown and shoe covers.
3. Keep room tidy, place all garbage and linen in proper bags immediately.

Pathology Specimen

1. Double bag, keeping outside bag clean. Mark "Contaminated."

Post-op Routine

1. Circulating nurse should open and apply any outer dressing.
2. Scrub person and surgeon must remove contaminated gown and gloves before moving the patient from the table, so as not to contaminate the patient's extremities.
3. If anesthesia personnel are present, they should wear gown and shoe covers.
4. All persons leaving the room should remove their shoe covers.
5. Decontaminate *all* items contaminated during the case.

THE SURGICAL SCRUB

Objective

To help prevent possibility of contamination of the operation wound by bacteria on the hands and arms. *Note:* fingernails should be kept short.

Procedure

The surgical scrub is the removal of as many bacteria as possible from arms and hands by mechanical washing before taking part in a surgical procedure.

A. Check to make sure all necessary equipment is available.
B. Preliminary wash-wet hands and arms with water. Wash hands and arms to 3" above the elbow with soap and water for 1 minute with brush.
C. Clean under nails with plastic nail cleaner, under the flow of water.
D. Rinse hands and arms slanting at fingertips using an upward-outward motion.
E. Obtain a sterile brush from the dispenser, open it (before the preliminary wash), wet the scrub brush. Begin with scrub brush by scrubbing fingernails on the left hand vigorously.
F. Then scrub each finger individually as if it had four (4) sides. Continue by scrubbing left hand to wrist. Repeat same procedure on other hand. (Scrub nails then fingers and hand to wrist).
G. Continue scrub, moving from wrist to mid-arm (half-way to elbow). Repeat same procedure on other arm, so level of progression remains even. Doing this on both arms scrub from mid-arm to one (1) inch above elbow. Drop scrub brush.
H. Rinse hands and arms. (Be careful to hold hand higher than elbow to keep water from dripping down arms.)

Proceed to the operating room, holding the fingertips and hands above elbow.

Avoid dripping contaminated water from the arms to back table.

Carefully take sterile towel from back table. One end of towel is used to dry the right hand and arm, the other end for drying left hand and arm.

Note: First scrub of each day should last a minimum of ten (10) minutes. Each consecutive scrub that day should be three (3) minutes.

Points to Remember

1. Never shake hands.
2. Do not touch anything while scrubbing.
3. You must not run arms back and forth through the water.
4. Hold hands up above the waist, fingertips above the elbows.
5. Do not touch arms to scrub suit.
6. Never hold hands near your mask.
7. Do not wet your scrub suit while you are scrubbing.
8. Pay particular attention to the crevices, fingernails and in between the fingers.

Develop a Surgical Conscience

9. More time should be spent on the hands than any other area.

10. Do not go over an area already scrubbed.

If you accidentally touch something, you must start the scrub again.

CLEANING THE OPERATING ROOMS BETWEEN CASES

Policy

To provide a safe environment for the patient undergoing surgery.

Procedure

A. Remove all dirty linen from room.
B. All trash removed from room—new trash liners in cans.
C. All dirty instruments removed from room.
D. Wipe table with solution to remove any blood or fluids.
E. Wipe Mayo stand and back table with antiseptic solution—(all equipment which was used).

PROCEDURE: CARE & DISPOSAL OF SURGICAL SPECIMEN

Objectives

A. To properly prepare tissue and material submitted by the surgeon, for gross and histological examination by the surgical pathologists.
B. To eliminate error by providing proper identification of materials submitted.
C. To help facilitate efficient and rapid control of the submitted material from the operating suite to the pathology department.

Equipment

A. Small plastic container with formalin, a dry culture tube or Saline in container or dry container.
B. Rubber band.
C. Masking tape.
D. Pen.
E. Proper pathology form.

General Instructions for Specimen Going to Pathology

A. When the scrub nurse receives the specimen of tissue from the surgeon, she places it in the specimen cup.
B. The circulating nurse will obtain the specimen of tissue the scrub nurse. Place in proper media. Label with patient's name.
Specimen-name-area specimen removed date Surgeons' name—fill out the proper pathology form. Apply label to specimen container. If more than one specimen these should be labeled as #1–#2.

Purpose

A. To sterilize all equipment and supplies needed for operating room and nursing units.
B. To assure the safety of the patient.
C. To protect against cross-contamination.
D. To provide a means by which *all* forms of microbial life is killed.

Steam Sterilization

A. All used equipment is brought into Central Supply and placed in the dirty area (right of door at sink) to be prepared for sterilization.
B. Wash all equipment with detergent, rinse well with distilled water three times.
C. Equipment is then checked for breakage and placed in the clean area of Central Supply.
D. Wrapping of equipment
   1. Disposable wrappers should be double thickness and indicators should be placed in the middle of the package. Tape with autoclave tape.
   2. Heat sealed packages should be checked for creases and indicators placed inside if there are no indicators on the outside of the wrapper.
E. Mark each package with what is inside and date of expiration.
   1. Disposable wrapped packages are dated to expire in one month.
   2. Properly sealed heat sealed packages are dated to expire six months after sterilization.
F. All outdated equipment is returned to Central Supply to be washed, rewrapped and resterilized. This is the responsibility of Operating Room personnel.

WASTE DISPOSAL PROTOCOL

GLOVES—gloves should be worn by medical staff when handling blood, tissue specimens, during vena puncture and cleaning.

PROTECTIVE GLASSES/FACE SHIELDS—should be worn during dermabrasions and any procedure when an aerosol of blood products could be created or when there is a possibility of contamination due to aerosol sprays or blood.

NEEDLES AND OTHER SHARPS—all should be disposed of in red sharps container.

GLASS TUBES AND BLOOD DRAWING PARAPHERNALIA—dispose in red sharps container.

BLOOD-SOAKED GAUZES AND GARMENTS—should be disposed of in "kick bucket" in the operating room. After surgery the material should be placed in the compactor and compacted.

DAILY WASTE FROM EXAM ROOMS—should be placed in compactor and compacted on a daily basis.

The contents of the compactor should be compacted and placed in a red hazardous waste contamination sack, boxed in a hazardous waste box, the box should be sealed, dated, office name placed on box.

The waste disposal company should be called for pick-up.

When pick-up company arrives, the pick-up should be logged in the data sheet indicating date, time, who made the pick-up, and the initial of the person authorizing the pick-up.

Prior to waste pick-up, the hazardous waste containers should be stored in a secured area away from public access.

Waste cartons and bags should be ordered such that at least three such containers are on premises at all times.

Sharp containers should be re-ordered so that one extra container is available in the office at all times.

Disinfecting Procedures

Blood-contaminated areas should be cleaned with a 1:10 dilution of bleach and water in a spray bottle. Following this, the areas should be cleansed with the antiseptic sprays used in our normal protocols.

- Wash hands with soap and water immediately after contaminated with blood or blood products.
- Report any episodes of contamination or injury such as needle sticks immediately to doctor and complete an incident report.

Gas Sterilization

A. All used eiquipment is to be cleansed and prepared for sterilization. Wash all equipment with detergent and rinse well with distilled water three times. Dry.
B. Equipment is then checked for breakage before wrapping.
C. Wrapping of equipment
   1. Paper disposable wrappers should be double thickness and indicators are placed in the middle of the package. Tape with Ethylene Oxide Tape.
   2. Heat sealed package should be checked for creases and indicators placed inside packages.
D. Mark each package with what is inside and the date of expiration.
   1. Disposable wrapped packages are dated to expire in one month after sterilization.
   2. Properly sealed heat sealed packages are dated to expire six months after sterilization.
E. Aeration of gas sterilization
   All gas sterilized equipment is placed in the aeration cabinet for a minimum of 12 hours.
F. All outdated equipment is to be disassembled and re-wrapped before re-sterilizing. This is to be the responsibility of the Operating Room personnel.

Sterilization by Emersion—Cidex

A. Throughly clean, rinse, and rough dry objects before immersing them in full strength cidex.
B. Flush and fill cleansed lumen of any hollow instrument.
C. Immerse completely for a minimum of *TEN HOURS* to destroy resistant pathogenic spores.
D. Remove instruments from Cidex using sterile techniques and rinse thoroughly with sterile water.

Appendix 6: Employee Forms

EMPLOYEE PHYSICAL EXAM AND MEDICAL PROFILE

Date _____

Name _____ Age _____

Address _____ Date of birth _____

City _____ State _____ Zip _____ Telephone _____

Marital status: M __ S __ D __ SEP __

Name of Spouse _____

Number of children and ages _____

NO	YES	Are you allergic to any medications?

List them if you can: _____

| NO | YES | Are you now taking any drugs or medications? |

List them if you can: _____

| NO | YES | Have you ever had surgery? |

If so list what was done and when: _____

| NO | YES | Have you ever been hospitalized for treatment of any problem other then surgery listed above or childbirth? |

If so list reason and when _____

When was your last physical exam? _____

Who is your family doctor? _____

Address _____

Who should we contact in case of emergency? (Family Member)

_____ Telephone (home) _____
                                       (work) _____

| NO | YES | Have you had "female" or GYN problems? Explain _____ |

| NO | YES | Men Only: Have you ever had prostate problems? |
| NO | YES | Do you have any other medical problems that have not been covered? Explain _____ |

Physical Exam

Pulse _____ B.P. _____ Respiration _____

Normal   Abnormal   Explain

Head-
Eyes-
Ears-
Nose-
Mouth-
Neck-
Chest-
Heart-
Abdomen-
Extremities-
Nervous system-
Other _____

LABORATORY

CBC   —   Normal/Abnormal
U/A   —   Normal/Abnormal
Chem profile — Normal/Abnormal
Serology   —   Normal/Abnormal

Summary comments: _____
_____
_____

                                      Physician's Signature _____
                                      Date _____

EMPLOYEE DATA RECORD

Name _____ Age _____ Date _____
Date of birth _____ Place _____
Address _____
    City _____ State _____ Zip _____
Telephone _____
Marital status M __ S __ D __ SEP __ Spouse _____
Present position: _____

Education

High School _____ Date graduated _____
Address _____
College _____ Degree _____
Address _____
College _____ Degree _____
Address _____
College _____ Degree _____
Address _____

Post graduate/Technical school

Name _____ Degree _____
Address _____ Date _____
Name _____ Degree _____
Address _____ Date _____
OTHER (Including BCLS or ACLS Certification, etc.)
_____

Do you or any family members have: (indicate who)
    Heart trouble _____ Excessive bleeding tendencies _____
    Tuberculosis _____ High blood pressure _____
    Diabetes _____ Psychiatric or "nerve problems" _____
    Excessive bruisability _____ Thyroid problems _____
    Excessive scarring _____

Do you have any history of bleeding:
    From the nose _____ In the urine _____ Vomiting blood _____
    From the rectum _____ Coughing up blood _____ Other? _____

No Yes Do you have hay fever, nasal allergies or asthma?
          Explain _____
No Yes Do you have or have you had any problems with your eyes?
          Explain _____
No Yes Do you have frequent pains in the chest?
No Yes Has a doctor ever said you had "heart trouble?"
          Explain _____
No Yes Do you have "stomach trouble" or ulcers?
          Explain _____
No Yes Do you have or have you had chest or lung problems?
          Explain _____
No Yes Have you ever had liver, gall bladder trouble or "yellow jaundice"? (circle which one)
No Yes Do you or any family members suffer from arthritis?

No	Yes	Do you have frequent skin infections, irritations or rashes (circle which one)
No	Yes	Do you often have severe headaches or dizzy spells? (circle which one)
No	Yes	Has any part of your body ever been paralyzed or numb? Explain _____
No	Yes	Did you ever have a convulsion or seizure?
No	Yes	Have you ever received treatment for your genital area? Explain _____
No	Yes	Were you ever treated for any venereal disease?
No	Yes	Are you frequently sick or ill?
No	Yes	Were you ever treated for anemia or any problems with your blood? Explain _____
No	Yes	Have you ever taken hormones or thyroid medications? (circle which one)
No	Yes	Do you smoke more than 10 cigarettes a day?
No	Yes	Do you drink more than 6 cups of coffee a day?
No	Yes	Do you usually take two or more alcoholic drinks a day?
No	Yes	Do you often get depressed?
No	Yes	Do you usually feel unhappy or depressed?
No	Yes	Does criticism always upset you?
No	Yes	Are you considered a nervous person?
No	Yes	Did you ever have a "nervous breakdown"?
No	Yes	Have you ever received medical treatment for a "nervous condition"?
No	Yes	Are you easily upset or irritated?
No	Yes	Have you ever been under the care of a psychiatrist or psychologist? Explain _____

POLICY STATEMENT ON PATIENT CONFIDENTIALITY AND CONFIDENTIALITY OF OFFICE FINANCES AND AFFAIRS

As an employee of Beeson Facial Plastic and Reconstructive Surgery I promise to maintain in the strictest confidence the names and identity of patients seen and treated. This confidentiality of patients will extend to their medical records and photographs. No patient information will be released without prior written consent by that patient and/or by direct permission from Dr. William Beeson.

As an employee of Beeson Facial Plastic and Reconstructive Surgery I also promise to maintain strict confidentiality in regard to all office operations and all financial affairs. I am also aware that any use of illicit drugs or excessive use of alcohol will not be tolerated. Any violation of the above stated items will be grounds for immediate termination of employment.

_____
(Employee Signature)

_____
(Witness)

_____
(Date)

Appendix 6: Employee Forms 183

JOB PERFORMANCE APPRAISAL

Office/Clerical Personnel

Employee's Name _____
Job Title _____ Soc. Sec. Number _____
Function _____
Date of Employment _____ (_____)

For personnel use only
_____ 90-Day Appraisal   Current Status
_____ 6-Month Appraisal   _____ Full Time   _____ Part Time
_____ Annual Appraisal   _____ Permanent   _____ Other
_____ Other

DATE: _____

Performance Rating Codes

To evaluate the performance level, the evaluator should begin with the definition of competent performance and determine if performance is better or less than competent. Listed below are the levels of performance and their general definitions. (Outstanding and unsatisfactory require specific justification under "Comments.")

Outstanding–Overall performance is conspicuously and uniquely above that of peers; truly exceptional level of accomplishment; always exceeds expectations; individual demonstrates full mastery in the factor.

Above Average–Overall performance is noticeably better than competent; frequently exceeds expectations; individual demonstrates a thorough knowledge of the function.

Competent–Overall performance is good; meets expectations and occasionally may exceed them in certain areas of performance.

Needs Improvement–Overall performance does not meet expectations; individual requires close monitoring and supervision; needs improvement to meet requirements.

Unsatisfactory–Overall performance is clearly below an acceptable level. Individual lacks ability to meet the overall requirements on a consistent basis.

Overall general statement of position responsibility:_____
_____

Performance Rating Factors

Job Knowledge: Consider the individual's familiarity with and application of position requirements; consider background experience and training.

__ Unsatisfactory __ Needs Improvement __ Competent __ Above Average __ Outstanding

Comments: _____

Skills: Consider the demonstration of the general skills necessary for the completion of assignments. Circle skills necessary.

     Filing   Typing   Reception   Dictaphone   Shorthand

__ Unsatisfactory __ Needs Improvement __ Competent __ Above Average __ Outstanding

Comments: _____

Quality of Work: Consider accuracy, completeness and thoroughness.

__ Unsatisfactory __ Needs Improvement __ Competent __ Above Average __ Outstanding

Comments: _____

Productivity: Consider the volume of work produced; the application of time, interest and energy to the completion of assignments; include promptness.

__ Unsatisfactory __ Needs Improvement __ Competent __ Above Average __ Outstanding

Comments: _____

Cost Containment: Consider the effective and efficient use of department resources and supplies; efficient use of time and priority setting.

__ Unsatisfactory __ Needs Improvement __ Competent __ Above Average __ Outstanding

Comments: _____

Initiative: Consider the willingness to do what is necessary for efficient operation without being asked or reminded.

__ Unsatisfactory __ Needs Improvement __ Competent __ Above Average __ Outstanding

Comments: _____

Cooperation: Consider the willingness to assist others in accomplishing inter-departmental and hospital goals.

__ Unsatisfactory __ Needs Improvement __ Competent __ Above Average __ Outstanding

Comments: _____

Appearance: Consider the overall presentability of the individual.

__ Unsatisfactory __ Needs Improvement __ Competent __ Above Average __ Outstanding

Comments: _____

Attendance: Consider the ability and willingness to conform to work schedules, including starting and quitting times, breaks and faithfulness in coming to work daily.

__ Unsatisfactory __ Needs Improvement __ Competent __ Above Average __ Outstanding

Comments: _____

Interpersonal Skills: Consider the ability to work with peers, superiors, and patients and visitors if applicable.

__ Unsatisfactory __ Needs Improvement __ Competent __ Above Average __ Outstanding

Comments: _____

Attitude/Awareness: Demonstrates sensitivity, concern and awareness of the needs of other individuals, including patients, visitors and fellow employees and staff consistent with the philosophy of Beeson Facial Plastic and Reconstructive Surgery.

Comments: _____

_____

Additional rating factor(s) relevant to position: _____

_____

__ Unsatisfactory __ Needs Improvement __ Competent __ Above Average __ Outstanding

Comments: _____

_____

Overall Performance

__ Unsatisfactory __ Needs Improvement __ Competent __ Above Average __ Outstanding

Comments: _____

_____

I have reviewed and discussed this job performance appraisal with my supervisor and I _____ agree _____ disagree with the appraisal. (Employee may comment below or use additional sheets, if necessary.)

Employee's Signature: _____ Date: _____

Comments: _____

_____

Recommendation

_____ Move to Permanent Status   _____ DO NOT move to Permanent Status
                                                         (Indicate action to be taken)

_____ Salary Increase Approved When Due

           Grade_____ Current Rate_____ Percent_____
           New Rate_____

__ Place on Performance Probation; will reevaluate on _____
                                                              (Date)

__ Remove from Performance Probation: _____
                                              (Effective Date)

_____   _____
(Supervisor/Appraiser Signature)   (Date)

_____   _____
(Administrative Signature)   (Date)

I have read the action taken.

_____ I agree with action taken
_____ I disagree with action taken as stated above, my statement is as follows:

_____

_____

_____   _____
Employee's Signature   Date

JOB PERFORMANCE APPRAISAL

Technical/Professional Personnel

Employee's Name _____

Job Title _____ Soc. Sec. Number _____

Function _____ Date of Employment _____

☐ 90-Day Appraisal
☐ 6-Month Appraisal
☐ Annual Appraisal
☐ Other

Current Status
☐ Full Time   ☐ Part Time
☐ Permanent   ☐ Other

_____
DATE

Performance Rating Codes

To evaluate the performance level, the evaluator should begin with the definition of competent performance and determine if performance is better or less than competent. Listed below are the levels of performance and their general definitions. (Outstanding and unsatisfactory require specific justification under comments.)

Outstanding—Overall performance is conspicuously and uniquely above that of peers; truly exceptional level of accomplishment; always exceeds expectations; individual demonstrates full mastery in the factor.

Above Average—Overall performance is noticeably better than competent; frequently exceeds expectations; individual demonstrates a thorough knowledge of the function.

Competent—Overall performance is good; meets expectations and occasionally may exceed them in certain areas of performance.

Needs Improvement—Overall performance does not meet expectations; individual requires close monitoring and supervision; needs improvement to meet requirements.

Unsatisfactory—Overall performance is clearly below an acceptable level. Individual lacks ability to meet the overall requirements on a consistent basis.

Overall general statement of position responsibility: _____

Performance Rating Factors

Technical Skills: Consider the necessary overall skills associated with accomplishing the position responsibility.

___ Unsatisfactory ___ Needs Improvement ___ Competent ___ Above Average ___ Outstanding

Comments: _____

Quality of Work: Consider the ability to provide an efficient discharge of tasks, coordination and follow through on responsibilities, the avoidance of errors.

___ Unsatisfactory ___ Needs Improvement ___ Competent ___ Above Average ___ Outstanding

Comments: _____

Productivity: Consider the efficient use of time, completion of assignments.

___ Unsatisfactory ___ Needs Improvement ___ Competent ___ Above Average ___ Outstanding

Comments: _____

Judgement: Consider the ability to translate knowledge into practice; effectiveness in evaluating practical solutions to problems.

___ Unsatisfactory ___ Needs Improvement ___ Competent ___ Above Average ___ Outstanding

Comments: _____

Written Documentation: Consider the ability to maintain necessary reports, records, charts, instructions; wording is clear, concise and appropriate for situation.

___ Unsatisfactory ___ Needs Improvement ___ Competent ___ Above Average ___ Outstanding

Comments: _____

Cost Containment: Consider the efficient use of supplies, equipment and/or patient care items; make conscious effort to reduce costs for department.

___ Unsatisfactory ___ Needs Improvement ___ Competent ___ Above Average ___ Outstanding

Comments: _____

Dependability: Consider the ability to adapt to hours, shifts; good use of work hours; ability to respond to situation at hand.

___ Unsatisfactory ___ Needs Improvement ___ Competent ___ Above Average ___ Outstanding

Comments: _____

Safety: Consider ability to follow procedures set up for employee and patient safety.

___ Unsatisfactory ___ Needs Improvement ___ Competent ___ Above Average ___ Outstanding

Comments: _____

Interpersonal Skills: Consider ability to be sensitive to varying individual needs; peers, subordinates, superiors and patients and visitors when applicable.

___ Unsatisfactory ___ Needs Improvement ___ Competent ___ Above Average ___ Outstanding

Comments: _____

Continuing Education: Consider participation in and contribution to education activities in order to increase understanding of responsibilities and makes effort to maintain and update necessary skills and knowledge.

___ Unsatisfactory ___ Needs Improvement ___ Competent ___ Above Average ___ Outstanding

Comments: _____

Attitude/Awareness: Demonstrates sensitivity, concern and awareness of the needs of other individuals, including patients, visitors, fellow employees and staff consistent with Beeson Facial Plastic and Reconstructive Surgery Standards.

___ Unsatisfactory ___ Needs Improvement ___ Competent ___ Above Average ___ Outstanding

Comments: _____

Additional Rating Factor(s) Relevant to Position: _____

___ Unsatisfactory ___ Needs Improvement ___ Competent ___ Above Average ___ Outstanding

Comments: _____

Summary of Past Goal Setting and Achievement/Progress Toward Those Goals:

_____

Future Goal Expectations:

_____

Overall Performance:

___ Unsatisfactory ___ Needs Improvement ___ Competent ___ Above Average ___ Outstanding

Comments: _____

I have reviewed and discussed this job performance appraisal with my supervisor and I ____ agree ____ disagree with the appraisal. (Employee may comment below or use additional sheets, if necessary.)

Employee's Signature: _____ Date: _____

Comments: _____

Recommendation

____ Move to Permanent Status   ____ DO NOT move to Permanent Status
                                                      (Indicate action to be taken)

____ Salary Increase Approved When Due

        Grade_____ Current Rate_____ Percent_____

        New Rate_____

___ Place on Performance Probation; will reevaluate on _____
                                                              (Date)

___ Remove from Performance Probation: _____
                                              (Effective Date)

_____   _____
(Supervisor/Appraiser Signature)   (Date)

_____   _____
(Administrative Signature)   (Date)

PERSONNEL ACTION FORM

Department Name: _____ Date: _____

EMPLOYEE NAME: _____ EMPLOYEE SOCIAL SECURITY NO. _____

TITLE: _____

Personal Data Changes:
NAME CHANGE: _____
                 (Last)   (First)   (Middle)

ADDRESS CHANGE: _____
                (Street)   (Apt.)   (City)   (State)   (Zip)

TELEPHONE NUMBER: _____

Change of Employment Status: POSITION
    FROM: _____ To: _____ Eff. Date: _____
          Title Code P.C. #   Title Code P.C. #

Status:
    From: ____ Full Time   To: ____ Full Time
                   ____ Part Time   ____ Part Time
                   ____ Permanent   ____ Permanent
                   ____ Temporary   ____ Temporary
                   ____ Summer Help   ____ Summer Help

Leave of Absence: (Refer to Employee Manual)
                  ____ Medical   ____ Maternity
                  ____ Military   ____ Marriage
                  ____ Personal   ____ Other
                     Attach Justification

____ Resignation   ____ Termination   Last Day Worked: _____

OVERAL PERFORMANCE EVALUATION: _____
_____

____ Eligible for Rehire   ____ Reevaluation Required for Rehire

Reasons: Work Related   Unrelated to Work

              ____ Nature of work   ____ Family reasons
              ____ Supv. or human relations problem ____ Leaving area
              ____ Dissatisfied with wages/benefits   ____ Returning to school
              ____ Unsatisfactory work performance   ____ Health reasons
              ____ Policy violations   ____ Travel problems
              ____ No call no show   ____ Temporary position
              ____ Layoff   ____ Accepted other position
              ____ Scheduling problems
              ____ Staffing problems

Other: (Explain) _____
_____

(Attach Resignation Letter)

                                                               Exit Interview Date: _____

Approved by: _____ Date: _____

POLICIES AND PROCEDURES FOR BEESON FACIAL PLASTIC AND RECONSTRUCTIVE SURGERY
8803 N. Meridian Street
Indianapolis, IN 46260

The ultimate purpose of all work in a medical office is to help people. Beeson Facial Plastic and Reconstructive Surgery is somewhat unique in that it exists to provide services to patient sin regard to the practice of aesthetic and reconstructive surgery of the face. In this connection, we strive for perfection in all facets of our work and in our contacts with our patients by phone, mail, and face-to-face communication. A medical office must adapt operating policies and rules to aid in reaching that ultimate objective or providing the highest quality of medical care in the most cost effective and appropriate surrounding.

Beeson Facial Plastic and Reconstructive Surgery is a sole proprietorship with William H. Beeson, M.D. being the sole proprietor.

Many of the rules and policies of a medical office are intended to build the confidence a patient feels in the physician and supporting personnel who work in the medical office. A strong doctor-patient relationship is necessary if the patient is to receive the full benefits from the physicians' service. The patient must feel sure that he or she can talk freely to the doctor, that the doctor and staff are knowledgeable and conscientious, and that the medical office is well managed. Only if these attitudes prevail will the patient be likely to adhere to the doctor's advice and perform his or her share of care during their convalescence. The physician's employees play a vital role in building this confidence by being cheerful, friendly tactful, neat, and industrious.

In order to facilitate and coordinate efforts, **Beeson Facial Plastic and Reconstructive Surgery** shall adopt the following guidelines:

1. Working days are Monday through Friday with postoperative rounds being made on Saturday mornings in the office and in the hospital.

2. The working day begins at 8:00 AM and ends at 5:00 PM unless otherwise specified.

    a. Nursing personnel working hours may extend beyond these routine hours.

    b. Nursing personnel will be required to take calls during their evening hours and on weekends.

    c. Nursing personnel will assist with postoperative rounds on weekends and early morning rounds in the hospital prior to 8:00 AM when necessary.

    d. On occasion, work may require office personnel to work beyond routine hours.

3. Lunch may be provided in this office for employees.

4. The lunch break will be taken at a time least likely to interfere with patient care.

5. Employees choosing to eat lunch away from the office shall arrange this at the beginning of the working day, shall limit the lunch break to thirty minutes, and shall assume the expenses incurred.

6. Any errands which require an employee's absence from the office shall be performed between the hours of 3:00 PM and 5:00 PM unless otherwise specified.

Telephone Calls

Personal telephone calls are strongly discouraged during working hours. This does not mean emergency or important telephone calls are not allowed. Please advise your family and acquaintances of this policy.

When personal phone calls are necessary, they should be made and received from the telephone in the employee lounge area. In order to keep our telephone lines available for business, the time of these calls should be kept to a minimum.

Pay Day

Regular full-time employees will be paid every other Monday.

Regular part-time and extra part-time employees will be paid every other Monday.

Holidays

Full-time employees will be paid for each of the following holidays:

New Year's Eve (1/2 day)	New Year's Day	Memorial Day
Independence Day	Labor Day	Thanksgiving
Christmas Eve (1/2 day)	Christmas Day	

An employee must work the business days preceding and following the holiday, or have a doctor's approval of absence in order to be paid for a holiday.

Vacations

Vacations shall consist of five (5) paid vacation days (non-accumulative) for first year employees. All other full-time employees are entitled to ten (10) vacations days (non-accumulative). After five years of employment, a regular full-time employee is entitled to fifteen (15) paid vacation days (non-accumulative).

To be eligible for a paid vacation, an employee must be employed full-time with Beeson Facial Plastic and Reconstructive Surgery for a minimum of nine (9) months.

Vacations must be approved and arranged at least one month in advance. An employee's request for vacation will be considered by the management of Beeson Facial Plastic and Reconstructive Surgery against its staffing requirements. Every effort will be made to accommodate the employee's request. In the event that a request can not be approved, acceptable alternatives will be provided based on employee seniority.

The date of employment will be used to determine eligibility for paid vacations.

Vacation time is to be taken yearly before the next anniversary date of employment.

Because vacations provide a period of rest and relaxation, each employee is expected to take his/her full allotted time during the year it is earned. Vacation time can not be carried into subsequent years, nor will an employee receive pay in lieu of vacation.

In the event of termination or resignation, an employee will be paid for accumulated and unused vacation time for the year up to the time of termination at accrued rate of .04167 days per month worked.

Bereavement

Regular full-time employees are entitled to three paid days in the event of the death of an employee's father, father-in-law, mother, mother-in-law, sister, brother, spouse, child, grandparents or grandchild.

One day with pay will be granted in the event of the death of other relatives of the employee's immediate family for the day of the funeral.

Sick Leave

An employee is eligible for sick leave with pay after six months of employment. Twelve (12) days of sick leave are allotted per year. In order to receive full pay, written documentation is required as to the nature of the illness. It will be each employee's responsibility to give the written documentation to Dr. Beeson or the office manager. Extra time off is not granted for illness during a vacation or on a holiday.

If not more than six (6) days of sick leave have been taken when the employee has completed three years of employment, the employee is granted an extra week of vacation. This extra week of vacation will only be available once every fourth year. Any sick leave taken must be recorded in the employee's record. Sick leave which exceeds the allotted amount will be regarded as time off without pay.

In the case of any absence, please notify the doctor as far in advance as possible, and each day of absence.

Maternity Leave of Absence

Regular full-time employees may be granted maternity leave of absence. However, if the employee has not returned to full employment within ten weeks, employment may be terminated at the discretion of the employer.

Medical Benefits

Full-time employees who have completed one month of employment are entitled to join the health insurance program of **Beeson Facial Plastic and Reconstructive Surgery** on the first day of the month following approval.

Employee families may be enrolled in the program in accordance with the rules and regulations of the insurance program. Family coverage is paid by the employee.

Medical Care

Each employee shall have a physician <u>other</u> than the physician in this office, in order that complete and objective treatment can be given without interference with the employer-employee relationship. If you have no family physician at present, we will be happy to suggest several to you.

Employees are encouraged to seek medical advice and treatment quite early at the onset of an illness or suspected illness to avoid the development of a more serious problem. Visits to a doctor other than in an emergency, shall be arranged through the office manager, and made at a time when Dr. Beeson is either out-of-town, or when no patients are scheduled.

Duties of Your Job

You position at **Beeson Facial Plastic and Reconstructive Surgery** is described by a summary of your main duties. Each summary is broad in its scope and is not intended to describe all that you do.

You will be expected to assume a variety of supportive responsibilities along with your main duties. These will be assigned as time and necessity determine.

In all cases, it is expected that each employee use his or her time to assist co-workers whenever possible. It is expected that this cooperation be carried out with a congenial attitude.

Salary Review

Three to six months after employment begin, Dr. Beeson will carefully review your performance in the various areas of responsibility included in your job. To the best of his ability, he will evaluate your performance and then discuss with you your strengths and weaknesses.

The Employee Performance Appraisal is designed to take a personal inventory of each employee's performance. The quality of work, quantity of work, job knowledge, cooperation, attitude, dependability, reliability, patient rapport, attendance, personal appearance, and other job-related skills will be evaluated in an objective manner.

If economic conditions an the quality of your work performance justify a salary increase, one may be given at this time. Similar salary review will be held at the end of one complete year of employment and each year thereafter, or when deemed appropriate by Dr. Beeson.

Personal Appearance and Cleanliness

Good grooming and an attractive appearance are especially important for health care personnel and for the overall impression of **Beeson Facial Plastic and Reconstructive Surgery**.

1. Dress: Attractive, well fitted, and non-offensive clothing should be worn in the office. Jeans, tennis shirts, or other casual sportswear are not appropriate office attire. White clinical lab coats may be worn by the nursing staff over their street attire.

2. Hair: Hair should be groomed and neat. Elaborate hairdos and beards are not appropriate.

3. Makeup: Makeup should not be obtrusive. If "touch-up" of makeup is needed during working hours, it should be attended to in the restroom.

4. Smoking: Smoking is prohibited in all areas of **Beeson Facial Plastic and Reconstructive Surgery**.

5. Eating and Drinking: Consumption of food and beverage is restricted to employee kitchen. Food and beverage should be consumed at time which will not interfere with your job responsibility.

6. Employee Kitchen/Lounge: Employee kitchen/lounge is to be maintained in a neat and clean manner by those who use it. All employees are expected to strictly adhere to this rule and to clean up appropriately after themselves.

7. Personal Activities: The standards of efficiency are necessarily very high for personnel in a medical office. There seldom are moments when all work is done. There is always some area of the office that needs cleaning, some stack of paper or photographs that need to be filed, and other work which should be attended to.

Outside Employment

Employees are expected to have employment with **Beeson Facial Plastic and Reconstructive Surgery** as their sole vocation. Additional or part-time employment is not allowed unless specifically approved by Dr. Beeson.

Confidential Information

Information about patients, their illnesses, or personal lives, must be dept completely confidential. When talking with the patient about any matter, it is essential that it be done in such a way as to prevent other patients from hearing such discussions.

Case histories, confidential papers, and appointment book should be kept in such a manner as to be out of view of the patients or other individuals visiting the office. Employees are not allowed to advise patients on personal matters. It is improper for us to reveal information on a patient even to another member of the patient's family (other than mother or father if the patient is a minor). If the patient asks questions about his or her own case, he or she should be referred to the doctor.

Information regarding office finances, salaries, and other personal office affairs are strictly confidential.

All business records of the employer shall be the sole and permanent property of **Beeson Facial Plastic and Reconstructive Surgery**. All other asset, including copies of those assets in the case of written material, shall remain within the premises of **Beeson Facial Plastic and Reconstructive Surgery** at all times.

The employee recognizes and acknowledges that, in the course of his or her employment, he or she will become acquainted with confidential information belonging to **Beeson Facial Plastic and Reconstructive Surgery** concerning business operations and that this information is a valuable, special, and unique asset of **Beeson Facial Plastic and**

Reconstructive Surgery. The employee will not, during or after the term of his or her employment, without the written consent of Dr. William Beeson, disclose this information to any person, firm, corporation, or association, or other entity for any reason or purpose whatsoever. All records, files, manuals, lists of patients, forms, materials, supplies, computer programs, lists of customers, and other materials furnished to the employee by the employer, used by the employee or generated or obtained by the employee during the course of their employment, shall be and remain the property of **Beeson Facial Plastic and Reconstructive Surgery**. The employee shall be deemed the bailee thereof for the use and benefit of **Beeson Facial Plastic and Reconstructive Surgery** and shall safely keep and preserve such property, except as consumed in the normal business operations of **Beeson Facial Plastic and Reconstructive Surgery**. Upon termination of employment, the employee shall immediately deliver to Dr. William Beeson all such property, including all copies, remaining in the employee's possession or control.

In the event of a breach or threatened breach by the employee of the aforenoted provisions, or of any other term of this agreement, the employer (**Beeson Facial Plastic and Reconstructive Surgery**) shall be entitled to an injunction restraining the employee from disclosing, in whole or in part, the information, or from rendering any services to any person, firm, corporation, association, or other entity to whom such information, in whole or in part, has been disclosed or has threatened to be disclosed, or from breaching the terms and conditions of this agreement. Nothing herein shall be construed as prohibiting **Beeson Facial Plastic and Reconstructive Surgery** from other remedies for such breach or threatened breach, including the recovery of damages from the employee. The employer shall be entitled to recover all costs incurred including reasonable attorney fees.

Non-Competitive Agreement

During the period of employment, the employee shall not undertake any service, except for the benefit of **Beeson Facial Plastic and Reconstructive Surgery**, unless Dr. William Beeson shall consent thereto, and shall not engage in any principle business or profession other than the rendition of services to the employer for and on behalf of the employer.

During the period of employment, the employee shall not undertake the planning or organization of any business activity competitive with the work he or she performs. The employees agrees that he or she will not, for a period of two (2) years following termination of his or her employment, directly or indirectly, solicit any of the employer's/employee's to work for the employee or any other competitive entity or person.

The employee agrees that for a period of two (2) years following termination of his or her employment with the employer, he or she will not directly or indirectly, as an employee, shareholder, or in any other capacity, become an employee of, invest in or otherwise become affiliated with any other facial plastic and reconstructive surgeon within a fifty (50) mile radius of any business location of the employer. The employee further agrees that during such two (2) year period, he or she will not, without the written consent of Dr. William Beeson, directly or indirectly, solicit or accept facial plastic and reconstructive surgery business from, or perform any of the services included within the employer's business for, any customer of the employer with whom he or she has had business or personal relations during the period of his or her employment with the employer.

It is the belief of the parties that the best protection which can be given to the employer and which does not in any way infringe upon the right of the employee to conduct any unrelated business is to provide for the restrictions described above. In the even that any of the said restrictions shall be held unenforceable by any court of competent jurisdiction, the party hereto agree and it is their desire that such court shall substitute a reasonable judicially enforceable restriction in place of any restriction deemed unenforceable and that as so modified, the restrictions shall be fully enforceable as if it had been set forth herein by the parties. In determining any restriction hereunder, it is the intent of the parties that the court recognize that the parties hereto desire that this agreement be imposed and maintained to the greatest extent possible.

In the even of a breach of these provisions, the employer shall be entitled to injunctive relief to protect his interests hereunder and in addition may recover its other losses, including damages. In the even the employer must enforce this agreement in court, the employee agrees to pay the reasonable attorney fees of the employer, including through the appellate process.

Travel

If the performance of your job requires that you drive (not commuting to or from home), the cost of your travel will be reimbursed by **Beeson Facial Plastic and Reconstructive Surgery**, based on generally accepted mileage costs. Toll fees and parking will be provided. The van owned by **Beeson Facial Plastic and Reconstructive Surgery** should be used as much as possible and should be used in preference of your personal vehicle.

Licensing and Certification

Nursing personnel must obtain certification in advanced cardiac life support within a time deemed appropriate by Dr. William Beeson in order to maintain and continue employment. All other employees must obtain basic cardiac life support within a time deemed appropriate by Dr. William Beeson in order to continue and maintain employment.

Bonding

All employees must be bondable by the bonding agency secured by **Beeson Facial Plastic and Reconstructive Surgery** in order to continue and maintain employment.

Civic Responsibility of Employees

When an employee is called for jury duty, his or her full salary will be paid by the doctor during the time of jury duty service for a maximum of two weeks. An amount will be subtracted, however, for all fees received by the employee from the government for jury duty. The employee will keep any payments received for transportation in connection with jury duty.

On election day, working hours will begin at 8:30 AM. Employees are expected to vote prior to beginning the work day.

Probation and Termination

It is understood that an employee is hired on a probationary status during the first ninety (90) days. During this period we shall try to determine whether the employee is adequately suited for employment in this office. (Not every individual fits easily in to the setting of a facial plastic surgery office, and yet might work perfectly and competently in some other kind of job). An employee having difficulty with some aspects of their work is expected to ask for assistance. If serious problems seem to exist at the end of ninety (90) days, a decision may be made to terminate employment.

If dismissal is necessary, either during or after the probationary period, the employee may be asked to work a period of two weeks before the termination point. In a few instances, however, severance pay may be given in the lieu of notice if the doctor feel it is desirable.

If an employee has committed a gross violation of rules, or has been dishonest, he or she will be discharged immediately without notice or severance pay.

If an employee decides to terminate his or her own employment, a written resignation at least fifteen (15) days prior to the resignation date shall be submitted. Employees who resign will be compensated for any accumulated vacation time due to them as noted in prior section.

Payment of an employee's final pay check will be withheld pending return of all keys and property of **Beeson Facial Plastic & Reconstructive Surgery**.

We recognize you as an employee have the right to terminate employment at will for any reason. This organization reserves the same right to dismiss employees at will.

Employee Physicals

Employment at **Beeson Facial Plastic & Reconstructive Surgery** requires successful completion of a pre-employment physical, which may include laboratory, x-ray, and physical examination. The results of the physical examination are confidential and will only be used to determine the candidate's ability to safely and efficiently perform the duties of the position for which they are being considered, without jeopardizing the health and recovery of patients.

Employee's Conduct

In all phases of human relations, certain rules and exceptional conduct must be observed. If rules are carefully defined and understood by all employees, the organization will maintain a high standard of patient care, cleanliness, and employee morals.

Employee misconduct, such as but not limited to the following, may result in disciplinary action.

1. Unexcused absences or tardiness.

2. Using obscene or abusive language towards employees or supervisors.

3. Reporting for duty in such condition as to be unable to perform work.

4. Violation of special office rules and regulations.

5. Violation of the rules regarding no soliciting or distribution of literature or merchandise to patients.

6. Any conduct, action, or lack thereof which would be in violation of Accreditation Association of Ambulatory Healthcare accreditation standards.

Gross misconduct will be cause for immediate discharge. Gross misconduct is defined as, but not necessarily limited to:

1. Mistreatment of patients, including neglect and using abusive language.

2. Violation of a patient's privacy by an unauthorized release of confidential information, such as the details of a patient's condition, either to employees not in the course of **Beeson Facial Plastic & Reconstructive Surgery** business, or to persons other than employees.

3. Stealing, or the unauthorized removal of property that belongs to **Beeson Facial Plastic & Reconstructive Surgery**, patients, visitors, or fellow employees.

4. Unauthorized handling, possession, or use of drugs, including marijuana and alcoholic beverages on office premises, or reporting to work under the influence of intoxicants or narcotics.

5. Deliberate destruction of property that belongs to **Beeson Facial Plastic & Reconstructive Surgery**, patients, visitors, or fellow employees.

6. Forging, altering, or deliberately falsifying any document, authorization, or record that is to be used by **Beeson Facial Plastic & Reconstructive Surgery**.

Complaints and Questions

Any employee who has questions concerning the matters outlined in our Policies and Procedures Manual should submit them in writing. An appointment time shall then be set for discussion with Dr. William Beeson at an appropriate time.

Problems should not be discussed among employees while at work. Should an employee become unhappy or dissatisfied with a particular situation, he or she should speak with his or her supervisor or Dr. William Beeson.

Suggestions

Suggestions and criticisms which will lead to improvement in achieving our goals and objective are to be encouraged. Consideration will be given to every concern by Dr. William Beeson.

As an employee of **Beeson Facial Plastic & Reconstructive Surgery**, I have read, understand, and agree to abide by the foregoing policies and procedures of this office.

_____   _____
(Date)   (Signature of Employee)

_____
(Witness)

_____
William H. Beeson, M.D.
(Employer)

DATE:_____

PERSONAL:

Name_____ Social Security No._____
      (Last)   (First)   (M.I.)

Present Address_____
               No.   Street   City   State   Zip

How many years have you lived at this address?_____Telephone No. (   )_____

Previous address_____How long?_____
                No.   Street   City   State   Zip

Job(s) applied for 1._____Rate of pay expected_____

                   2._____Rate of pay expected_____

How did you learn of this opening?_____

Do you want to work _____Full time or_____Part time. Specify days and hours
if part time_____

Have you worked for us before?_____If so, when?_____

List any friends or relatives working for us_____

If hired, on what date will you be available to start work?_____

Are there any other experiences, skills, or qualifications which you feel would especially
fit you for work with this Clinic_____
_____
_____

If hired, do you have a reliable means of transportation to get to work?_____

Do you have any physical handicaps which would prevent you from performing specific kinds
of work?_____If yes, describe the defect(s) and explain the work limitations__
_____

Have you had a serious illness in the past 5 years?_____No_____Yes (describe)
_____

Have you ever received compensation for injuries?_____No_____Yes (explain)_____
_____

Have you ever been <u>convicted</u> of a crime, excluding misdemeanors and summary offenses?
_____No _____Yes (describe in full)_____
_____

Person to be notified in case of accident or emergency
Name_____Phone Number_____
Address_____

EDUCATIONAL BACKGROUND

TYPE OF SCHOOL	NAME & ADDRESS	YEARS ATTENDED	GRADUATED	COURSE/MAJOR
GRAMMAR OR GRADE				
HIGH SCHOOL				
COLLEGE				
POST GRADUATE				
BUSINESS OR TRADE				
OTHER				

MILITARY SERVICE RECORD

Have you ever served in the armed forces?_____ If yes, what branch?_____

Dates of duty: From_____ To_____ Rank at discharge_____

What were your duties in the service (include special training and duty station)?_____

_____

Have you had any schooling under the G.I. Bill of Rights?_____ If yes, describe_____

_____

Are you over 21 years of age?_____

Birthdate_____
       Month   Day   Year

How old are you?_____

Sex:_____ Male _____ Female

Height_____ ft. _____ in.

Weight_____ lbs.

Marital status_____ Single _____ Engaged _____ Married _____ Separated _____ Divorced
                _____ Widowed

When were you married?_____
                      Month   Day   Year

How many dependents do you have (including yourself)?_____

Are you a United States citizen?_____

Have you registered for the draft?_____

What is your Selective Service classification?_____

Please tell us when you attended school.

    Elementary...From_____ to_____

    High School...From_____ to_____

    College...From_____ to_____

    Other...From_____ to_____

Have you ever been bonded?_____ If yes, for what job?_____

REFERENCES

(Excluding former employers or relatives)

Name and Occupation	Address	Phone Number
1.		
2.		
3.		

PRIOR WORK HISTORY (LIST IN ORDER, LAST OR PRESENT EMPLOYER FIRST)

DATES FROM	TO	NAME & ADDRESS OF EMPLOYER	RATE OF PAY START	FINISH	SUPERVISOR'S NAME AND TITLE	REASON FOR LEAVING

Describe in detail the work you did.

DATES FROM	TO	NAME & ADDRESS OF EMPLOYER	RATE OF PAY START	FINISH	SUPERVISOR'S NAME AND TITLE	REASON FOR LEAVING

Describe in detail the work you did.

DATES FROM	TO	NAME & ADDRESS OF EMPLOYER	RATE OF PAY START	FINISH	SUPERVISOR'S NAME AND TITLE	REASON FOR LEAVING

Describe in detail the work you did.

May we contact the employers listed above?_____ If not, which one(s) you do not wish us to contact_____

Occasionally the form of an application blank makes it difficult for an individual to adequately summarize his complete background. To assist us in finding the proper position for you in this Clinic, use the space below to summarize and additional information necessary to describe your full qualifications.

Thank you for completing this application form and for your interest in employment with us. We would like to assure you that your opportunity for employment with us will be based only on your merit and on no other considerations.

PLEASE READ CAREFULLY

APPLICANT'S CERTIFICATION AND AGREEMENT

I hereby certify that the facts set forth in the above employment application are true and complete to the best of my knowledge. I understand that if employed, falsified statements on this application shall be considered sufficient cause for dismissal. You are hereby authorized to make any investigation of my personal history and financial and credit record through and investigative or credit agencies or bureaus of your choice.

Signature of Applicant_____

DO NOT WRITE BELOW THIS LINE

Interview:_____Yes _____No   Date:_____Hour_____

Result of interview_____
_____
_____

Acceptable for employment?_____Starting rate_____Starting date_____Shift_____

Occupation_____Dept_____Clock No._____

Interviewed by_____Employed by_____
_____Approved by_____

CORRECTIVE ACTION NOTIFICATION

EMPLOYEE NAME _____ DATE _____

Action Taken

_____ 1st Formal Counseling Session
_____ 2nd Formal Counseling Session
_____ 3rd Formal Counseling Session
_____ Suspension for _____ days
                         1–15
         from _____ to _____ inclusive
_____ These actions require notification of automatic disciplinary probation for _____ months from _____ to _____

Previous Action Taken

	DATE	ACTION	REASON
1.	_____	_____	_____
2.	_____	_____	_____
3.	_____	_____	_____

Cause for Present Action Being Taken

(Be specific: Date, Time, Location, Witness(es), etc.)
_____
_____
_____

Required Improvement Goals for Employee

1. _____
2. _____
3. _____

_____   _____   _____
Signature of Person Initiating   Title   Date
       Form

_____   _____
William Beeson, M.D.   Date

Appendix 7: Patient Care Forms

Date _____

Name _____   Date of Birth _____

Address _____   Home Number _____
        _____   (May we contact you at this number?)

City _____ State _____ Zip Code _____

EMPLOYMENT INFORMATION

Name of Employer _____   Position _____

Business Telephone Number _____
(May we contact you at this number?)

RESPONSIBLE PARTY INFORMATION

Responsible Party _____   Relationship _____

Address _____   Telephone _____

REFERRAL INFORMATION

How did you hear of Dr. Gilmore? (Please give name)

Friend _____   Patient _____   M.D. _____

May we send a thank you note? _____

Please give address _____

Please check any of the following sources from which you may have heard of Dr. Gilmore:

Magazine Advertising   _____   Office Contact: Staff or Brochure _____
News Publications   _____   Radio Interview   _____
Television Interviews   _____   Staff Speaking Engagement   _____
Imager Presentation   _____   Dr. Gilmore Speaking Engagement   _____
Dallas Institute of Cosmetic Surgery _____
Other (Please specify) _____

EMERGENCY INFORMATION

Please provide a name and telephone number of someone we could reach in case of an emergency.

Name _____   Telephone _____

Relationship _____

SURGICAL FEE AGREEMENT

PROPOSED SURGICAL PROCEDURE(S) _____

_____

THE FEE FOR THE ABOVE-MENTIONED PROCEDURE(S) IS $_____. THIS FEE WILL REMAIN AS SUCH FOR ONE (1) YEAR FROM THE SIGNING OF THIS AGREEMENT. SHOULD YOU DECIDE NOT TO HAVE SURGERY UNTIL AFTER THAT DATE, ANOTHER CONSULTATION WILL BE REQUIRED AND THE FEE MAY BE CHANGED.

OUR POLICY FOR THIS TYPE OF SURGERY IS TO REQUIRE THAT THESE CHARGES BE PAID AT LEAST TWO WEEKS IN ADVANCE OF THE DATE OF SURGERY. SHOULD YOU HAVE INSURANCE, WE SHALL BE HAPPY TO COMPLETE THE NECESSARY FORMS FOR YOU AFTER SURGERY. IF YOUR INSURANCE COMPANY MAKES AN ALLOWANCE FOR YOUR SURGERY WE WILL REIMBURSE THE AMOUNT OF PAYMENT UP TO THE AMOUNT NOTED ABOVE.

I UNDERSTAND AND AGREE TO THE ABOVE.

DATE:_____ SIGNED:_____

WITNESSED:_____

PATIENT NAME _____ CHART NUMBER _____
PROPOSED SURGERY _____ DATE _____
PRE-OP APPOINTMENT _____
PLACE OF SURGERY _____ TIME _____
TIME PATIENT IS TO BE AT OFFICE/HOSPITAL _____
POST OPERATIVE ACCOMMODATIONS _____

PRESCRIPTIONS   ALLERGIES _____
    ___ AMPICILLIN   ___ COMPAZINE SUPPOSITORY
    ___ TETRACYCLINE   ___ NOVAFED
    ___ KEFLEX   ___ VALIUM
    ___ DARVOCET N 100   ___ OTHER _____
    ___ PERCOCET   ___ OTHER _____
    ___ TYLENOL #4   ___ OTHER _____

LABS
    ___ CBC   ___ PTT   DATE OF MOST CURRENT LABS ON CHART _____
    ___ SMA 12   ___ BETA SUB   DATE REQUEST WAS GIVEN _____
    ___ PT   ___ U/A   PLACE LABS DRAWN _____
                                 DATE LABS DRAWN _____

CURRENT EKG ON CHART _____
CURRENT EYE EVALUATION ON CHART _____
CURRENT OPTHALMOLOGY EXAM: DATE _____ DOCTOR _____
CONSENT SIGNED: BEESON FACIAL _____ HOSPITAL _____
PREOPERATIVE PHOTOS/SLIDES: DATE TAKEN _____ BY WHOM _____
HAS FEE BEEN RECEIVED: AMOUNT PAID _____ DATE PAID _____

HOSPITAL SCHEDULING
    DATE SCHEDULED WITH HOSPITAL _____ SPOKE WITH _____
    TIME REQUESTED _____ LENGTH OF PROCEDURE _____
    TYPE OF ANESTHESIA _____ IN/OUT PATIENT _____
    WAS CASE PLACED ON WAIT LIST _____ IF YES, WHAT NUMBER ARE WE _____
    RN WHO SCHEDULED SURGERY _____
    IF INPATIENT: DATE ADMITTING CALLED _____ SPOKE WITH _____
    TYPE OF ACCOMMODATIONS _____ RN INITIALS _____
    NOTES _____
    _____
    _____

INSURANCE PRECERTIFICATION
    NAME OF INSURANCE COMPANY _____
    TELEPHONE # _____ SPOKE WITH _____
    HE/SHE STATES _____
    _____
                                                                   RN INITALS _____
    IS SECOND OPINION REQUIRED _____
    NOTES _____
    _____
    _____

SITTING SERVICE
    AGENCY _____ SPOKE WITH _____ DATE _____
    DATE AND TIME OF COVERAGE _____
    PLACE OF SERVICE _____ RN INITIALS _____
    NOTES _____
    _____
    _____

Beeson Facial Surgery
Treatment Record

Name _____ Age _____ Date _____ Chart # _____

    Consent signed _____   Face washed _____

    Photo taken _____   Questions answered _____

Allergies _____ Medication _____

Temp _____ BP _____ Pulse _____ Resp _____

Hx: _____
_____

P.E.   Normal   Abnormal

    Head   _____   _____   _____

    Eyes   _____   _____   _____

    Ears   _____   _____   _____

    Nose   _____   _____   _____

    Mouth   _____   _____   _____

    Neck   _____   _____   _____

    Chest   _____   _____   _____

    Cardiac   _____   _____   _____

    ABD   _____   _____   _____

    EXT   _____   _____   _____

    Neuro   _____   _____   _____

Pre-Op Dx: _____ Procedure: _____

Post-Op Dx: _____ Surgeon: _____

Condition: _____ Comp: _____

Start Time _____   Finish Time _____

    Time   Medication

    _____   _____

    _____   _____

    _____   _____

    _____   _____

Post-Op instructions given verbally _____ All questions answered _____

Post-Op sheets given _____

RX given:

- _____ Tylenol #4
- _____ Pecocet
- _____ Darvocet
- _____ Novafed
- _____ ¼% E Sol
- _____ Seldane
- _____ Ampicillin
- _____ Tetracycline
- _____ Keflex
- _____ Zovirax Pills
- _____ Zovirax Ointment
- _____ Hytone 1%
- _____ Hytone 2½%
- _____ Westcort
- _____ Retin-A

Other _____

Return Appointment _____ Released to: _____

BP _____ Pulse _____ Resp _____ Time _____

Path Specimen labeled and recorded in book _____

Charge Slip filed _____

Nurse _____

Doctor _____

Beeson Facial Plastic and Reconstructive Surgery
8803 North Meridian Street
Indianapolis, Indiana 46260

Name_____ Date of Birth_____ Today's Date_____

Address: Home_____
                street   city   state   zip   telephone

        Business_____
                street   city   state   zip   telephone

Marital Status: S, M, D, Sep. Occupation_____ Ages of Children_____

How were you referred to us?_____

In which surgical procedure(s) are you interested? (please circle)

    Rhinoplasty (nose)................... Chin................... Face or Neck Lift.................... Eyelids...................

    Chemical Peel.................... Dermabrasion................... Scar Revision................... Protruding Ears..................

    Removal of Cysts, Warts, Moles, Etc..................... Hair Transplantation.................... Other...................

What **specifically** do you wish to have corrected: (i.e. what don't you like about the above condition(s)?)_____
_____

When did you begin to consider surgical correction?_____

Why have you decided to have it done at this point in time?_____

Have you consulted any other doctor about this? (when?)_____
Have you discussed this surgery with your family? **Yes No**   Are they agreeable? **Yes No**

Have you had any previous cosmetic surgery? **Yes No**   When, and what, if anything was done?_____
_____

        Who performed the surgery?_____ Where was it performed?_____

        Were you satisfied with the results?_____ If not, why?_____

Have you had **any** other surgery, or an **injury,** to the face, nose, neck or eyes?_____

    When?_____ Describe, as best you can_____

Has anyone in your family or a close friend had cosmetic or reconstructive surgery?_____

    What was done?_____ By whom?_____

Have you had **any other** prior surgery? (What was done & when was it performed?) In the head & neck area?_____, On

your skin?_____, On your teeth or gums?_____, In your chest?_____, In your abdomen?_____,

On the reproductive system?_____, On your back, arms, or legs?_____ Were there any complications?
_____

        Did you have a normal recovery?_____

        Were you satisfied with the results?_____ If not why?_____

                            MEDICAL HISTORY   (circle appropriate response)

No   Yes   Are you now taking **any** drugs or medications? (How Often?)
                List them if you can_____

No   Yes   Are you allergic to any medications?
                List them if you can_____

When was your last physical examination?_____

Who is your family doctor?_____ Address_____

No   Yes   Would you object to our contacting him in regard to any medical problem that might arise?

No	Yes	Have you ever received local anesthesia ("Novacaine or Xylocaine") by a dentist or doctor? (circle appropriate response)
No	Yes	Did you have any "reaction" to the anesthesia? Explain _____
No	Yes	Are you considered a healthy person?
No	Yes	Do you take vitamins regularly?

Do you or any family members have: (indicate who)
Heart trouble_____ Excessive bleeding tendencies_____ Tuberculosis_____
High blood pressure_____ Diabetes_____ Psychiatric or "nerve" problems_____
Excessive bruisability_____ Thyroid problems_____ Excessive scarring_____

Do you have any history of bleeding:
From the nose_____ In the urine_____ Vomiting blood_____
From the rectum_____ Coughing up blood_____ Other?_____

No	Yes	Do you have hay fever, nasal allergies or asthma? Explain _____
No	Yes	Do you have or have you had any problems with your eyes? Explain _____
No	Yes	Do you have frequent pains in the chest?
No	Yes	Has a doctor ever said you had "heart trouble?" Explain _____
No	Yes	Do you have "stomach trouble" or ulcers? Explain _____
No	Yes	Do you have or have you had chest or lung problems? Explain _____
No	Yes	Have you ever had liver, gall bladder trouble, hepatitis or "yellow jaundice"? (circle which one)
No	Yes	Do you or any family member suffer from arthritis?
No	Yes	Have you ever received x-ray (radiation) "treatments" to any area in the head and neck?
No	Yes	Do you have frequent skin infections, irritations or rashes (circle which one)
No	Yes	Have you in the past or do you currently use steroid (cortisone) creams frequently?
No	Yes	Do you ever have "cold sores" or fever blisters?
No	Yes	Do you often have severe headaches or dizzy spells? (circle which one)
No	Yes	Has any part of your body ever been paralyzed or numb? Explain _____
No	Yes	Did you ever have a convulsion or seizure?
No	Yes	Have you ever received treatment for your genital area? Explain _____
No	Yes	Were you ever treated for any venereal disease?
No	Yes	Are you frequently sick or ill?
No	Yes	Do you worry about your health?
No	Yes	Were you ever treated for anemia or any problems with your blood? Explain _____
No	Yes	Have you ever taken hormones or thyroid medication? (circle which one)
No	Yes	Do you smoke more than 10 cigarettes a day?
No	Yes	Do you drink more than 6 cups of coffee a day?
No	Yes	Do you usually take two or more alcoholic drinks a day?
No	Yes	Do you often get depressed?
No	Yes	Do you usually feel unhappy or depressed?
No	Yes	Does criticism always upset you?
No	Yes	Are you considered a nervous person?
No	Yes	Did you ever have a "nervous breakdown"?
No	Yes	Have you ever received medical treatment for a "nervous condition"?
No	Yes	Are you easily upset or irritated?
No	Yes	Do you tend to hold a "grudge" when someone angers you?
No	Yes	Have you ever considered consulting a psychiatrist?
No	Yes	Have you ever been under the care of a psychiatrist or psychologist? Explain _____
		Women Only: When was your last menstrual period?
No	Yes	Are your periods often irregular?
No	Yes	Have you had "female" or GYN problems? Explain _____
No	Yes	**Men Only:** Have you ever had prostate problems?
No	Yes	Do you have any other medical problems that have not been covered?

Explain _____

Signed _____ Date_____

Thank you,
  The information you have provided us is essential in our comprehensive evaluation in your case. Please read the consultation booklet and write down any questions you may have so that we may discuss them in detail during your consultation period. If you do not have the booklet please ask for one.

William H. Beeson, M.D.

Beeson Facial Surgery
Pre-Operative History and Physical Exam

Date _____
Name _____
Marital Status: Single   Married   Widowed   Divorced   Separated
Age _____
Sex _____
Race _____
Date of Birth _____
Occupation _____

CHECK THE FOLLOWING:

YES	NO	
___	___	Any questions
___	___	Read consultation book
___	___	Read post-operative book

FAMILY HISTORY   AGE   MEDICAL PROBLEMS
Father _____
Mother _____
Brothers _____
Sisters _____

YES	NO	
___	___	Any family history for problems with anesthetics?
___	___	Any family history for bleeding disorders?
___	___	Any family history for hypertension?
___	___	Any family history for glaucoma or eye diseases?
___	___	Any family history for hyperthermia?

PAST MEDICAL HISTORY
Prescription Medications:

NAME	DOSAGE	FREQUENCY
_____	_____	_____
_____	_____	_____
_____	_____	_____

Over the Counter Medications: (Aspirin, Contact, Vitamins, etc.)
_____
_____
_____

Allergies:
_____
_____
_____

Last Tetanus Shot: Date _____

PRIOR HOSPITALIZATION FOR MEDICAL REASONS

DATE	PROBLEM	HOSPITAL
_____	_____	_____
_____	_____	_____
_____	_____	_____
_____	_____	_____

PRIOR SURGERIES

PROCEDURE	DATE
_____	_____
_____	_____
_____	_____

Name of personal physician _____
Date last seen _____
Reason seen _____
Ophthalmologic Exam _____
Ophthalmologist _____ Date _____
Do you smoke? _____ Packs per day? _____ How long? _____
Alcohol (How many drinks per day/week?) _____

HISTORY OF PRESENT PROBLEM
Chief complaint (what bothers patient the most and any functional problem?)
_____
_____
_____
_____
_____

REVIEW OF SYSTEMS

YES	NO	

SCALP:
___ ___ Any history of scalp problems requiring medical treatment? (severe dandruff, psoriasis, etc.)

SKIN:
___ ___ Any history of cuts to face/neck area requiring stitches?
___ ___ Any history of facial fractures or severe trauma to face or neck?
___ ___ Any history of skin problems? (hives, rashes, psoriasis, eczema, dermatitis)
___ ___ Have you ever been on Accutane or had x-ray treatments to face for acne?
___ ___ Ever had collagen or silicone injections in face?
___ ___ Do you bruise easily or take aspirin or vitamin E?
___ ___ Any history of blood clotting problems?
___ ___ Any history of anemia?

EYE:
___ ___ Any history of glaucoma?
___ ___ History of eye diseases or eye injuries?
___ ___ History of chalazia or stye or other eye infections within the past five years?
___ ___ Wear contacts or glasses?
___ ___ Any problems with dry eyes?
___ ___ History of problems with allergies affecting eyes?
___ ___ Date of last eye exam? _____

NOSE:
___ ___ History of prior injury to nose?
___ ___ History of frequent nose bleeds?
___ ___ History of chronic congestion?
___ ___ History of sinus problems?
___ ___ History of inhalation allergies?
___ ___ History of prior nasal surgery?

MOUTH:
___ ___ Wear dentures or have partial plate?
___ ___ Have cracked, broken or loose teeth?
___ ___ History of TMJ problems?
___ ___ Problems with occlusion?
___ ___ Problems with sores or ulcers in mouth?
___ ___ History of fever blisters or cold sores?

NECK:
___ ___ History of thyroid problems?
___ ___ History of neck pain?
___ ___ History of "whip-lash" to neck or other trauma?

CHEST:
___ ___ History of bronchitis or pneumonia?
___ ___ Shortness of breath with exertion?
___ ___ Smoking history?
___ ___ History of T.B.?
___ ___ History of emphysema?
___ ___ Problem with asthma?
   Last episode: _____
   Last time had to be treated by doctor? _____
   Last time hospitalized? _____

CARDIAC:
___ ___ History of heart murmur?
___ ___ History of heart disease?
___ ___ History of hypertension?
___ ___ History of chest pain?
___ ___ Must sleep elevated?
___ ___ Has swelling in legs/ankles?

YES	NO	
		ABDOMEN:
___	___	History of ulcer disease?
___	___	History of hepatitis?
___	___	History of G.I. problems such as pancreatitis, diverticulosis, or colitis?
___	___	History of diabetes?
___	___	History of hernia?
___	___	History of hemorrhoids?
		GYN:
___	___	Any history of gyn problems? (remember to check surgery list - hysterectomy, etc.)
___	___	History of irregular periods?
___	___	Is there any chance you could be pregnant?
		Last menstrual period? _____
		G.U.:
___	___	History of genito-urinary problems?
___	___	History of prostate problems?
___	___	History of kidney stones/frequent kidney infections?
		NEUROLOGICAL:
___	___	History of seizures/epilepsy?
___	___	History of migraine headaches?
___	___	History of stroke?
___	___	History of numbness to extremities?
___	___	History of prior head injury?
___	___	History of nervous breakdown in past?
___	___	Are you seeing a psychiatrist or psychologist presently? If so, who? _____
___	___	History of facial paralysis (Bell's palsy) When? _____ How long did it last? _____ What percent of recovery? _____ Which side of face was affected? _____
___	___	History of other neurological problems? (describe) _____

PHYSICAL EXAM

_____ Blood Pressure   _____ Respirations
_____ Temperature   _____ Weight
_____ Pulse   _____ Height

	NORMAL	ABNORMAL	REMARKS
Head:	☐	☐	
Eyes:	☐	☐	
Nose:	☐	☐	
Mouth:	☐	☐	
Neck:	☐	☐	
Skin:	☐	☐	
Chest:	☐	☐	
Cardiac:	☐	☐	
Abdomen:	☐	☐	
Neuro:	☐	☐	

POST-OPERATIVE CARE REVIEW
1. Need for responsible adult to stay first night.
2. Need for ice compresses to be applied.
3. Activity restrictions.
4. Medication directions.
5. Post-operative instructions:
   —wound care
   —activity restrictions
   —how to reach us in an emergency
   —always call or come in if any questions or concerns
   —how and when to take medications

SITTER
☐ Sitter Needed
Hours: _____
Date(s): _____
☐ Sitting service not needed (indicate who will stay with patient)
_____

SURGERY SCHEDULED
PROCEDURE: (circle)

FL	Bleph	FH	Brown lift	NSR
H.T.	SML	MLI	Mentoplasty	Otoplasty
Peel	D.B.	Scar Revision	Scalp Reduction	

PLACE: (circle one)
Office   Riverview
St. Vincent's (86th)
St. Vincent's (Carmel)
ASI
Methodist
Community North
Date: _____
Anesthesia (circle one)   LSB   GEN   Our anesthetic
Time to arrive at office _____
Time to take medications _____

PATIENT REVIEW
YES	NO	
___	___	Have you read the consultation book?
___	___	Reviewed post-operative instructions with patient/told to read booklet also?
___	___	Do you have any questions?
___	___	Do you feel Dr. Beeson has explained the treatment, the options, the risks of surgery, and the post-operative care to your satisfaction? Initial _____

CHECK LIST
Eye sheet completed (plus visual acuity) _____
Ophthalmologic exam completed/dated _____
Prescriptions given, Meds. Dispensed (circle which ones)
Tylenol #4   Ampicillin   Novafed
Percocet   Keflex
Darvocet   Tetracycline
Vitamins   Erythromycin
Tigan   Zovirax Pills
Valium   Zovirax Ointment

YES	NO	
___	___	Post-operative instruction booklets given?
___	___	Pre-operative sheets given?
___	___	Consent form signed?
___	___	Supply list given?
___	___	Supply pack given?
___	___	EKG obtained?
___	___	Labs drawn? SMA-12 CBC U/A PT PTT UA BETA-SUB
___	___	Outside labs received?
___	___	Outside EKG received?
		Photos:
___	___	Slides checked
___	___	Prints checked

Insurance numbers (if applicable) _____
Insurance company number _____
Name of insured _____
Fee paid _____   Amount _____
Cash _____   Check _____   Visa _____

Nurse _____
Date _____   Time _____
Doctor _____

TO THE PATIENT: You have the right, as a patient, to be informed about your condition and the recommended surgical, medical, or diagnostic procedure to be used so that you may make the decision whether or not to undergo the procedure after knowing the risks and hazards involved. This disclosure is not meant to scare or alarm you; it is simply an effort to make you better informed so you may give or withhold your consent to the procedure.

I voluntarily request Dr. Howard A. Tobin as my physician, the staff of the Facial Plastic & Cosmetic Surgical Center, and such associates, technical assistants, and other health care providers as they deem necessary, to carry out the following surgery:

_____

_____

I understand that Dr. Tobin may discover other or different conditions which require additional or different procedures than those planned. I authorize him, and such associates, technical assistants, and other health care providers to perform such other procedures which are advisable in their professional judgment.

I consent to the use of blood and blood products as deemed necessary.

I understand that no warranty or guarantee has been made to me as to result or cure.

I understand that external incisions may leave scars that are visable. The location of these incisions have been described to me. I realize that occasionally, scars may have to be revised because of unsatisfactory appearance.

Just as there may be risks and hazards in continuing my present condition without treatment, there are also risks and hazards related to the performance of the surgical procedures planned for me. I realize that common to surgical procedures is the potential for infection, blood clots in veins and lungs, hemorrhage, allergic reactions, and even death. I also realize that the following risks and hazards may occur in connection with this procedure: Unsatisfactory appearance, poor healing, skin loss, nerve damage, painful or unattractive scarring, impairment of organs such as eye or lip function.

I also realize that the following additional risks and hazards may occur in connection with the following procedures:

Dermabrasion or Chemical Peel: Pigment changes in the skin.

Breast Augmentation: Leakage from the implant may occur and require replacement. Bleeding or infection may require removal of the implant. Although every attempt will be made to make both breasts exactly the same following surgery, their appearance may not be identical in size or shape. Breast implants may wrinkle, and the wrinkles could be palpable or even visible in cases where there is a limited amount of breast tissue to cover the implant. Numbness of parts of the breasts and nipples can occur, and although usually temporary, it can be long lasting or permanent. Fibrous tissue may cause unnatural firmness around the implants and this could require further surgery or removal of the implants. Breast feeding may not be possible after surgery. Polyurethane covered implants may be used. Although present evidence indicates that these implants are as safe as conventional silicone implants, they have not been used with the same frequency and for the same length of time as conventional silicone implants. This has been discussed with me._____

(pt's initials)

Liposuction Surgery: Indentation, waviness or unsatisfactory contouring may result.

Nasal Surgery: Deformity of skin, bone or cartilage, perforation of the nasal septum, breathing obstruction, recurrence or worsening of the condition may occur. Additional surgery may be required for correction.

Breast Elevation or Reduction: The breasts may be of different size or shape. There may be numbness of the breast or nipple which could be permanent. There may be loss of all or part of the nipple. Breast feeding may not be possible after surgery. Further surgery may be needed in the future.

Other risks include: _____

_____

THIS PARAGRAPH PERTAINS TO SMOKERS - Smokers are recognized to have a significantly higher risk of post operative wound healing problems as well as operative and post operative bleeding. Patients should discontinue smoking for two weeks after surgery. Although it helps to stop smoking for several weeks before and after surgery, this does not eliminate the increased risk resulting from long term smoking.

I understand that anesthesia involves additional risks and hazards but I request the use of anesthetics for the relief and protection from pain during the planned and additional procedures. I realize the anesthesia may have to be changed possibly without explanation to me .

I understand that certain complications may result from the use of any anesthetic including respiratory problems, drug reaction, paralysis, brain damage, or even death. Other risks and hazards which may result from the use of general anesthetics range from minor discomfort to injury to vocal cords, teeth, or eyes.

THIS PARAGRAPH PERTAINS TO FEMALE PATIENTS ONLY - Anesthetic agents can be harmful to the fetus of a pregnant woman. General anesthesia should be avoided during pregnancy whenever possible. I hereby state that I am not pregnant and accept the responsibility of making this determination.

I hereby give permission to Dr. Tobin or any assistant he may designate to take photographs for diagnostic purposes and to enhance the medical record. I agree that these photographs will remain his property and he may use them for medical, scientific or other presentations and publications.

I have been given an opportunity to ask questions about my condition, alternative forms of anesthesia and treatment, risks of nontreatment, the procedures to be used, and the risks and hazards involved, and I believe that I have sufficient information to give this informed consent.

{ } If initialed, I have been told that a medical grade synthetic implant may be used in the above mentioned operation and have been advised of the risks as well as alternative methods of treatment. I understand that on occasion, implants are rejected by the body.

I certify that Dr. Tobin has discussed the operation with me to my satisfaction, this form has been fully explained to me, that I have read it or have had it read to me, that the blank spaces have been filled in, and that I understand its contents.

I certify that I have read and filled out the patient registration and medical history form fully and correctly to the best of my knowledge, and that the information that I have supplied is complete and correct.

I agree to follow the instructions given to me by Dr. Tobin to the best of my ability before, during and after the above mentioned surgical procedure, and will notify Dr. Tobin of any problems following my surgery.

DO NOT SIGN THIS FORM UNLESS YOU HAVE READ IT AND FEEL THAT YOU UNDERSTAND IT. ASK ANY QUESTIONS YOU MIGHT HAVE BEFORE SIGNING.

_____
PATIENT OR OTHER LEGALLY RESPONSIBLE PERSON SIGN

_____
WITNESS:

DATE: _____ TIME: _____ A.M./P.M.

CONSULTATION AND MEDICAL QUESTIONNAIRE

Name _____ Date of Birth _____ Today's Date _____

Address: Home _____
                 STREET   CITY   STATE   ZIP

Address: Business _____
                     STREET   CITY   STATE   ZIP

Marital Status: S, M, D. Sep. Occupation _____ Ages of Children _____

How were you referred to us? _____

In which surgical procedure(s) are you interested? (please circle)
    Rhinoplasty (nose)   Chin   Face or Neck Lift   Eyelids   Chemical Peel   Dermabrasion   Scar Revision
    Protruding Ears   Removal of Cysts, Warts, Moles, Etc.   Hair Transplantation   Collagen Injection   Liposuction
    Other _____

What **specifically** do you wish to have corrected: (i.e. what don't you like about the above condition(s)? _____

When did you begin to consider surgical correction? _____
Is having surgery your idea or is it someone else's idea? _____
Why have you decided to have it done at this point in time? _____
Have you consulted any other doctor about this? (when?) _____
Have you discussed this surgery with your family? Yes / No   Are they agreeable Yes / No
Do you understand that the object of any cosmetic operation is improvement in appearance, not perfection? Yes / No
Are you aware that the results of the operation might not fully meet your expectations? Yes / No
Have you had any previous cosmetic surgery? Yes / No.   When, and what was done?

    Who performed the surgery? _____ Where was it performed? _____
    Were you satisfied with the results? _____ If not, why? _____
Have you had **any** other surgery, or an **injury,** to the face, nose, neck or eyes? _____
    When? _____ Describe, as best as you can _____
Has anyone in your family or a close friend had cosmetic or reconstructive surgery? _____
    What was done? _____ By whom? _____
Have you had **any** prior surgery? (what was done?): On your skin? _____, On your teeth or gums? _____,
    In the head & neck area? _____, In your chest? _____, In your abdomen? _____, On the reproductive
    system? _____, On your back, arms, or legs? _____, Were there any complications? _____
Did you have a normal recovery? _____
Were you satisfied with the results? _____ If not, why? _____
Have you ever been dissatisfied with the treatment you received from a doctor or dentist?   Yes / No

MEDICAL HISTORY (Circle apppropriate response)

No Yes Are you now taking **any** drugs or medications?
            How Often? _____
            List them if you can _____
No Yes Do you take aspirin or any aspirin containing medications?
No Yes Are you allergic to any medications?
            List them if you can _____

Who is your family doctor? _____
Address _____
No Yes Would you object to our contacting him in regard to any medical problem that might arise?
            When was your last physical examination?
            _____
No Yes Was eveything O.K.?

No Yes Have you ever received local anesthesia ("Novocaine or Xylocaine" by a dentist or doctor)?
No Yes Did you have any "reaction" to the anesthesia?
No Yes Are you considered a healthy person?
No Yes Do you take vitamins regularly?
No Yes Do you suffer with recurring fever blisters?

Do you or any family members have:
(circle if yes and indicate who)

Heart trouble _____
High blood pressure _____
Excessive bruisability _____
Excessive bleeding tendencies _____
Diabetes _____
Thyroid problems _____
Tuberculosis _____
Psychiatric or "nerve" problems _____
Excessive scarring _____

Do you have any history of bleeding: (circle if answer yes)
From the nose   In the urine
Vomiting blood   From the rectum
Coughing up blood
Other _____

No Yes Do your cuts bleed longer than those other people have?
No Yes Have you ever had any bleeding episode that required the attention of a doctor?
No Yes Have you ever had excessive bleeding on more than one occasion?
No Yes Do you have hay fever or asthma?(circle which one)
No Yes Do you have frequent pains in the chest?
No Yes Has a doctor ever said you had "heart trouble?"
No Yes Do you have "stomach trouble" or ulcers?
No Yes Have you ever had liver, gall bladder trouble or "yellow jaundice?" (circle which one)
No Yes Do you or any family members suffer from arthritis?
No Yes Do you have frequent skin infections, irritations or rashes? (circle which one)
No Yes Do you often have severe headaches or dizzy spells? (circle which one)
No Yes Has any part of your body ever been paralyzed or numb?
No Yes Did you ever have a convulsion or seizure?

No Yes Have you ever received treatment for your genital area? Explain _____
No Yes Have you ever had loss of vision?
No Yes Do you suffer with blurred vision?
No Yes Are you being treated for glaucoma?
No Yes Are you frequently sick or ill?
No Yes Do you worry about your health?
No Yes Were you ever treated for anemia?
No Yes Have you ever taken hormones or thyroid medication? (circle which one)
No Yes Were you ever treated for any venereal disease?
No Yes Do you smoke more than 10 cigarettes a day?
No Yes Do you drink more than 6 cups of coffee a day?
No Yes Do you usually take two or more alcoholic drinks a day?
No Yes Do you often get depressed?
No Yes Do strange places or people make you afraid?
No Yes Do you usually feel unhappy or depressed?
No Yes Does criticism always upset you?
No Yes Do you wish you always had someone to advise you?
No Yes Are you considered a nervous person?
No Yes Did you ever have a "nervous breakdown?"
No Yes Have you ever received medical treatment for a "nervous condition?"
No Yes Are you easily upset or irritated?
No Yes Are you constantly keyed up and jittery?
No Yes Do you tend to hold a "grudge" when someone angers you?
No Yes Have you ever considered consulting a psychiatrist?

Women Only: When was your last menstrual period? _____

No Yes Are your periods often irregular?
No Yes Have you had "female" or GYN problems? Explain _____
No Yes **Men Only:** Have you ever had prostate problems?
No Yes Do you have any medical problems that have not been covered? Explain _____
No Yes Are there any reasons you should not have an operation at the present time?
No Yes Have you read the Consultation booklet sent to you?

Signed _____   Date _____

Thank you,

The information you have provided us is essential in our comprehensive evaluation in your case. Please read the booklet "Cosmetic and Reconstructive Surgery of the Face" and write down any questions you may have so we may discuss them in detail during your consultation period.

Appendix 8: Patient Instruction Forms

Beeson Facial Plastic and Reconstructive Surgery
8803 North Meridian Street
Indianapolis, Indiana 46260

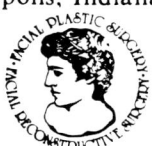

PRE-OPERATIVE INSTRUCTION SHEET FOR OUTPATIENT SURGERY

Your surgery will be performed as an outpatient at our office or at the outpatient surgery section either Methodist or St. Vincent Hospital.

You may be asked to have lab work done prior to your surgery. If this should be necessary in your case, please have the tests done **within** two weeks **prior** to your surgery date.

In order to help diminish the amount of swelling and discoloration following surgery, we request that you purchase several items at your drug store and take them as follows:

> Theragran M (to be taken once daily)
> Vitamin C (500 milligrams - to be taken once daily)

Start these medications approximately 24 hours prior to your surgery and take them before 7:00 AM of the day of your surgery. You might receive some additional prescriptions when you schedule your surgery, if so you need to have them filled and begin taking them as prescribed.

Do not take Vitamin E, Aspirin (acetylsalicylic acid) or products containing Aspirin (Bufferin, Anacin, Empirin, Stanback, Excedrin, Fiorinal, Darvon Compound, APC, etc.) during the week before or after your operation; we will be happy to prescribe a pain remedy not containing Aspirin if you need one,(Tylenol or Percogesic may be purchased at the drug store without a prescription).

Please contact us immediately for instructions if you develop a cold, sore throat, fever blisters, or any skin eruption of the face. None of these necessarily mean that your surgery would have to be cancelled but we may wish to give you some additional instructions.

Wash your hair thoroughly the night before or morning prior to surgery; do not reapply hair spray.

Men should shave closely the morning of surgery.

If your surgery is scheduled after 12:00 noon (as it is in most cases) we encourage you to have coffee, hot tea, juice and dry toast for breakfast prior to 7:00 AM but do not eat or drink anything except the medications we prescribe for you after that time.

You should have someone drive you to the hospital or office the morning of surgery and arrange for someone to pick you up and plan to stay with you the night of surgery. You may take a cab to the hospital or office on the morning of surgery but it still will be necessary to have someone with you the night of your surgery. If you have no one to stay with you, we will be happy to help arrange a sitter for you. It is **imperative** that you not be alone following surgery.

On the day of surgery before coming to the hospital or office, please remove make-up, false eyelashes, wigs, hairpieces, and jewelry. We prefer you leave these items at home. Plan to wear something that buttons up the front rather than clothing that pulls over the head.

You may bring a scarf, sun glasses, or other articles to cover your dressings when leaving the office.

It is best not to have a permanent or hair coloring within 7 days prior to surgery.

Also ...... Please be good enough to contact us **immediately** if you should need to postpone your surgery so that we may have opportunity to fill the vacancy in our surgery schedule.

Please keep these suggestions and bring them with you the morning of surgery. Write down any questions you have on this sheet so that our staff can answer them for you. Post-operative instructions will be given to you following surgery.

Be assured that we will do everything within our power to make your surgical experience as convenient and comfortable as possible.

Thank you for your confidence in us,

William H. Beeson, M.D.

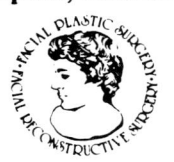

Beeson Facial Plastic and Reconstructive Surgery
8803 North Meridian Street
Indianapolis, Indiana 46260

RHINOPLASTY

1. It is important for your family to read the Nasal Surgery booklet to familiarize themselves with your surgery. They can read it to you or you can wait and read it the day following your surgery. It will answer some very important questions that you may have regarding your post-operative care.

2. Sleep with the head of your bed elevated 30 to 40 degrees for one week, by putting two pillows at the head of the bed.

3. Apply ice compresses made of face cloths to your eyes for 20 minute periods every two hours during the first three days after surgery.

4. Stay up as much as possible after the first 24 hours, but rest when you become tired.

5. Avoid bending or lifting heavy things for a week after surgery, and avoid bumping your nose.

6. Take only prescribed medications or Tylenol, not Aspirin, as it promotes bleeding.

7. When bathing, avoid getting the nasal dressing wet. If it becomes loose let us know.

8. Report any excessive bleeding that persists after pressure and lying down for 15 minutes.

9. Report any persistent temperature above 100 degrees.

10. Don't blow the nose at all for 10 days after surgery.

11. You may clean the outside of the nose with a Q-tip moistened with peroxide, very gently.

12. Nose drops should not be used as they might delay healing.

13. Avoid foods that are hard to chew.

14. Avoid sniffing, because the suction will cause swelling.

15. Avoid sneezing, but if you must try to sneeze with mouth open.

16. Avoid rubbing nostrils with a Kleenex, instead use a drip pad at the base of the nose, when needed.

17. Again, it is very important to read the booklet to answer any questions that you might have regarding your post-operative care. If you do not find the answer, do call us at 846-0846.

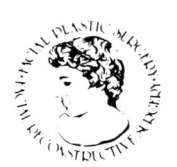

Beeson Facial Plastic and Reconstructive Surgery
8803 North Meridian Street
Indianapolis, Indiana 46260

HAIR TRANSPLANT POST-OPERATIVE CARE

1. Sleep with the head of the bed elevated.

2. The first day after your surgery, shower 2-3 times a day with warm water.

3. Starting on the second day after surgery shower 3-4 times a day and begin using baby shampoo.

4. Starting the first day after surgery gently clean grafts with hydrogen peroxide and Q-tips.

5. Please read the Hair Transplant Booklet carefully for complete instructions.

6. Please call us if you have any questions.

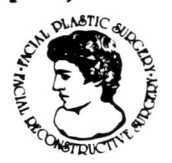

Beeson Facial Plastic and Reconstructive Surgery
8803 North Meridian Street
Indianapolis, Indiana 46260

POST-OPERATIVE INSTRUCTIONS FOR WOUND CARE

- If wounds are covered with a tape dressing, leave in place until dressing comes off on its own.

- When wound is exposed, clean gently with hydrogen peroxide soaked Q-tips, four to five times daily, followed by application of Bacitracin ointment.

- Continue above process until wounds are completely healed (usually 10-14 days).

BE SURE TO CALL US IMMEDIATELY TO REPORT:

1. Temperature over 101°F (temperature of 100°F is normal with wound healing)

2. Sudden swelling or discoloration

3. Hemorrhage

4. Discharge from wound or other evidence of infection

5. Development of any drug reaction

*If you have any further questions, you are urged to call us at our office number (846-0846). If after hours, we can be reached through the Medical Exchange at 926-3466.

We will see you on _____ for your first **post-operative visit.**

POST-OPERATIVE INSTRUCTIONS FOR DERMABRASION

1. At the conclusion of the dermabrasion a dressing was applied to the areas which were treated. Try to leave this dressing in place and on the morning following your surgery wash the abraded area with tap water only.

2. Use your fingertips or cotton balls to wash and be very gentle. Pat the area dry and apply a **thick** coat of _____ .

3. Repeat the washing and dressing procedures each morning and each night for seven days.

4. The weeping coming from under the dressing during the first few hours after surgery is serum. It may be profuse in the beginning and should subside in one or two days.

5. Keep the dermabraded areas covered with a thick coat of _____ at **all** times to avoid crusting.

6. NEVER PICK AT CRUSTS THAT DO NOT LOOSEN EASILY. Apply the softening creams or ointments to them and they should come off easily with time. You may trim the gauze carefully with scissors as it loosens but do not pull at the portions that are not loose.

7. After your first post-operative visit to our office we can advise you about the continued care in your particular case.

8. **Remember** each case is different and some people may tend to heal faster than others.

GENERALLY

A. The intense pink color will fade within five to seven days and a light pink will replace it for several days.

B. Persons who are prone to have cold sores (fever blisters) may have a flare-up following dermabrasion. If this should happen notify us immediately so that we may recommend treatment.

C. Occasionally small "white heads" may appear in the treated areas; these usually disappear within two to three weeks — occasionally longer.

D. The skin may feel somewhat tense and dry during the healing period but cold cream, Crisco vegetable shortening, or _____ ointment may be used as a moisturizer. Do not use anything else without first checking with us.

E. In most cases makeup may be used to cover the treated areas within seven to fourteen days.

F. In most cases you may be able to return to school or work as soon as the weeping has subsided.

G. The skin will retain swelling or edema for several weeks following dermabrasion so be patient since continued improvement in the texture of the skin may occur up to six to twelve months in some cases.

H. Try to avoid direct rays of sun for at least six to eight weeks since your "new" skin will be more sensitive and will have a tendency to burn and tan more easily. The dermabraded areas should be protected with a sunscreen product (U-VAL, SHADE, etc.) for three to six months and you should wear a large brimmed hat to shade the face during this interval.

I. Prolonged exposure to the sun (sunbathing, golfing, fishing, tennis, or similar activities) during the sunny parts of the day should be avoided during this six to eight week period.

FINALLY

If any other questions arise or anything should develop that you are uncertain about, do not hesitate to telephone us anytime.

We want to see you again on _____ ; please make every attempt to keep this and all subsequent appointments since it is vitally important that we monitor your healing.

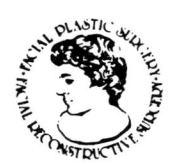

Beeson Facial Plastic and Reconstructive Surgery
8803 North Meridian Street
Indianapolis, Indiana 46260

BLEPHAROPLASTY

1. Sleep with the head of the bed elevated for one week, by elevating the head with two pillows.

2. Apply ice compresses every 20 minutes following your surgery. Continue ice compresses two days after surgery for 20 minutes every two hours.

3. Apply peroxide 3-4 times a day with Q-tips, but be very careful not to get any in the eye.

4. Apply a small amount of vaseline to the sutures at the outer corners of the eye only. Be very careful not to use too much as it may cause eye irritation.

5. Take only prescribed medications or Tylenol for pain.

6. When you shower the day after your surgery be careful to keep the force of the shower from beating directly on the suture lines, but it is alright for them to get wet.

7. Report any excessive bleeding that persists after holding pressure for 15 minutes.

Beeson Facial Surgery

Retin-A

Retin-A is a form of vitamin A. It has been used for a number of years in the treatment of acne because of its beneficial exfoliative (skin peeling) action, especially on plugged oil glands (comedones). It also has been noted to be useful in the treatment of thickened skin disorders (hyperkeratosis). However, its ONLY FDA approval is for the treatment of acne.

In recent months considerable attention has been given Retin-A as an anti-aging agent. Excessive exposure to sunlight prematurely ages skin. Sun damaged skin may appear wrinkled, yellowed, blotchy, coarse, rough, leathery and dry. Often times these changes do not appear until ten to twenty years following excessive sun exposure. Retin-A was found to be helpful in treating sun aging damage to the skin. Primarily the improvements were noted to be:

1. Exfoliation and increased epidermal turnover. These actions increased the turgor (fullness) of the skin and reduced the appearance of fine wrinkling.

2. New blood vessel formation and increased blood flow (a more helpful color).

3. More uniformed pigmentation.

4. Increased collagen formation in the deeper skin layers.

While Retin-A may be helpful in eliminating fine wrinkling (rhytids), it will not remove deep wrinkling or expression lines. As we age, a number of things happen to our face. Our skin loses moisture, it loses elasticity, the fat will re-distribute, and the muscles deteriorate or atrophy. Face lift surgery tightens muscles, removes extra fatty tissue, and re-positions and removes excess skin. A phenol chemical peel removes the superficial layer of the skin. It penetrates into the deeper layers of the skin to provide a rejuvenation of the skin and a "tightening" effect. It is very effective in removing deep wrinkles and is more permanent in its effect than Retin-A. However, there is a two week "convalescent" period before one can usually resume normal social activities following a phenol chemical peel.

Retin-A is not a replacement for face lift surgery or phenol chemical face peeling. However, it can be an effective, adjunctive agent in maintaining a youthful, freshened appearance to the skin, if used correctly.

Recommended Use

1. Apply a pea size amount of Retin-A to the palm of your hand. Add a small amount of water to form a pasty consistency. Apply to all areas of face. (Retin-A can also be applied to the neck and hands).

2. Wait approximately one hour after washing face before applying Retin-A.

3. Do not wash the skin or apply any other medication for at least two hours after application. It is best to leave the treated area undisturbed overnight.

4. Apply Retin-A initially one time every other day with a maximum of three applications per week. (Over a period of time you may be able to apply Retin-A more frequently and possibly even use a stronger concentration.)

Precautions

1. Retin-A may be drying to your skin. For that reason you may need to use a moisturizer more frequently. The moisturizer which you normally use will probably be satisfactory. However, some individuals with sensitive skin find that Eucerin lotion or Complex-15 lotion is more satisfactory for sensitive skin.

2. Because Retin-A is removing the "filtering layers" of the skin, you may burn more easily when exposed to the sun. For this reason it is recommended that a sun-screen rated 15 or higher be used. Such a sun-screen should be applied to the skin the night before planned sun exposure and then again approximately one hour before going out into the sun. This will help you to obtain a tan but avoid a sunburn. There are many excellent over-the-counter sun-screens. A sun-screen should be rated "15". This will provide you with the maximum amount of sun block. No studies have been performed which show that sun-screens higher than "15" are anymore effective. Many individuals find that they are sensitive to PABA which is contained in many sun-screens. Sun-screens can be obtained which do not contain PABA and are recommended for more sensitive skin.

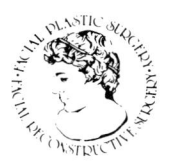

Beeson Facial Plastic and Reconstructive Surgery
8803 North Meridian Street
Indianapolis, Indiana 46260

PREOPERATIVE INSTRUCTION SHEET FOR HOSPITAL PATIENTS

IN PREPARATION FOR YOUR OPERATION ....

Please contact us immediately for instructions if you develop a cold, sore throat, fever blisters, any skin eruption of the face the week before proposed surgery.

In order to help diminish the amount of swelling and discoloration following surgery, we request that you purchase several items at your drug store and take them as follows:

>   Theragran M (to be taken twice daily)
>   Vitamin C (500 milligrams — to be taken twice daily)

You might receive some additional prescriptions when you schedule your surgery, if so you need to have them filled and begin taking them as prescribed.

Do not take Vitamin E, Aspirin (acetylsalicylic acid) or products containing aspirin (Bufferin, Anacin, Empirin, Stanback, Excedrin, Fiorinal, Darvon Compound, APC, etc.) during the week before or after your operation; we will be happy to prescribe a pain remedy not containing Aspirin if you need one. (Tylenol or Percogesic may be purchased at the drug store without a prescription).

Wash your hair thoroughly the night before your surgery; **do not** reapply hair spray. Patients being admitted for face lifts should wash their hair the morning of surgery.

Men should shave closely the day of surgery, particularly in the upper lip area.

Women should remove all cosmetics (including fingernail polish, mascara, eyebrow pencil, eye liner, etc.) the morning of surgery: if admitted to the hospital the morning of your operation, you should remove the cosmetics immediately upon arriving at your room.

If you are to be admitted to the hospital, bring the following with you:

1. The envelope given to you in the office — it contains the instructions to the nursing staff in preparation for your surgery. Give it to the nurse when you arrive on the floor.
2. Materials to remove cosmetics — mineral oil is helpful in removing mascara.
3. Bath robe and slippers
4. Toothbrush and toothpaste
5. Night gown or pajamas (optional)
6. Blouse or shirt with buttons down the front
7. (optional) A pair of sunglasses to wear home
8. A head scarf to wear home (optional for women) — a loosely fitting wig may be worn.

If your surgery is scheduled after 12:00 noon, we encourage you to have coffee, hot tea, juice and dry toast for breakfast prior to 7:00 AM, but do not eat or bring anything else except the medications we will prescribe for you.

Gowns furnished by the hospital must be worn to surgery. Something fancier may be worn afterwards if you desire; however garments that slip over the head should not be used.

Rings, watches, and other valuables should be left at home or with a relative or close friend at the hospital.

Special nurses are usually not necessary. However, if one is desired, we will try to help you arrange for one.

If you want a relative or friend to remain with you at night, please check with the clerk who admits you regarding hospital policy, since the policy in your case will depend upon the type of room accommodations you have.

Please do not take any medications without our knowledge while confined to the hospital — they may conflict with something we have ordered for you.

You will not be permitted to drive home when discharged; therefore, you should make plans to have someone drive you or take a taxi, which the hospital personnel will be glad to obtain for you.

ALSO ....

Please be good enough to contact us **immediately** if you should need to postpone your surgery so that we may have an opportunity to fill the vacancy in our surgery schedule, thank you for your confidence in us.

William H. Beeson, M.D.

NOTE: Please keep these suggestions and bring them to the hospital with you.

Instructions for Patients After Surgery

Medications: In most cases, we will provide you with medications required. Instructions will be included with the medicines. Some are to be taken for a specific period of time, while others are to be used only as required - i.e. for pain or rest. Please do not begin any other medications. <u>Do not take any medications containing aspirin for vitamin E for two weeks after surgery.</u>

Activity: Most patients will rest the day of surgery, sleeping much of the time. After facial surgery, it is best to keep the head elevated 30 degrees to help minimize swelling. Progressive activity is encouraged as tolerated, but do not drive for 24 hours. Remember, it is quite common to feel fatigue following surgery. If there is bleeding from the surgical site, rest quietly until it subsides, using mild pressure. Call, of course, if bleeding persists or is heavy.

Diet: In general, a diet of choice is allowed after surgery. There are a few exceptions. When incisions have been made inside the mouth, patients should remain on clear liquids for a full day after surgery. It is best to avoid a lot of chewing for several days following rhinoplasty, chemical peel or dermabrasion.

Heat & Cold: Cold tends to prevent formation of swelling or edema, while heat tends to hasten its resolution. Therefore, we recommend cold packs or iced compresses during the day of surgery and perhaps the first post operative day. After that, warm (not hot) packs can be used as desired. Iced compresses are especially important after eyelid surgery and should be kept in place continuously for the first 8 hours after surgery.

Swelling: Swelling is a normal sequel to surgery and must be expected. Resolution takes time and may not be complete for several weeks to a few months depending on the exact type of surgery and the individual patient. This is especially true after rhinoplasty, were the last bit of swelling may not resolve until more than six months have elapsed. Of course we should be notified if swelling is excessive.

Dressings: You will be given any specific instructions required concerning dressings. Generally, face lift and otoplasty dressings are removed one to two days after surgery. Rhinoplasty casts stay in place for about a week. Elastic tape used after facial or implant surgery is usually removed two to three days after surgery. When used on the breast or body, it generally should remain in place for a week or until suture removal. Once dressings are removed, they rarely need to be replaced unless there is drainage.

Incisions: Incisions are closed with either suture or staples. When sutures are used, we generally prefer absorbable material since it requires no removal. Staple removal is really quite painless. A special device carefully unfolds the staple allowing simple extraction. It is always much easier than expected and is usually carried out about ten days after surgery.

When incisions are covered with steristrips, they should be left in place as long as possible, since they help to support the wound, and minimize scar formation.

Incisions can be gently washed at any time after surgery, even if covered with steristrips or elastic tape. They can also be cleaned with either hydrogen peroxide or alcohol. If desired, open incisions can be covered with a light coating of an antibiotic ointment such as Neosporin, Polysporin or Bacitracin. Of course, it is most important to keep incisions clean and free of tension. Avoid picking at them. Beginning two weeks after surgery, application of cocoa butter or vitamin E may help to promote better healing with softer scars.

Incisions can be covered with make up about five days after surgery. Make up can be placed over steristrips.

Eventually, all incisions heal by scar formation. Scars will normally be red at first, but will gradually fade. Scars that begin to thicken may require injections of kenalog - a simple painless office procedure.

Additional Instructions:

_____
_____

Rhinoplasty: Bloody drainage is normal for a day following surgery. Keep a clean dry pad taped in place as needed. Beginning two days after surgery, clean the nostrils frequently by gently swabbing with a Q tip saturated with hydrogen peroxide. This should be followed with an application of an antibiotic ointment such as Neosporin, Polysporin, Neomycin etc., again using a Q tip to apply. Vaseline can also be used. This will help to minimize crusting in the nose. It will not hurt to get the splint wet. Expect to be unable to breathe through your nose for several days.

Occasionally, bleeding will occur about a week after surgery. If it does, first blow the clots out of the nose, then sit quietly with ice pack on the the face and back of the neck allowing the blood to flow freely until it clots. If it does not stop within an hour or so, call the office.

After splint removal, be careful not to allow eyeglasses to cause ridges on the side of the nose. If they do, tape the glasses to your forehead to prevent this. Contact lenses can be worn as soon as they can comfortably be removed. Avoid contact physical activity for six weeks. Avoid sunburn on the nose for six months after surgery.

Face Lift: Avoid unnecessary turning of the head and neck for six weeks. Expect numbness of the face and ears for several weeks. Treat incisions as described above. It is fine to gently wash your hair. If a hair dryer is used, avoid hot settings since numbness could allow the skin to burn.

Eye Lid Surgery: Tearing and intermittent swelling is common for a few weeks after surgery. Bruising around the eyes usually subsides within a week, but can be covered with make up on the third day. Blood may streak the eyeball itself but this will clear without treatment. Occasionally the lower lid will droop a bit for a few weeks as a result of swelling. If small whiteheads occur along the incision, they can be opened with the point of a fine needle. Contact lenses should not be worn for a week. A mild drop such as Visine can be used if the eye feels dry or slightly irritated.

Chemical Peel & Dermabrasion: Open areas of treatment can be washed with cool to slightly warm water and a glycerine base soap. Very frequent washing is helpful (hourly, if possible, while awake) starting the day after surgery. A bland ointment or plain vegetable shortening can be used to soften the skin and help separate scabs. For severe itching, a cortisone cream can be used. Do not peel adherent scabs! This can promote scarring. After the scabs have separated, make up can be used. Cocoa butter or vitamin E is felt by some to promote better healing after scab separation. Occasionally, milia (whiteheads) will have to be opened with the point of a needle.

It is very important to protect the new skin from sun for a minimum of six months after treatment to minimize the possibility of pigmentary change. When exposed to sun, a factor 15 or above sunscreen must be used.

Breast Surgery: Wear a soft firm bra without an underwire for the first two weeks after surgery, unless instructed otherwise. If standard implants have been inserted, you will be instructed in massage technique. If the newer, polyurethane covered implant is used, massage is not necessary. Avoid heavy exercise for about two weeks after surgery, but normal light activity can be resumed within a day or so. After breast *reduction*, drainage through the incision is not uncommon, and is no cause for concern, but we should be notified of any significant swelling, tenderness or drainage.

Otoplasty: An elastic band should be worn over the ears for one week, and while sleeping for at least three more weeks.

Liposuction. Wear your elastic garment all of the time for the first three weeks after surgery (removing it only to wash and dry it). Wear it about half of the time for the next three weeks. Expect significant soreness and bruising for a week or so. Some bloody drainage through the incision is to be expected for a day or so after surgery. Your activity can progress to normal within a few days, although you should not push yourself for a day or so after surgery.

Do not hesitate to contact us if you have any problems that are not covered by these instructions. We are here to help you! If you cannot reach us, 915-695-3630 is answered 24 hrs. a day.

INSTRUCTIONS FOR PATIENTS HAVING SURGERY AT THE FACIAL PLASTIC & COSMETIC SURGICAL CENTER

1. Please report to the Cosmetic Surgical Center _____, at _____ o'clock.

2. If outside lab work has been requested, please be sure it has been sent to the Center, or bring it with you. If checked be sure & bring: ( ) Urine specimen   ( ) EKG tracing & report   ( ) Vision report
   ( ) Blood test report   ( ) Chest x-ray report   ( ) _____

3. Be sure to stop products conatining **aspirin & vitamin E** for two weeks prior to surgery. Read the labels carefully of any medications you take. (Remember many pain medicines & cold capsules contain aspirin, check if unsure.)

4. Wear comfortable clothing. Avoid pull over shirts. Women should not wear pantyhose or make-up. Please leave your valuables at home. You may bring some tennis socks or footies for your feet.

5. If you are having facial surgery, cleanse your face & wash your hair the night prior & the morning of surgery. If you are having body surgery you should shower the night prior & the morning of surgery, in some cases you will be given a special soap to shower with.

6. Most importantly, you should have **NOTHING TO EAT OR DRINK AFTER MIDNIGHT,** unless otherwise specified.

7. You will need someone to drive you home and stay with you the first 24 hours. You should not drive for 24 hours after surgery.

8. General anesthesia is given by a Certified Registered Nurse Anesthetist. The anesthetist requests that the anesthesia fees be paid on the day of surgery. Anesthesia fee: $_____.

9. The balance of your surgery charge is $_____ and is due_____. We are here to serve. If you have any questions about your instructions or surgery, please feel free to call.

INSTRUCTIONS FOR MEDICATIONS

The medications checked below apply to you.

The night before surgery
[ ] 1. **Halcion** .5 mg. A sleeping pill for you to take, if you need it. You should take it 15-20 minutes before going to bed.
[ ] 2. **Prednisone** 5 mg. Will help keep the swelling and bruising to a minimum. You should take **three** the night before surgery. Then starting the night of surgery or the following morning take one three times a day, until all are taken.

After surgery
[ ] 3. **Keflex** 250 mg. (an antibiotic) Take one every six hours until all are taken.
[ ] 4. **Propoxyphene Compound** (an equivalent of Darvon compound) For any discomfort that you might have. You may take one capsule every 3-4 hours as needed. If you are allergic to it you will be given another type of medication.
[ ] 5. **Chlordiazepoxide hydrochloride** 5 mg. (an equivalent of Librium) To help you relax and sleep. You may take one every 4-6 hours as needed. At night you may take two to help you sleep.
[ ] 6. **Additional Medications:**

You may be given other medications and they will be explained to you. Please contact us if you have any questions.

PRE-OPERATIVE INSTRUCTIONS: FACIAL COSMETIC SURGERY

1. Avoid exposure to strong sunlight one week prior to surgery.

2. No alcohol for 24 hours prior to surgery.

3. No Vitamin E for one week before surgery and one week after surgery. Recommended dosage for Vitamin E is 100 Units daily.
   CAUTION: DO NOT EXCEED 300 UNITS.

4. No aspirin for two weeks prior to and following surgery. You may use acetaminophen (i.e., Tylenol, Anacin 3 or generic acetaminophen).

5. You may have a regular diet the night before surgery. (Avoid highly seasoned food.)

6. Nothing by mouth after midnight the night of surgery; this means NO BREAKFAST OR COFFEE THE MORNING OF SURGERY UNLESS SPECIFIED ON YOUR SURGERY CHECK-LIST.

7. Shampoo your hair the night before surgery. Do all tinting procedures at least one week before the surgery date. Facelift patients may have no perms or hair coloring until Dr. Gilmore says it is O.K. (Approximately one (1) month).

8. Wash face well the day of surgery. DO NOT WEAR FACE OR EYE MAKEUP THE DAY OF SURGERY. DO NOT WEAR FALSE EYELASHES THE DAY OF SURGERY.

9. Do not wear CONTACT LENSES the day of surgery.

10. Dress comfortably the day of surgery. No pullover shirts, high heels, pantyhose or binding clothes. (Jogging suits are comfortable.)

11. YOU MAY NOT DRIVE THE DAY OF SURGERY. AN ADULT MUST BE WITH YOU AT ALL TIMES THE FIRST 24 HOURS AFTER SURGERY. THIS IS EXTREMELY IMPORTANT! NO EXCEPTIONS!

12. Important medical information should be in our office two weeks prior to surgery, unless other arrangements have been made.

13. Remember to take 2 antibiotic tablets (Vibramycin or Velosef) the night before surgery.

14. Reconfirm surgery time and phone number, where you can be reached, prior to surgery.

*** PLEASE LEAVE ALL VALUABLES AT HOME. DO NOT WEAR ANY JEWELRY. WE WILL NOT BE RESPONSIBLE FOR ANY VALUABLES BROUGHT TO THE OFFICE.

POST-OPERATIVE INSTRUCTIONS FOR BLEPHAROPLASTY (EYELIDS)

ITEMS YOU MUST HAVE ON HAND:

a. Hydrogen Peroxide
b. Cotton tip applicators (i.e. Q-tips)
c. Lacrilube (prescription not needed)
d. Artificial tears, Tears Plus, or Hypotears (prescription not needed)
e. Oval eye pads

INSTRUCTIONS

1. The day of surgery go immediately to bed and rest with your head elevated on two pillows. The following day rest as often as necessary but do not stay in bed. A normal amount of activity will help reduce swelling.

2. Apply cold compresses to eyes until bedtime. Compresses can be discontinued the following day or continued, if desired, for comfort. Cold compresses should be discontinued after the second day. (Oval eye pads soaked in a small bowl of ice water. Squeeze out excess water.)

3. Start with a light diet. 7-up, crackers, clear soups, etc., then, perhaps, a baked potato later in the day as tolerated. Return to normal diet the next day.

4. Take medications as directed.
   (a) Chart medication and time taken for easy reference.
   (b) Pain medication should not be taken more frequently than three hours apart unless instructed by our office.
   (c) Medication taken with a small amount of food is better tolerated.

5. Clean the suture lines twice daily. The day of surgery clean only as needed (for cleaning use a Q-tip dipped in Hydrogen Peroxide, being careful not to get peroxide into your eyes).

6. Use artificial tears for eye irritation or eye dryness (Tears Plus, Hypotears).

7. Lacrilube on a Q-tip may be applied gently to the incision lines if they feel tight or itchy.

8. Do not use eye makeup until you have checked with our office.

9. After the first week gently massage upper and lower eyelids with cream, as instructed, twice daily for a few minutes; upper lid from inner to outer and lower lid from inner and sweep upward (Lacrilube or comparable).

10. Return to our office at appointed time for your check-up after your surgery.

NOTES:

1. Suture lines will be removed in stages (three to seven days before complete.

2. Some people will experience more bruising and swelling than others. This takes from several hours to days to peak before it begins to subside. This is normal.

3. Puffiness in the lids, especially the lower lids, may remain for several weeks before it disappears. This is normal.

4. Eyes can be dry on some patients for a period of time before the dryness disappears. This is normal.

5. Vision may be blurred slightly in some patients for a short time. This will disappear and is normal.

6. Do not exercise unless it has been cleared with the doctor.

7. Best results cannot be determined immediately. It sometimes takes from weeks to months before your healing process is completed. Try not to compare results immediately after your surgery.

* Please call the office immediately if:
  1. Extreme pain under dressing or excessive bleeding should occur.
  2. There is a drastic change in vision.
  3. You have a persistent temperature over 100 degrees.

EMERGENCY NUMBERS TO CALL:

Office: 960-0950 (answered 24 hours) If you reach the answering service, inform them that you are a surgery patient and that it is an emergency.

Emergency Room - Medical City Dallas Hospital: 661-7200
Paramedics and Ambulance: 911 or call your local emergency number

Appendix 9: Administrative Forms

Beeson Facial Surgery
Patient Telephone Log

Name _____ Date _____ Time _____ A.M.
P.M.
Mon. Tues. Wed. Thurs.
Fri. Sat. Sun.

☐ Post Op. — Question/Problem
☐ Rx Renewal
☐ Pre-Op Question
☐ Scheduling Change
☐ Cancellation
☐ New Consult

Problem: _____
_____
_____

Action: _____
_____
_____
_____
_____

☐ Told to come in today if desires/we will be happy to see/if not, call if any questions or changes.

☐ Rx Renewal Called In (Med.): _____
(Disp.) _____
(Sig.) _____
(Pharmacy): _____

Nurse _____

Doctor _____

EQUIPMENT REPAIR

Date: _____ Equipment: _____
Nature of Breakage or Malfunction: _____
_____

Sent Out to Repair: _____
Date: _____ Company: _____ Carrier: _____
Inv. #: _____ Est. Cost: _____ Actual Cost: _____
Date Returned: _____ Repaired: _____ Unable to Repair: _____

Repaired on Premises: _____
Date: _____ Company/Service: _____ Repaired: _____ Unable to Repair ___
Inv. #: _____ Est. Cost: _____ Actual Cost: _____
                                        Signature: _____

PURCHASE AUTHORIZATION

BEESON FACIAL PLASTIC AND
RECONSTRUCTIVE SURGERY

PURCHASE AUTHORIZATION

ITEM	CAT. NO	ITEM COST	QTY.	COST

TOTAL COST: $ _____

COMPANY: _____

PERSONNEL TAKING ORDER: _____

TELEPHONE: _____

ORDER PLACED BY: _____

DATE: _____ TIME: _____

AUTHORIZED BY: _____

DATE: _____

PURCHASE RECEIPT

ORDER RECEIVED AND VERIFIED BY: _____

DATE: _____

CRASH CART CHECK SHEET

Drawer #1

Adrenalin 1mg 1:1000 _____
Aminophylline 500mg/20ml _____
Ammonia, Aromatic _____
Apresoline HCL 20mg/ml _____
Aqua Mephyton 10mg/ml _____
Aramine 10mg/ml _____
Atropine 1mg/ml _____
Benadryl 50mg/ml _____
Bretylium 50mg/ml _____
Calcium Chloride _____
Decadron Phosphate 4mg/ml _____
Digoxin 0.5mg/2ml _____
Dilantin 259mg/5ml _____
Dopamine HCL 200mg/5ml _____
Dramamine 50mg/ml _____
Isuprel 0.2mg/ml _____
Meperidine 100mg/ml _____
Morphine 15mg/ml _____
Narcan 0.4mg/ml _____
Nitrostat 0.4mg/tab _____
Phenobarbital 130mg/ml _____
Physostigmine 1mg/ml _____
Potassium Chloride 20meq/10ml _____
Pronestyl 500mg/ml _____
Propanolol 1mg/ml _____
Quinidine Gluconate _____
Sodium Chloride Injection _____
Verapamil _____

Drawer #2

Sodium Bicarbonate 44.6meq/50ml _____
Epinephrine 1mg 1:10,000 _____
Dextrose 500mg/ml _____
Hyperstat _____
Lidocaine 1% 100mg/10ml _____
Lasix 20mg/ml _____
Mannitol 12.5g/2ml _____
Intercaths _____
Angiocaths _____
Tubex _____
Butterfly Needles _____

Drawer #3

Tracheal Tubes _____
Suction Kits _____
Airways _____
Brook Airway _____
Laryngoscope (bulbs & batteries) _____
Tongue Depressor (bite block) _____
Nasogastric Suction Tips, 1 ea.: size 14, 16, 18 french _____

Drawer #4

Syringes _____
Needles _____
Blood Tubes _____
Yankauer Suction Tip _____
Cautery, Disposable _____
Adrenalin Chloride Solution 1mg/ml _____
Tigan Inj. 200mg/ml _____
Xylocaine HCL 1% _____
K-Y Jelly _____
Ophthalmic Solution _____

Drawer #5

Drug Sign Out Sheet _____
Emergency Flashlight _____
IV Solutions & Tubing _____
Trach Set _____
Extra Sponges _____
Extra Suture _____
Oxygen Mask _____

Defibrillator (check & charge) _____

Respirator Bag & Ambu Mask _____

Oxygen Tank (check Guage) _____

Date Checked _____

Signature _____

INVENTORY SHEET

	Stor.	OR		Stor.	OR
Acetone			Hydrogen Peroxide		
Allergy Labels			Indicator Strips (gas)		
Alcohol, Isopropyl			Instrument milk		
Alcohol wipes			IV set, tubing 96″		
Ammonia ampules			Kay Fee Towels 13½″ × 18″		
Angiocaths 20g 1½″			Kerlix 3″ × 5 yds		
Applicators 6″ wood			Kling 3″ × 5 yds		
Autoclave wrap 25″ × 25″			Lactated Ringers 500ml		
Autoclave tape 1″			Dextrose 5% 500ml		
Bandaids 1″			Latex suction tubing		
Basic sterile pack			Merseline Mesh 12″ × 12″		
Barrier sterile			Micropore tape ½″ (flesh tone)		
Benzoin, tincture of			Micropore tape 1″, ½″ (white)		
Blades, surgical #10			Methylene Blue 1% inj. 10mg/ml		
Bulbs, headlight			Medicine droppers		
Caviclean			Mineral oil		
Chromic, 3-0 suture			Needles 18g 1½″		
Chromic, 6-0 suture			Needles 21g 1½″		
Dexon, 4-0 S suture			Needles 25g 1½″		
Dexon, 5-0 Plus suture			Needles 27g 1½″		
Dexon, 6-0 suture			Normal Saline, sterile		
Ethibond, 2-0 suture			Nu Gauze, sterile sponge, 1½″ × 3″		
Plain, 4-0 Septal suture			O Syl disinfectant		
Plain, 5-0 suture			Penlight, diagnostic		
Plain, 5-0 Ophthalmic			Septisol Foam		
Prolene, 3-0 suture			Septisol Solution		
Prolene, 4-0 suture			Silver Nitrate sticks		
Prolene, 5-0 suture			Skin-stapler 25 regular		
Prolene, 5-0 blue suture			Skin-stapler 12 wide		
Prolene, 6-0 suture			Skin Scribes		
Coban wrap			Specimen cup, sterile, clear, 4oz		
Cool Soak Kleener			Sporicidin Solution		
Distilled water			Surgi-peel 5″ × 200″		
Foam Cleaner Disinfectant			Suction tubing, sterile, 10′ roll		
ECG Electrodes			Surgical hats		
Edsonite			Surgical masks		
Eye pads oval, sterile			Surgical shoe covers		
Fluro Ethyl			Surgicel 2″ × 3″		
Gauze Sponges 4×4 sterile;12 ply 10/box			Syringe, TB 25g ⅝″		
Gauze Sponges 4×4 non-ste 12 ply 200/pkg			Syringe, 3cc		
			Syringe, 5cc		
Gauze Sponges 2×2 non-ste 12 ply 200/pkg			Syringe, 10cc		
			Scrub brushes, chloroxylenol		
Gelfoam 1″ × 3″			Telfa pads, 8″ × 3″, 4″ × 3″		
Gloves, sterile #6			Tongue Depressor		
Gloves, sterile #6½			Thermometer sheath		
Gloves, sterile #7			Sterile water		
Gowns, sterile, large			Xeroform gauze 3″ × 9″		
Metal cleaner			Xylocaine 0.5% w/epi 1:100,000		
Metal polish			Xylocaine 1% w/epi 1:100,000		
Vapo-Solution			Xylocaine 2% w/epi 1:100,000		
Head drape			Xylocaine Jelly		

IN-SERVICE RECORD

Date: _____   Time: _____   Location: _____

Topic: _____
_____

Purpose: _____
_____
_____

Content: _____
_____
_____

Attendance: _____
_____
_____
_____
_____

DRUG DESTRUCTION FORM

Drug:
Date:
Description:
Signature _____
Witness _____

DRUG DESTRUCTION FORM

Drug:
Date:
Description:
Signature _____
Witness _____

DRUG DESTRUCTION FORM

Drug:
Date:
Description:
Signature _____
Witness _____

CONSULTS FOR THE WEEK OF _____

Name _____
Referred by _____
Address _____
City _____
Home # _____ Work # _____
Consult Date _____ Time _____
Reason _____ Chart # _____

_____
_____
_____
_____
Cancelled: _____
No Show: _____
Surgery Scheduled: _____

Name _____
Referred by _____
Address _____
City _____
Home # _____ Work # _____
Consult Date _____ Time _____
Reason _____ Chart # _____

_____
_____
_____
_____
Cancelled: _____
No Show: _____
Surgery Scheduled: _____

Name _____
Referred by _____
Address _____
City _____
Home # _____ Work # _____
Consult Date _____ Time _____
Reason _____ Chart # _____

_____
_____
_____
_____
Cancelled: _____
No Show: _____
Surgery Scheduled: _____

Name _____
Referred by _____
Address _____
City _____
Home # _____ Work # _____
Consult Date _____ Time _____
Reason _____ Chart # _____

_____
_____
_____
_____
Cancelled: _____
No Show: _____
Surgery Scheduled: _____

Name _____
Referred by _____
Address _____
City _____
Home # _____ Work # _____
Consult Date _____ Time _____
Reason _____ Chart # _____

_____
_____
_____
_____
Cancelled: _____
No Show: _____
Surgery Scheduled: _____

	NAME	REASON	RESCHEDULED
CONSULT SCHED			
CONSULT CX'd			
SXies SCHED			
SXies Cxed			
SXies Re-sched			
Missed Appts			

Appendix 10: Perioperative Patient Care Quality

Preamble

One of the founding premises of AORN is that it is the responsibility of the registered professional nurse to ensure high-quality nursing care to patients undergoing surgery. The Association has repeatedly demonstrated its ongoing commitment to the premise through promulgation of standards of practice, a certification program, and competency statements.

The Association's first *Standards of Nursing Practice: OR* were developed with the American Nurses' Association (ANA) Division on Medical Surgical Practice and printed in 1975. Subsequently, AORN provided its membership with a variety of programs and activities to assist nurses in the operating room to be aware of and to use the standards to evaluate their professional practice. These standards were revised after data was collected from practicing nurses to determine the applicability and usefulness of the standards. The resulting revision, entitled, "Standards of Perioperative Nursing Practice," was published in 1981. These standards were joined by "Standards of Administrative Nursing Practice: OR" in 1982 and "Patient Outcome Sandards for Perioperative Nursing" in 1985. In addition to standards of nursing practice, the Association began publishing recommended practices in the technical aspects of perioperative nursing in March 1975.

The certification program was ultimately approved by the House in 1978 ". . . to enhance quality patient care" and to ". . . demonstrate accountability to the general public for nursing practice." Certification demonstrates the perioperative nurse's individual commitment to excellence in practice in the clinical setting as well as the Association's ongoing commitment to fostering excellence in the clinical setting.

Perioperative nurses may now better validate and measure the quality of their practice by use of the *"Competency Statements in Perioperative Nursing."* These were published by AORN in 1986.

Further, resolution and statements adopted by the House of Delegates consistently reiterate the primacy of the concern for quality. The commitment to quality has remained constant as each resolution or statement includes reference to the clients' entitlement to and the nurse's obligation to provide quality care.

Quality may take on new parameters in light of limited resources and no longer be defined as the best money can buy. However, quality, as the best it can be, will be the focal point of consideration. Quality of care has two fociquality of the service provided, which means the care given meets the expressed needs of the consumer; and quality of process, meaning conformance to specifications or performance that demonstrates adherence to established standards. Nurses have developed a scope and definition of practice that embraces those elements of health care that have been mandated by the consumer. The scope of practice includes independently assessing patient needs; making collaborative decisions relative to intraoperative care; contributing to the patient's safety; and evaluating and monitoring care provided. In addition to striving for excellence in practice, the perioperative nurse actively participates in shaping the practice environment and identifies clinical and organizational indicators of quality.

Present fiscal and personnel resource limitations have precipitated the suggestion that in 1989 and beyond we can regress and allow lesser qualified personnel to perform nursing services. This perception is inaccurate and the suggestion is misguided. The acuity of the perioperative patient in the acute-care setting requires more intensive application of technology and nursing care. The less acutely compromised perioperative client is receiving care as an ambulatory patient, who still requires intensive application of nursing knowledge in the realms of teaching, assessing, and fostering selfcare potential.

As perioperative nurses address the uncertainties and anxieties of the future, the guided constant will continue to be their commitment to quality. To that end, perioperative patient care quality has been operationally defined for use.

Operational Definition of Perioperative Patient Care Quality

Perioperative patient care quality is based on a professional nursing practice that encompasses accepted components of analysis and inter-

---

Reprinted with permission from *AORN Standards and Recommended Practices for Perioperative Nursing*, 1991. Copyright © AORN Inc, 10170 East Mississippi Avenue, Denver, CO 80231.

pretation. These include the following components:

Structure—providing patient care within an environment that is conducive to its effective and efficient administration as outlined in the *"AORN Standards of Administrative Nursing Practice: OR."* [1]

Process—meeting the needs of the patient in a caring manner and conforming to established standards of nursing practice as outlined in the *"AORN Standards of Perioperative Nursing Practice"* and *"AORN Recommended Practices for Aseptic and Technical Pactices: OR."* [2]

Outcome—achieving a desired conclusion and/or reducing the probability of undesired outcomes as perceived by the patient and according to a well-defined and properly implemented practice as outlined in the "AORN Patient Outcome Standards for Perioperative Nursing." [3]

Notes

1. "Standards of administrative nursing practice: OR," in *AORN Standards and Recommended Practices for Perioperative Nursing* (Denver: Association of Operating Room Nurses, Inc., 1991) II: 4-1 — 4-7.

2. "Standards of Perioperative Nursing Practice," II: 3-1 — 3-4.

3. "Patient Outcome Standards for Perioperative Nursing," II: 5-1 — 5-2.

Appendix 11: Recommended Practices for Laser Safety in the Practice Setting

The following recommended practices were developed by the Technical Practices Coordinating Committee and have been approved by the Board of Directors. They were published as proposed recommended practices in the January 1989 *AORN Journal* for comment by members and others. They are intended to represent a consensus of AORN members and others.

These recommended practices are intended as achievable recommendations representing what is believed to be an optimal level of practice. Policies and procedures will reflect variations in practice settings and/or clinical situations that determine the degree to which the recommended practices can be fulfilled.

AORN recognizes the numerous different settings in which perioperative nurses practice. The recommended practices are intended as guidelines adaptable to various practice settings. These practice settings include traditional operating rooms, ambulatory surgery units, physicians' offices, cardiac catheterization laboratories, endoscopy rooms, radiology departments, and all other areas where surgery may be performed.

Purpose

These recommended practices provide guidelines to assist perioperative nurses in the safe use of lasers in their practice settings. Nationally accepted standards for laser safety are incorporated in these recommendations. There are several types of lasers currently available. Health care workers educated in laser safety should be familiar with the unique features, specific operation, and safety measures for each type of laser used in their practice settings.

Recommended Practice I

All health care workers should be alerted to laser use areas and associated admittance restrictions.

Interpretive statement 1:
Appropriate warning signs should be conspicuously displayed at all entrances to the laser use area.

Rationale 1:
The placement of laser warning signs at all entrances to the surgical or treatment room during laser use alerts personnel to the need to implement laser safety requirements.[1]

Interpretive statement 2:
Designs, symbols, and wording of the warning signs should be specific for type of laser in use.

Rationale 2:
Warning signs and labels serve as control measures to reduce the possibility of exposure of the eye(s) and skin to hazardous levels of laser radiation and other hazards associated with the operation of laser devices during testing, normal operation, and maintenance.[2]

Recommended Practice II

Eyes of patients and health care workers should be protected from laser beams.

Interpretive statement 1:
Laser-safe eye protection with the appropriate wavelength and optical density should be used by health care workers and conscious patients.

Rationale 1:
Each type of laser light has a specific wavelength, thus requiring different types of eye protection.[3]

Interpretive statement 2:
Under anesthesia, patients' eyes should be protected from the laser beam. Their eyelids should be closed, taped, and/or covered with saline moistened pads. Protective eye shields should be used for procedures immediately around the eye or on the eyelid.

Rationale 2:
Eyes are particularly vulnerable to laser injury.[4]

Interpretive statement 3:
Laser-safe eye protectors should be available near the posted warning sign(s) that indicates the need for eye protection.

Rationale 3:
Readily available eye protectors help ensure compliance with eye safety procedures.[5]

Reprinted with permission from *AORN Standards and Recommended Practices for Perioperative Nursing*, 1991. Copyright © AORN Inc, 10170 East Mississippi Avenue, Denver, CO 80231.

Interpretive statement 4:
All viewing windows in the laser room should provide protection in accordance with the specific laser in use.

Rationale 4:
The use of "beamstop" material prevents laser beam transmission.[6]

Recommended Practice III

Skin and other tissues of patients and health care workers should be protected from aberrant and reflected laser beams.

Interpretive statement 1:
The laser should be in standby mode when not in use.

Rationale 1:
When the laser is set up and on but not being fired, the controls should be set to "standby," "wait," or "disable" to prevent inadvertent activation.[7]

Interpretive statement 2:
Exposed tissue around the operative field should be protected with saline or water-saturated towels and/or sponges, when using thermally intensive lasers.

Rationale 2:
The solution (saline or water) absorbs or disperses the energy of the beam in areas not intended for laser application.[8]

Interpretive statement 3:
Dulled, ebonized, or nonreflective anodized finished instruments should be used near the laser site.

Rationale 3:
Dulled, ebonized, or nonreflective anodized finished instruments decrease the amount of direct laser beam reflection and beam scatter.[9]

Interpretive statement 4:
Backstops or guards should be used during laser surgery where applicable.

Rationale 4:
Appropriate backstops prevent the beam from affecting nontargeted tissue.[10]

Recommended Practice IV

Patients and health care workers should be protected from inhaling fumes associated with laser use.

Interpretive statement 1:
Plume and noxious fumes should be evacuated through a filter device.

Rationale 1:
Plume and noxious fumes are irritating to the respiratory tract.[11] Some particles in the laser plume are classified as hazardous to breathe. Use of a mechanical smoke evacuator system, with a high-efficiency filter, during plume generating laser vaporization procedures decreases risk of plume inhalation.[12]

Interpretive statement 2:
Surgical high-filtration masks should be worn during procedures that produce a plume.

Rationale 2:
Surgical masks deter or delay inhalation of the larger carbonaceous particles.[13]

Recommended Practice V

Patients and health care workers should be protected from fire hazards associated with laser use.

Interpretive statement 1:
Flammable or combustible anesthetics, prep solutions, drying agents, ointments, plastic resins or flammable plastics, or other materials should not be used near the laser site.

Rationale 1:
The intense heat of the laser beam can ignite combustible/flammable solids, liquids, and gases.[14] Pooled prep solutions can retain laser heat and burn tissue.[15]

Interpretive statement 2:
Moistened reusable fabrics and/or laser-retardant drapes should be used to drape the operative site.

Rationale 2:
Wet sponges or towels and laser-retardant drapes around the laser interaction site decrease the potential of fire. Because the flammability of methane gas must be considered, moistened counted sponges may be inserted into the rectum when procedures are performed in the perianal area.[16]

Interpretive statement 3:
A basin of water or saline and a halon fire extinguisher should be readily available.

Rationale 3:
Water or saline is needed in case of accidental fire within the sterile field. The halon fire extinguisher is effective for laser fires as it does not harm the optics or delicate circuits of the laser.[17]

Interpretive statement 4:
An endotracheal tube used during laser surgery in the aerodigestive tract (ie, oral, nasopharyngeal, laryngotracheal, endobronchial) should be laser safe.

Rationale 4:
Endotracheal tubes can ignite and support combustion if not laser safe.[18]

Recommended Practice VI

Patients and health care workers should be protected from electical hazards associated with laser use.

Interpretive statement 1:
Electrical circuitry of the laser room(s) should have adequate amperage to meet the power requirements of the specific laser.

Rationale 1:
Some lasers have sizable power requirements. Failure to provide sufficient power can trip circuit breakers serving other outlets.[19]

Interpretive statement 2:
Liquids should not be placed on the laser unit.

Rationale 2:
Spilled liquid may act as a conductor and cause internal short-circuiting.[20]

Recommended Practice VII

Policies and procedures for laser safety should be developed within the practice setting.

Discussion:
Policies and procedures should include but are not limited to:
- laser safety,
- care and preventive maintenance of lasers,
- credentialing mechanisms,
- laser safety officer,
- documentation of laser use (eg, laser log), and
- medical surveillance of health care personnel.

These recommended practices should be used as guidelines for the development of policies and procedures for laser safety within the practice setting. Policies and procedures establish authority, responsibility, and accountability and serve as operational guidelines. An introduction and review of laser safety policies and procedures should be included in the orientation and ongoing education of personnel to assist in the development of knowledge, skills, and attitudes that affect patient care.

Glossary

Anodization: An electrolytic action that changes the whole molecular make-up of the metal before coating with a protective or color film.

Backstops/guards: Materials (eg, quartz rods, titanium rods) that will stop the laser beam from penetrating beyond the expected impact site.

Beamstops: Materials that will stop the reflection, transmission, and scatter of the laser beam.

Ebonized: Black nonreflective surface.

LASER: Acronym for light amplification by the stimulated emission of radiation.

Optical density: The light absorbing quality of a translucent substance.

Wavelength: The distance measured between two successive peaks of a wave.

Notes
1. K Ball, "Laser safety," *Today's OR Nurse* 8 (October 1986)11.
2. American National Standards Institute, *American National Standard for the Safe Use of Lasers* Z136.1, (New York City: American National Standards Institute, Inc, 1986) 11-12, 16, 22-23.
3. *Ibid*; Ball, "Laser safety," 12.
4. Laser Institute of America, *Laser Safety Guide,* sixth ed (Toledo: Laser Institute of America, 1987) 2-5.
5. D Lundergan, "Practice laser safety," in *Surgical Application of Lasers,* second edition, J A Dixon, ed (Chicago: Year Book Medical Publishers, Inc, 1987) 80-81.
6. *Ibid*; Ball, "Laser safety," 12.
7. J A Kneedler, G H Dodge, *Perioperative Patient Care,* second ed (St Louis: Blackwell Scientific Publications, 1987) 191.
8. *Ibid.*
9. *Ibid*; Lundergan, "Practical laser safety," 83-84.
10. T A Fuller, ed, *Surgical Lasers: A Clinical Guide* (New York City: Macmillan Publishing Co, 1987) 107.
11. K Ball, "Controlling smoke evacuation and odor during laser surgery," *Today's OR Nurse* 8 (December 1986) 4-12.
12. C Nezhat et al, "Smoke from laser surgery: Is there a health hazard?" *Lasers in Surgery and Medicine* 7 no 4 (1987) 376-382.
13. *Ibid.*
14. J Pfister, J Kneedler, "Laser safety," in *A Guide to Lasers in the OR* (Aurora, Colo: Education Design/Editorial Consultants, 1983) 33-35.
15. *Ibid*; Ball, "Laser safety," 12.
16. Ball, "Laser safety," 12-13.
17. *Ibid,* 13.
18. *Ibid.*
19. D Ayscue, "Operating room design: Accommodating lasers," *AORN Journal* 43 (June 1986) 1281.
20. *Ibid*; Ball, "Laser safety," 13.

Suggested reading
American National Standards Institute. *American National Standard for the Safe Use of Lasers* Z136.3. New York City: American National Standards Institute, Inc, 1988.

Apfelberg, D B, ed. *Evaluation and Installation of Surgical Laser Systems.* New York City: Springer-Verlag, 1987.

Ball, K. "Legal aspects of laser surgery." *Today's OR Nurse* 9 (February 1987) 23-28.

Bendick, P J. "Laser safety in the operating room." *American College of Surgeons Bulletin* 71 (July 1986) 10-12.

Cayton, M M. "Nursing responsibilities in laser surgery." *Medical Instrumentation* 17 (November 1983) 419-421.

Dixon, J A, ed. *Surgical Application of Lasers,* second ed. Chicago: Year Book Medical Publishers, Inc, 1987.

England, E P. "Lasers: Issues problems and implications for practice." *Perioperative Nursing Quarterly* 1 (June 1985) 29-38.

Faulconer, D R. "Nursing management: Lasers." *Today's OR Nurse* 6 (May 1984) 31.

Giangiordano, M H; Doiron, D R. "Lasers in outpatient surgery offer an alternative to conventional methods." *AORN Journal* 43 (January 1986) 336-343.

Gruendemann, B J; Meeker, M H. *Alexander's Care of the Patient in Surgery* eighth ed. St Louis, C V Mosby Co, 1987, 170-175.

Kapsar, P. "Hazard of laser plume question." *AORN Journal* 47 (February 1988) 462-466.

Klein, B R. *Health Care Facilities Handbook,* second ed. Quincy, Mass: National Fire Protection Association, 1987, 504-506.

Lundergan, D; Smith, S. "Nurses' administrative responsibilities for lasers." *AORN Journal* 38 (August 1983) 217-222.

Mackety, C J. *Perioperative Laser Nursing*. Thorofare, NJ: Charles B Slack, Inc, 1984.

Mackety, C J, ed. *Laser Nursing*. New York City: Mary Ann Liebert, Inc. Quarterly publication.

Murphy, E. "Legal implications of OR laser use." *Today's OR Nurse* 6 (June 1984) 29.

Pfister, J, ed. *Laser Network*. Aurora, Colo: Education Design/Editorial Consultants. Quarterly publication.

Trevor, M. *A Laser Safe Environment*. Danbury, Conn: Davis + Geck Film Library, 1987, film and film study guide.

Wells, M P, ed. *Decision Making in Perioperative Nursing*. Philadelphia: B C Decker, Inc, 1987, 160-163.

Originally published in September 1989 *AORN Journal*.

Appendix 12: Recommended Practices for Operating Room Environmental Sanitation

The following recommended practices were developed by the AORN Recommended Practices Subcommittee and have been approved by the Technical Practices Coordinating Committee and the Board of Directors. They were published as proposed recommended practices in the August 1988 *AORN Journal* for comment by members and others. They are intended to represent a consensus of AORN members and others.

These recommended practices are intended as achievable recommendations representing what is believed to be an optimal level of practice. Policies and procedures will reflect variations in practice settings and/or clinical situations that determine the degree to which the recommended practices can be fulfilled.

AORN recognizes the numerous different settings in which perioperative nurses practice. The recommended practices are intended as guidelines adaptable to various practice settings. These practice settings include traditional operating rooms, ambulatory surgery units, physicians' offices, cardiac catheterization laboratories, endoscopy rooms, radiology departments, and all other areas where surgery may be performed.

Purpose

These recommended practices provide a guideline for environmental sanitation within the surgical suite in all health care settings. Sanitation practices should provide a safe, clean environment for the surgical patient and personnel. A basic premise of these practices is that all surgical cases should be considered potentially contaminated.

Recommended Practices

Recommended Practice I
Patients should be provided with a safe, clean environment free from dust and organic debris.

Interpretive statement 1:
Before the first scheduled procedure of the day, furniture, surgical lights, and equipment should be damp dusted. Damp dusting should be done with a clean, lint-free material moistened with a hospital-grade disinfectant.

Rationale 1:
Studies have shown that 90% to 99% of viable microbial contaminants from the air and other sources are deposited on horizontal surfaces in the operating room.[1]

Proper cleaning of these surfaces will help to control airborne microorganisms that travel on dust and lint.[2]

Interpretive statement 2:
Preparation of the operating room should include a visual inspection of the room for total cleanliness by the perioperative nurse before the case cart/supplies and instrument sets are brought into the room.

Rationale 2:
Some recommendations are based on a reasonable theoretical rationale; for many of these practices, little or no scientifically valid evidence is available to permit evaluation of their effect on the incidence of infection.[3]

Recommended Practice II
During the surgical procedure, efforts should be directed at confining contamination.

Interpretive statement 1:
Areas outside the sterile field contaminated by organic debris should be cleaned promptly.

Rationale 1:
Prompt cleanup of organic debris and blood contamination using a tuberculocidal, hospital-grade disinfectant or a 1:10 dilution of household bleach prepared daily helps maintain a safe, clean environment.[4]

Interpretive statement 2:
Contaminated disposable items should be discarded into an impervious container.

Rationale 2:
Soiled disposable articles are placed into impervious containers to prevent exposure of personnel to articles contaminated with potentially infectious material and to prevent contamination of the environment.[5]

Interpretive statement 3:
Contaminated items should be handled using protective barriers.

Rationale 3:
Because one is never certain which patients may harbor blood-borne viruses or pathogenic bacteria,

---

Reprinted with permission from *AORN Standards and Recommended Practices for Perioperative Nursing*, 1991. Copyright © AORN Inc, 10170 East Mississippi Avenue, Denver, CO 80231.

the use of protective barriers prevents contamination of the health care worker.[6] Examples of protective barriers are gloves, gowns, masks, and protective eyewear.

Interpretive statement 4:
All blood, body fluids, and tissue specimens should be placed in a clean impervious container for transport. The exterior surfaces of specimen containers received from the operative field should be cleaned with a tuberculocidal hospital-grade disinfectant or a 1:10 dilution of household bleach before they are removed from the operating room.

Rationale 4:
Inanimate objects soiled with blood, blood products, and body fluid may potentially infect health care workers.[7]

Interpretive statement 5:
Contamination of documents such as laboratory slips, x-rays, and charts that will leave the patient care area should be prevented.

Rationale 5:
Objects soiled with blood, blood products, and body fluids may potentially infect health care workers.[8]

Recommended Practice III
After the procedure, all items that have come in contact with the patient and/or the sterile field should be considered contaminated, and their disposition should comply with local, state, and/or federal regulations for contamination control measures.

Interpretive statement 1:
Gowns and gloves are removed (inside out) and placed into impervious containers before leaving the operating room.

Rationale 1:
Gowns and gloves are removed in a manner that contains contamination. They are enclosed in impervious containers to prevent exposure of personnel to potentially infectious material and to prevent contamination of the environment.[9]

Interpretive statement 2:
Soiled linen (reusable textiles) should be handled as little as possible and with minimal agitation. It should be placed and transported in containers that prevent leakage.

Rationale 2:
Minimal handling of soiled linen prevents wide distribution of contaminated lint and debris into the environment.[10]

Interpretive statement 3:
All disposable sharps should be placed in puncture resistant containers.

Rationale 3:
Injuries caused by needles, scalpels, and other sharp devices are a source of transmission of human immunodeficiency virus (HIV), hepatitis B virus, and other contaminants.[11]

Interpretive statement 4:
Until terminally sterilized, disinfected, or disposed, contaminated instruments, basins, trays, and other items should be handled only by gloved personnel.

Rationale 4:
Gloves reduce the risk of gross contamination of hands when handling items or surfaces soiled with blood or body fluids.[12]

Interpretive statement 5:
Disposable suction tubing should be used.

Rationale 5:
Disposable suction tubing eliminates the difficulty encountered in cleaning the lumen of the reusable suction tubing.[13]

Interpretive statement 6:
If reusable suction containers are used, they should be emptied and disinfected.

Rationale 6:
Any item that has had contact with blood exudates, and secretions is potentially infective.[14]

Interpretive statement 7:
All other items for disposal should be enclosed in impervious containers.

Rationale 7:
Contaminated articles are enclosed in impervious containers to prevent inadvertent exposure of per-

sonnel to infective material and contamination of the environment.[15]

Interpretive statement 8:
All equipment and furniture used during the surgical procedure should be cleaned with a hospital-grade disinfectant. Mechanical friction should be used.

Rationale 8:
Equipment and furniture used for the surgical procedure are considered contaminated.[16]

Interpretive statement 9:
Transport vehicles should be cleaned with a detergent disinfectant after each use.

Rationale 9:
Patient transport vehicles are considered contaminated because of patient contact.[17]

Interpretive statement 10:
Floors should be cleaned using a detergent disinfectant.

Rationale 10:
Sanitation in the operating room is essential to remove organic debris and dust.[18]

Recommended Practice IV
At the conclusion of the day's schedule, operating rooms, scrub/utility areas, corridors, furnishings, and equipment should be terminally cleaned.

Interpretive statement 1:
Furniture and equipment should be thoroughly cleaned with a disinfectant. Mechanical friction should be used.

Rationale 1:
Sanitation in the operating room is essential to reduce the possibility of contamination of patients and health care personnel.[19]

Interpretive statement 2:
Handles of cabinets and push plates of doors should be cleaned.

Rationale 2:
Contamination is more likely to occur around handles and push plates.[20]

Interpretive statement 3:
Refillable soap dispensers should be disassembled and cleaned before being refilled.

Rationale 3:
Liquid soap containers can become contaminated and serve as reservoirs for microorganisms.[21]

Interpretive statement 4:
Floors should be flooded with a fresh hospital-grade detergent disinfectant, mechanically scrubbed, and the solution removed.

Rationale 4:
Sanitation in the OR is essential to remove organic debris and dust.[22]

Interpretive statement 5:
Cleaning equipment should be disassembled, cleaned with a detergent disinfectant, and dried thoroughly before storage.

Rationale 5:
Cleaning equipment is cleaned to prevent growth of microorganisms during storage and to prevent subsequent contamination of the operating room.[23]

Recommended Practice V
All areas and equipment in the surgical suite should be cleaned according to an established routine.

Interpretive statement 1:
Areas and equipment to be cleaned should include, but are not limited to, air conditioning grills/filters, cabinets, shelves, walls, ceilings, overhead tracks, offices, lounges, and locker rooms.

Rationale 1:
Sanitation is essential to reduce the possibility of contamination of the patient, personnel, and operating room.[24]

Recommended Practice VI
Policies and procedures on operating room environmental sanitation should be written, reviewed annually, and readily available within the health care setting.

Interpretive statement 1:
These policies and procedures should include au-

thority, responsibility, and accountability for the enforcement of operating room environmental sanitation.

Rationale 1:
Policies and procedures serve as operational guidelines.[25]

Interpretive statement 2:
Information on operating room environmental sanitation should be included in the staff orientation and ongoing education of personnel in the operating room practice setting.

Rationale 2:
Staff orientation and education assist in the development of job knowledge, skills, and attitudes that affect direct patient care.[26]

Interpretive statement 3:
Policies and procedures establish guidelines for quality improvement activities to be used when monitoring operating room environmental sanitation.

Rationale 3:
Quality improvement activities acts as a tool to monitor operating room environmental sanitation in the practice setting.[27]

Glossary
Disinfectants: Agents that kill all growing or vegetative forms of microorganisms, thus completely eliminating them from inanimate objects. Germicide is a synonym for disinfectant. The three levels of disinfectants are:
  low-level: An agent that kills most vegetative bacteria, fungi, and lipoprotein (lipid- and protein-coated) viruses.
  intermediate or hospital grade: An agent that kills the tubercle bacilli and nolipid viruses.
  high-level: An agent that kills vegetative bacteria, tubercle bacilli, some spores, fungi, lipid and nonlipid viruses.
Impervious: Incapable of being passed through, as by a liquid.
Sterilization: Processes by which all pathogenic and nonpathogenic microorganisms, including spores, are killed. This term refers only to a process capable of destroying all forms of microbial life, including spores.
Terminal sterilization and disinfection: Procedures carried out for the destruction of pathogens at the end of operative procedures in the operating room or in other areas of patient contact.

Notes:
1. G F Mallison, "Housekeeping in operating suites," *AORN Journal* 21 (February 1975) 213-220.
2. P Wells, "'Confine and contain approach' to OR cleanup," *AORN Journal* 25 (January 1977) 60-65.
3. J S Garner, M S Favero, "Guideline for handwashing and hospital environmental control, 1985," in *Guidelines for the Prevention and Control of Nosocomial Infections* (Atlanta: Centers for Disease Control, 1985) 5.
4. Centers for Disease Control, "Recommendations for prevention of HIV transmission in health-care settings," *Morbidity and Mortality Weekly Report* (MMWR) 36 (2S) (Aug 21, 1987) 10S-11S.
5. *Ibid,* 6S.
6. *Ibid,* 7S.
7. *Ibid,* 6S.
8. *Ibid,* 6S.
9. L J Atkinson, M L Kohn, eds, *Berry and Kohn's Introduction to Operating Room Technique,* sixth ed (New York City: McGraw-Hill, 1986) 158, 184-185; Centers for Disease Control, "Recommendation for Prevention of HIV transmission in health-care settings," 11S.
10. Centers for Disease Control, "Recommendation for prevention of HIV transmission in health-care settings," 11S.
11. Centers for Disease Control, "Update: Universal precautions for prevention of transmission of human immunodeficiency virus, hepatitis V virus, and other bloodborne pathogens in health-care settings," MMWR 37 (24) (June 24, 1988) 380. Centers for Disease Control, "Recommendations for prevention of HIV transmission in health-care settings," 3S-6S.
12. Centers for Disease Control, "Recommendations for prevention of HIV transmission in health-care settings," 6S.
13. L K Groah, *Operating Room Nursing: The Perioperative Role* (Reston, Va: Reston Publishing

Co, 1983) 160; Atkinson, Kohn, eds, *Berry & Kohn's Introduction to Operating Room Technique,* 183.

14. Centers for Disease Control, "Recommendations for prevention of HIV transmission in healthcare settings," 12S.

15. *Ibid,* 9S.

16. Groah, *Operating Room Nursing: The Perioperative Role.* 159, 170; Atkinson, Kohn, eds, *Berry & Kohn's Introduction to Operating Room Technique,* 184.

17. Atkinson, Kohn, eds, *Berry & Kohn's Introduction to Operating Room Technique,* 184.

18. C Spry, *Essentials of Perioperative Nursing: A Self-Learning Guide* (Rockville, Md: Aspen Publishers, 1988) 102.

19. *Ibid,* 102.

20. Atkinson, Kohn, eds, *Berry & Kohn's Introduction to Operating Room Technique,* 186.

21. Garner, Favero, *Guideline for Handwashing and Hospital Environmental Control,* 1985, 8.

22. Spry, *Essentials of Perioperative Nursing: A Self-Learning Guide,* 102.

23. Groah, *Operating Room Nursing: The Perioperative Role.* 172.

24. Spry, *Essentials of Perioperative Nursing: A Self-Learning Guide,* 102-103.

25. "Standards of administrative nursing practice: OR," *AORN Standards and Recommended Practices for Perioperative Nursing* (Denver: Association of Operating Room Nurses, Inc., 1987) II:3-3.

26. *Ibid,* II:3-4.

27. *AMH/88, Accreditation Manual for Hospitals* (Chicago: Joint Commission on the Accreditation of Healthcare Organizations, 1987) 2:95.

Suggested Readings

"Acquired immune deficiency syndrome (AIDS): Precautions for clinical and laboratory staffs," *Morbidity and Mortality Weekly Report* 31 (Nov 5, 1982) 577-579.

AMH/88, Accreditation Manual for Hospitals, Chicago: Joint Commission on the Accreditation of Healthcare Organizations, 1987.

American Hospital Association, "A hospital-wide approach to AIDS: Recommendations of the advisory committee on infections within hospitals." *Infection Control* 5 (May 1984) 242-248.

Centers for Disease Control. "Recommendations for preventing the transmission of infection with human T-lymphotropic virus Type III/lymphadenopathy-associated virus during invasive procedures." *Morbidity and Mortality Weekly Report* 35 (April 11, 1986) 221-223.

Centers for Disease Control. "Recommendations for preventing the transmission of infection with human T-lymphotropic virus Type III/lymphadenopathy-associated virus in the workplace." *Morbidity and Mortality Weekly Report* 34 (Nov 15, 1985) 681-685.

Chiba, E. "Procedures for HB antigen carriers," in *Competent to Care – The World Over,* (World Conference of Operating Room Nurses IV). Denver: Association of Operating Room Nurses, Inc, 1985, 275-283.

Garner, J; Simmons, B. *Guideline for Isolation Precautions in Hospitals.* Atlanta: Centers for Disease Control, 1983.

Garner, J; Simmons, B. *Guideline for Prevention of Surgical Wound Infection.* Atlanta: Centers for Disease Control, 1985.

Gerberding, J L. "Recommended infection control policies for patients with human immunodeficiency virus infection: An update," *The New England Journal of Medicine,* 315 (Dec 11, 1986) 1562-1564.

Gruendemann, B; Meeker, M, eds. *Alexander's Care of the Patient in Surgery,* eighth ed. St. Louis: C V Mosby, 1987.

Hughes, J. "Epidemiology of nosocomial infections," in *Manual of Clinical Microbiology,* fourth ed, E H Lennette et al, eds, Washington, DC: American Society for Microbiology, 1985, 99-142.

Palmer, P N. "Nurses, surgeons, anesthesiologists meet to discuss operating room problems," *AORN Journal* 46 (July 1987) 28-31.

Reed, E; Applegeet, C. "Infection control: Aorn recommended practices in ambulatory surgery." *AORN Journal* 43 (May 1986) 1002-1005.

Ricards, J. "Clinical issues," *AORN Journal* 41 (May 1985) 920-922.

Scullin, D. "Anesthetic implications of the acquired immunodeficiency syndrome (AIDS): Part I." *American Association of Nurse Anesthetists (AANA) Journal* 54 (Oct 1985) 400-410.

Scullin, D. "Anesthetic implications of the acquired immunodeficiency syndrome (AIDS): Part II."

American Association of Nurse Anesthetists (AANA) Journal 54 (Dec 1986) 480-485.

Turner, J; Williamson, K. "AIDS: A challenge for contemporary nursing (Part II: Clinical AIDS)." *Focus on Critical Care* 13 (Aug 1986) 41-50.

Originally Published June 1975
Format revised March 1978, March 1982, and July 1982
Revision April 1984 *AORN Journal.*
Revised November 1988 *AORN Journal.*

Appendix 13: Recommended Practices for Selection and Use of Packaging Materials

The following recommended practices were developed by the AORN Recommended Practices Subcommittee and have been approved by the Technical Practices Coordinating Committee and the Board of Directors. They were published as proposed recommended practices in the November 1987 *AORN Journal* for comment by members and others. They are intended to represent a consensus of AORN members and others.

These recommended practices are intended as achievable recommendations representing what is believed to be an optimal level of practice. Policies and procedures will reflect variations in practice settings and/or clinical situations that determine the degree to which the recommended practices can be fulfilled.

AORN recognizes the numerous different settings in which perioperative nurses practice. The recommended practices are intended as guidelines adaptable to various practice settings. These practice settings include traditional operating rooms, ambulatory surgery units, physicians' offices, cardiac catheterization laboratories, endoscopy rooms, radiology departments, and all other areas where surgery may be performed.

Purpose
These recommended practices provide guidelines for selection and use of packaging materials used for items to be sterilized. These packaging materials include reusable fabrics, single-use disposables, and container systems. Packaging materials should ensure sterility of package contents until opened for use and should permit removal of contents without contamination.

Recommended Practice I
Materials used for packaging of sterile supplies should be compatible with the sterilization process.

Interpretive Statement 1
Materials used for packaging prior to steam sterilization should allow adequate air removal, steam penetration, and drying.

Rationale 1
Basic sterilization parameters for fabric-wrapped packs and packages are based on 140-thread count.[1] Sterilization parameters can vary according to humidity, altitude, fabric, wrap, load, and position for each sterilizer.[2] Sterilizer parameters for container systems currently are not standardized.[3]

Interpretive Statement 2
Materials used for packaging prior to gas sterilization should allow adequate penetration of sterilant and effective aeration.

Rationale 2
Toxic residues can be harmful to the patient and personnel.[4]

Interpretive Statement 3
Reusable fabrics should be laundered before each use to provide a hydrated wrapper.

Rationale 3
Laundering reusable fabrics provides the fibers with a relatively normal state of hydration before sterilization.[5]

Interpretive Statement 4
The surface area covered by heat-sealed patches on reusable fabric should be given consideration before the fabric is used.

Rationale 4
Reusable materials with heat-sealed patches can be effectively sterilized. The limit to the percent of exposed surface area that can be patched depends on mode of sterilizing, positioning in the sterilizer, and the number of layers of patched fabric.[6]

Interpretive Statement 5
Peel-pack pouches should have as much air removed as possible before sealing.

Rationale 5
Air acts as a barrier to heat and moisture and may cause rupturing of packages.[7]

Interpretive Statement 6
Like materials of penetrable surfaces of peel-pack pouches should touch when double packaged. The inner pouch should be sealed.

Reprinted with permission from *AORN Standards and Recommended Practices for Perioperative Nursing,* 1991. Copyright © AORN Inc, 10170 East Mississippi Avenue, Denver, CO 80231.

Rationale 6
Like materials of peel-pack pouches must be placed together to ensure penetration of sterilant, air, and/or moisture. Sealing the inner pouch facilitates delivery of multiple items to the sterile field. Proper packaging allows visualization of the item.[8]

Recommended Practice II
Materials used for packaging should contribute to the maintenance of sterility of contents.

Interpretive Statement 1
Loss of sterility of package contents is considered event related, not time related, and is dependent in part on the type of packaging used.

Rationale 1
Event-related factors include the following:
a. frequency and method of handling,
b. storage area conditions such as location, space, open/closed shelving, temperature, humidity, dust, insects, flooding, vermin, etc.[9]

Interpretive Statement 2
Packages wrapped in reusable fabrics or single-use disposable wrappers should be double-wrapped sequentially. Materials should be used according to manufacturer's recommendations.

Rationale 2
The sequential-wrapping method, covering the item once then wrapping it again, provides an improved barrier and allows for aseptic presentation.[10]

Interpretive Statement 3
Package integrity should be maintained.
a. Wrappers of all types should be free of holes.
b. Peel-packaging materials should be resistant to tears and punctures and should not delaminate when opened.
c. Container system filters should remain intact, and valves and/or gaskets should remain sealed following sterilization. Manufacturers' recommendations should be followed.

Rationale 3
Contamination of sterile contents can occur with ports of entry including holes, breaks, or ruptures in packages or faulty mechanical function of container systems.[11]

Interpretive Statement 4
Peel-packaging materials should provide a seal of proven integrity and not allow for resealing.

Rationale 4
Seal integrity relies on bonding the plastic portion to the paper portion to prevent contamination.[12]

Recommended Practice III
Materials used for packaging should permit ease in aseptic presentation.

Interpretive Statement 1
The wrapper or container system should permit opening without significant risk of product contamination or damage to the product.

Rationale 1
Only sterile items are used within a sterile field.[13]

Interpretive Statement 2
Double pouching or additional packaging of multiple items may be necessary.

Rationale 2
The inner pouch, or additional packaging, is used to keep multiple items together for ease in aseptic presentation.[14]

Recommended Practice IV
Policies and procedures for packaging selection and use should be written, reviewed annually, and readily available within the practice setting.

Interpretive Statement 1
Policies and procedures should establish authority, responsibility, and accountability for selection and use of packaging materials.

Rationale 1
Policies and procedures serve as operational guidelines.[15]

Interpretive Statement 2
This information should be included in the orientation and ongoing education of all appropriate personnel within the practice setting.

Rationale 2
Orientation and education facilitate interpretation and administration of policies and procedures.[16]

Interpretive statement 3:
Policies and procedures establish guidelines for quality improvement activities to be used when monitoring the selection and use of packaging materials.

Rationale 3:
Quality improvement activities acts as a tool to monitor the selection and use of packaging materials for the surgical suite.[17]

Glossary
Container system—Specifically designed metal or plastic receptacles used to package items for sterilization, usually surgical instruments.[18]
Double wrap—Sequential wrapping using two wrappers.
Heat-sealed patch—Patch sealed by heat and occasionally referenced as a vulcanized patch.
Packaging—A generic term meant to include all types of packaging such as plastic covers, woven or nonwoven wraps, pouches, container systems, etc.
Pouch—A flexible bag or receptacle used to package items for sterilization.[19]
Reusable wrappers—(a) Two layers of 140-thread-count woven fabric finished using a technique that contains raw edges and loose theads without cross-stitching, forming a blind hem; (b) one layer of 270-280-thread-count woven fabric without cross-stitching.
Single-use disposables—Materials made of nonwoven fabric and discarded after use.[20]

Notes
1. *Good Hospital Practice: Steam Sterilization and Sterility Assurance* (Arlington, Va: Association for the Advancement of Medical Instrumentation, 1988) 7.
2. J J Perkins, *Principles and Methods of Sterilization in Health Sciences*, second ed (Springfield, Ill: Charles C Thomas, 1982) 193-194; "Recommended practices for sterilization and disinfection," in *AORN Standards and Recommended Practices for Perioperative Nursing* (Denver: Association of Operating Room Nurses, Inc, 1988) III:14-1.
3. M C Reichert, "Innovations in sterilization technology for instrument processing," *Medical Instrumentation* 17 (January-February 1983) 88-89.
4. *Inhospital Sterility Assurance–Current Perspectives* (Arlington, Va: Association for the Advancement of Medical Instrumentation, 1982) 33.
5. Perkins, *Principles and Methods of Sterilization in Health Sciences*, 214.
6. V W Greene, G M Borlaug, E Nelson, "Effects of patching on sterilization of surgical textiles," *AORN Journal* 33 (June 1981) 1260.
7. N E Danielson, *Ethylene Oxide Use in Hospitals: A Manual for Health Care Personnel*, second ed (Chicago: American Hospital Publishing, Inc, 1986) 67.
8. *Ibid*, 73.
9. L K Groah, *Operating Room Nursing: The Perioperative Role* (Reston, Va: Reston Publishing Co, Inc, 1983) 179.
10. *Inhospital Sterility Assurance–Current Perspectives*, 31.
11. Danielson, *Ethylene Oxide Use in Hospitals*, 64; American Society for Hospital Central Service Personnel of the American Hospital Association (ASHCSP/AHA), *Training Manual for Central Service Technicians* (Chicago: American Hospital Association, 1986) 131.
12. ASHCSP/AHA, *Training Manual for Central Service Technicians*, 130; Danielson, *Ethylene Oxide Use in Hospitals*, 64.
13. *Inhospital Sterility Assurance–Current Perspectives*, 30-31.
14. "Questions," *Journal of Hospital Supply, Processing, and Distribution* 1 (September-October 1983) 68.
15. "Standards of administrative nursing practice: OR," in *AORN Standards and Recommended Practices for Perioperative Nursing* (Denver: Association of Operating Room Nurses, Inc, 1988) II:3-3.
16. B J Gruendemann, M H Meker, eds, *Alexander's Care of the Patient in Surgery*, eighth ed, (St Louis: C V Mosby Co, 1987) 7-8.
17. *AMH/88 Accreditation Manual for Hospitals* (Chicago: Joint Commission on Accreditation of Healthcare Organizations, 1987) 83.

18. ASHCSP/AHA, *Training Manual for Central Service Technicians,* 130.
19. *Ibid,* 247.
20. *Ibid,* 221.

Suggested Reading

Beck, W C. "Aseptic barriers in surgery: Their present status." *Archives of Surgery* 116 (February 1981) 240-244.

Belkin, N. "Finding the balance in packaging materials." *HPN Hospital Purchasing News* 10 (March 1986) 30-31.

Hogness, J R, et al. *International Conference on the Reuse of Disposable Medical Devices in the 1980's.* Washington, DC: Institute for Health Policy Analysis, Georgetown University Medical Center, 1984, 13.

Hoke, L. "Sterile packaging: A shared responsibility." *Journal of Hospital Supply, Processing and Distribution* 2 (September-October 1984) 89-91.

Klapes, N A, et al. "Effect of long-term storage on sterile status of devices in surgical packs," *Infection Control* 8 (July 1987) 289-293.

Standard, P G; Mackel, D C; Mallison, G F. "Microbial penetration of muslin- and paper-wrapped sterile packs stored on open shelves and in closed cabinets." *Applied Microbiology* 22 (September 1971) 432-437.

Originally published February 1983 *AORN Journal.*
Revised November 1988 *AORN Journal.*

Appendix 14: Recommended Practices for Sterilization and Disinfection

The following recommended practices were developed by the AORN Recommended Practices Subcommittee and have been approved by the Technical Practices Coordinating Committee and Board of Directors. They were originally published in the November 1985 *AORN Journal* for comment by members and others. They are intended to represent a concensus of AORN members and others.

These recommended practices are intended as achievable recommendations representing what is believed to be an optimal level of practice. Policies and procedures will reflect variations in practice settings and/or clinical situations that determine the degree to which the recommended practices can be fulfilled.

AORN recognizes the numerous different settings in which perioperative nurses practice. The recommended practices are intended as guidelines adaptable to various practice settings. These practice settings include traditional operating rooms, ambulatory surgery units, physicians' offices, cardiac catheterization laboratories, endoscopy rooms, radiology departments, and all other areas where surgery may be performed.

Purpose

These recommended practices provide guidelines to achieve sterilization and disinfection of supplies and equipment. The outcome of surgical intervention depends on the creation and maintenance of an aseptic environment. Measures to prevent surgical wound infection include provision of supplies and equipment free of contamination at the time of use. Sterilization and disinfection are methods utilized in this effort. Sterilization provides the highest level of assurance that an object is void of viable microbes while disinfection reduces the risk of microbial contamination but without the same level of assurance.

Recommended Practice I
All items to be sterilized should be prepared to reduce the bioburden.

Interpretive Statements:
1. All items should be thoroughly cleaned.
2. Items should be prepared in a clean, controlled environment.

Rationale
1. The reliability of sterilization is affected by the number, type, and inherent resistance of organisms on the items to be sterilized, (i.e., bioburden or bioload), as well as surrounding soil, crystals, oils, and other materials which may interfere with penetration of sterilant.[1]
2. Temperature, humidity, illumination, area design, attire of personnel, and cleaning procedures are some of the factors which should be regulated to assure appropriate presterilization processing.[2]

Recommended Practice II
All articles to be sterilized should be arranged so all surfaces will be directly exposed to the sterilizing agent for the prescribed time and temperature.

Interpretive Statements:
1. All jointed instruments should be open and/or unlocked. Instruments designed for disassembly should be disassembled. Instruments should not be held together with rubberbands. If lubrication is necessary, a nontoxic water soluble lubricant should be used.
2. Instrument sets should be placed in perforated wire mesh bottom trays or in instrument container systems. The total weight of the metal mass should not exceed approximately 16 pounds or a weight documented by the manufacturer of the sterilizer or container system or independent research.
3. When utensils are nested in one package, they should be separated by absorbent towels or other moisture absorbing material.
4. Nested items should be positioned in the same direction so that air pockets are not created, condensate can drain out and sterilant can circulate freely.
5. After laundering, textiles to be sterilized should be stored at a temperature of 65-72° F. (18-22° C.) and at a relative humidity of 35-75%.
6. Woven textile drape packs should not exceed 12" × 12" × 20", weigh more than 12 lbs. or exceed 7.2 lbs./cu. ft. pack density.
7. All articles should be aligned on sterilization carriers or in the sterilizer in a manner which does not interfere with air removal and introduction of sterilant.

Reprinted with permission from *AORN Standards and Recommended Practices for Perioperative Nursing*, 1991. Copyright © AORN Inc, 10170 East Mississippi Avenue, Denver, CO 80231.

Rationale
1. Reliable sterilization depends on contact of the sterilant with all surfaces.[3]
2. The conditions necessary for sterilization are difficult to achieve in excessively heavy instrument sets. Heavy sets may require longer time to attain sterilization temperature and drying may be delayed due to condensation and pooling of moisture.[4]
3. Placing absorbent towels or other moisture absorbent materials between nested utensils enhances passage of steam to all surfaces during the sterilization process and facilitates drying by preventing pooling of the condensate.[5]
4. Superheating occurs when dehydrated materials absorb the moisture from steam causing an increased release of heat. Superheating will cause deterioration of the textiles and may cause sterilization failure.[6]
5. Limiting the size and density of pack aids penetration of the sterilizing agent.[7]
6. Proper placement of packs and utensils in a steam sterilizer load facilitates displacement of air, contact of steam with all surfaces of containers and their contents and also facilitates drying. In combined loads of fabrics and hard goods, placing hard goods on the lowest shelves of the sterilizer rack prevents wetting of fabric packs from condensate dripping from hard goods surfaces.[8]

Recommended Practice III
All wrapped articles to be sterilized should be packaged in materials that meet the criteria in the AORN Recommended Practices for Selection and Use of Packaging Materials.[9]

Recommended Practice IV
Chemical indicators, also known as sterilization process indicators, should be used to indicate that items have been exposed to a sterilization process.

Interpretive Statements:
1. A chemical indicator should be clearly visible on the outside of every package to be sterilized.
2. A chemical indicator may be placed in packages or open trays to be sterilized.
3. Chemical indicator results should be interpreted according to manufacturer's written instructions and indicator reaction specifications.

Rationale
1. Chemical indicators show that items have been exposed to one or more specific physical conditions during a sterilization cycle but may not prove that sterilization has been achieved. Chemical indicators do not replace sterilization quality assurance measures, such as the monitoring of temperature, time and pressure; biological monitoring, proper sterilizer operation and proper packaging, storing and handling.[10]
2. Chemical indicators, when used within packages, should be placed in the position which is the most difficult for the sterilant to reach.[11]
3. A great deal of controversy exists regarding the use of chemical indicators in every package to be sterilized. The cost effectiveness of this procedure is not proven. Chemical indicators vary in their abilities to monitor sterilization parameters.[12] Indicators which measure more parameters are not necessarily better. The key parameters of steam sterilization include time, temperature, steam saturation and purity while the primary parameters for ethylene oxide sterilization are time, temperature, gas concentration, and relative humidity. Each practice setting should formulate its own policy regarding the use of chemical indicators. Factors to be considered should include their benefit vs. cost, performance limitations, and personnel knowledge of sterilization principles.[13]

Recommended Practice V
The efficacy of the sterilizing process should be monitored at regular intervals with reliable biological indicators.

Interpretive Statements:
1. Commercially manufactured biological indicators prepared in accordance with United States pharmacopoeia minimum performance criteria should be stored and used according to the indicator manufacturer's written instructions.
2. Measurements should be performed with a

biological indicator that employs spores of established resistance in a known population.
3. Biological indicator types and minimum recommended measurement intervals should be:
   a. Steam sterilizers — *Bacillus stearothermophilus*; weekly and as needed.[14]
   b. Ethylene oxide (EO) sterilizers — *Bacillus subtilis*, var. globigii, or var. niger; at least weekly, and as needed.[15]
4. Every sterilizer load containing implantable objects should be monitored with a biological indicator. These objects should not be used until the biological indicator test is negative at 48 hours.[16]
5. Biological indicators should be placed in a test pack. Biological indicator test packs should be utilized for routine monitoring and as a challenge test following any major redesign and relocation, suspected malfunction, major repair, and as needed. The following are examples of test packs that can be used:
   a. Steam Sterilizer
      Routine test pack: One biological test pack for steam sterilizers consists of three muslin surgical gowns, twelve towels, thirty 4" by 4" gauze sponges, five laparotomy sponges, and one muslin drape sheet, or equivalent linens. Two biological indicators separated by a towel should be placed in the center of the pack. Chemical indicators must also be placed in the center of the one towel above or below the biological indicators. The pack should be approximately 12" by 12" by 20" in size and should weigh 10-12 pounds.[17] (It should be noted that the Association for the Advancement of Medical Instrumentation (AAMI) is in the process of evaluating a towel test pack.)
   b. General Purpose EO Sterilizer
      1. The routine test pack should consist of the following items: Two biological indicators of the same lot number, one in the test pack, and one as a control. Place one biological indicator (BI) in a plastic (or glass) syringe of sufficient size that the plunger diaphram does not touch the BI when the plunger is inserted into the barrel of the syringe. The BI should not be removed from the protective covering supplied by the manufacturer. The instructions of the BI manufacturer should be consulted to ensure that the BI selected is appropriate for use in the specific sterilizer being monitored. The needle end of the syringe must be open (i.e., the tip guard must be removed). The syringe is placed in the folds of a clean surgical towel (30" by 18", huckaback). These items are contained in one peel pouch or nonwoven wrapper that is large enough to contain the test pack components which is typical of that customarily used in the health care facility. The contents of the test pack should be aerated. The BI can be removed before or after aeration.[18]
      2. Challenge test pack: This EO test pack presents a greater challenge to sterilizer and consists of materials, different than the routine test pack. This consists of four clean surgical huckaback towels 30" × 18", fan folded in thirds, not ironed or taken directly from the dryer. (If dried, hold in an area of controlled humidity 24 hours), 1 - 10" section of latex tubing $^{3}/_{16}$" inside diameter, $^{1}/_{16}$" wall thickness, 1 plastic airway or a plastic syringe containing a chemical indicator, three BI indicators, 2 in test pack and 1 of the same lot number for control and two plastic or glass syringes (12 or 20 cc) without protective caps of the size to accommodate BI. (Check BI indicator manufacturer recommendations.) Wrap in two 24" × 24" wrappers.[19]
6. The biological test pack should be placed in the area of the sterilizer that will most challenge all sterilization parameters.
   a. Steam sterilizers: On edge at the front bottom, near the door in a routinely loaded sterilizer.
   b. EO Sterilizers: Placement and number of test packs depend on the chamber size.[20]
7. A single positive spore test does not necessarily indicate sterilizer failure.
   a. If the test is positive, the sterilizer should immediately be rechallenged for proper use and function. Items, other than implantable

ones, do not necessarily need to be recalled unless a sterilizer malfunction is found.[21]

b. If a sterilizer malfunction is discovered, all available items from the suspect load(s) should be recalled and reprocessed. A malfunctioning sterilizer should not be put back into use until it has been serviced and successfully tested according to manufacturer's recommendations.

Rationale

1. The biological monitoring process is the best method presently at our disposal to confirm the effectiveness of a sterilizing process.[22]
2. Sources vary in their recommendations on the frequency of use of biological test packs. Individual policy, based on knowledge of data, should determine frequency.[23]
3. It is recognized that in an emergency situation it may not be possible to quarantine implantable items for 48 hours. This recommendation should be followed whenever possible.[24]
4. False positive biological indicators from properly functioning sterilizers are not uncommon.[25]

Recommended Practice VI
Saturated steam under pressure should be utilized for sterilization of heat and moisture stable items. Steam sterilizers should be used according to manufacturer's written instructions.

Interpretive Statements:

1. Items to be steam sterilized should be disassembled, thoroughly cleaned, rinsed, and wiped or air dried.
2. Items should be positioned in a steam sterilizer to enhance air removal, allow free circulation and penetration of steam and to prevent excessive condensation.
3. The time-temperature settings recommended by the device manufacturer should be followed.

Rationale

1. Thorough cleaning removes concealed organisms protected by dried organic material that render sterilization more difficult.[26]
2. Effective sterilization of items is not only dependent on conscientious operation of the sterilizer but also upon correct methods of packaging and arrangement of items in the sterilizer.[27]

3. The time-temperature relationship required to achieve sterilization by steam varies with the type of sterilizer, cycle design, bioburden, packaging, and the size and type of item(s) to be sterilized.[28]

Recommended Practice VII
EO sterilization should be used for processing heat and moisture sensitive items. EO sterilizers and aerators should be used and vented according to the manufacturer's written instructions.

Interpretive Statements:

1. Items to be EO sterilized should be disassembled, cleaned, rinsed and wiped or air dried until no visible water droplets remain.
2. Articles should be positioned in the EO sterilizer to allow free circulation and penetration of the sterilant.
3. All EO sterilized items should be aerated according to the device and aerator manufacturer's written instructions.
4. The sterilizer manufacturer's recommendations for door opening and transfer should be followed.
5. Personnel should avoid direct contact with items during the transfer from EO sterilizer to aerator. The EO sterilized items should remain on the cart or in the basket during transportation.
6. Inhalation of EO should be avoided or minimized.
7. The employer should provide for monitoring employee exposure to EO.
8. EO sterilizers and aerators should be vented to the outside atmosphere via an appropriate vent line.

Rationale

1. Heavily soiled items inhibit gas permeation. Excessive moisture inhibits sterilization and produces toxic byproducts not removed through aeration.[29]
2. EO sterilization depends upon a correct balance of the four essential parameters which are concentration of the sterilant, relative humidity, temperature, and exposure time. The operating manual should describe the required relationship of these parameters for proper operation of that sterilizer.[30]

3. Aeration of EO sterilized items essential to reduce the residue of EO which may be harmful to staff and/or patients. Length of aeration depends on many variables, including:
   a. Composition, form, density, and weight of the sterilized item.
   b. Type of EO sterilization system used.
   c. Temperature of aeration chamber, number of filtered air changes per hour and air flow characteristics, and
   d. Intended use of the item (e.g., external application or implantable).

   Polyvinyl chloride (PVC) is one of the most challenging materials from which EO residue must be eliminated. If the composition of an item is not known, it should be treated like PVC. Aeration required for PVC in a mechanical aerator is 8 hours at 60°C. (140°F.) or 12 hours at 50°C. (122°F.).[31]

4. Desirable EO sterilizer safety features include but are not limited to:
   a. Purge system at end of cycle.
   b. Door locking and sealing mechanisms.
   c. Audible alarm at end of EO cycle.
   d. Automatic door controls.[32]

5. The carts or baskets utilized to transfer items from the EO sterilizers to the aerator should be pulled rather than pushed. Pushing causes air to flow over the contents of the cart and the potential for inhalation of EO by the operator is increased.[33]

6. Excessive exposure to EO presents a health hazard to workers.[34]

7. EO sterilizer and aerator design and venting guidelines are extensive. Consult governmental regulations, (Occupational Safety and Health Agency (OSHA)), and the sterilizer and/or aerator manufacturer's recommendations for additional requirements.[35]

Recommended Practice VIII
Every package should be imprinted or labeled with a load control number that indicates the sterilizer used, the cycle or load number, the date of sterilization and an expiration date.

Interpretive Statement:
Load control numbers should be used for quality control to facilitate the identification and retrieval of supplies, inventory control, and stock rotation.

Rationale
Quality control records to insure sterility must be documented and records maintained.[36]

Recommended Practice IX
Sterilized articles should be carefully handled and only as necessary. They should be stored in a well-ventilated, limited access area with controlled temperature and humidity.

Interpretive Statements:
1. All wrapped sterilized items should remain untouched on the sterilizer rack or carriage until adequately cooled.
2. The contents of any sterilized package should be considered contaminated if the integrity of the packaging is visibly damaged.
3. All wrapped sterilized packages should be handled and stored in a manner which minimizes stress and pressure. The storage area should provide protection against dust, insects, vermin and temperature and humidity extremes.

Rationale
1. Placement of warm wrapped sterilized items on a cold surface can induce condensate formation resulting in contamination of the items.[37]
2. Cautious minimal handling of sterile packages reduces the possibility of microbial contamination.[38]

Recommended Practice X
Performance records for all sterilizers should be maintained for each cycle and retained for the period of time indicated by individual policy and/or the state's statute of limitations.

Interpretive Statements:
1. Mechanical control monitors such as the time-temperature recording device and temperature and pressure gauges should be monitored by the sterilizer operator at the beginning and end of each sterilizer cycle to verify function.
2. The time-temperature recording device indicat-

ing the load number of each steam sterilization cycle should be maintained and changed daily or more often as required by the sterilizer manufacturer's instructions.
3. A sterilizer performance record should include the sterilizer identification number, sterilization date, cycle number, contents of each load, duration and temperature of exposure phase (if not provided on sterilizer recording charts), identification of operator(s), results of biological tests and dates performed, time-temperature recording charts from sterilizers, and any other test results.

Rationale
Sterilizer performance records may be utilized for documentation for product recall and quality assurance.[39]

Recommended Practice XI
Flash sterilization should be used for emergency sterilization of clean, unwrapped instruments and porous items only.

Interpretive Statements:
1. Flash sterilization should be used only when time does not permit sterilization by the preferred wrapped procedure.
2. Implantable items should not be flash sterilized.
3. Specialty instrumentation or devices (i.e. drills) require different exposure times. The device manufacturer's recommendations should be followed.
4. The recording device should be checked to assure appropriate time and temperature exposure following each cycle.
5. The item(s) should be transferred in a manner to maintain sterility.

Rationale
1. Flash sterilization is defined as sterilization of unwrapped items in a gravity displacement or prevacuum sterilizer with recommended minimum exposure times and temperatures as follows:
   a. Gravity displacement
      1. Instruments, metal, 3 minutes at or above 132° C. (270° F.).
      2. Instruments, metal combined with porous items, 10 minutes at or above 132° C. (270° F.).[40]
   b. Prevacuum
      1. Instruments, metal, 3 minutes at or above 132° C. (270° F.).
      2. Instruments, metal combined with porous items, 4 minutes at or above 132° C. (270° F.).[40]
2. Speed works against reliability of sterilization. It reduces the margin of safety, the ability to accommodate operator error, increases the possibility of trapped air, and requires a high degree of reliability in the sterilizer.[41]

Recommended Practice XII
Preventive maintenance of all sterilizers should be performed according to individual policy on a scheduled basis by qualified personnel, using the sterilizer manufacturer's service manual as a reference.

Interpretive Statements:
1. Sterilizers should be inspected and cleaned daily or at the interval recommended by the manufacturer. Proper function of the recording chart and pen and integrity of door gasket should be included in this inspection.
2. The chamber discharge system should be cleaned at least weekly according to manufacturer instructions.
3. In a prevacuum sterilizer, a Bowie-Dick test should be carried out each day prior to the first sterilization cycle. If the sterilizer is in use 24 hours a day, the test should be run at the same time each day. The Bowie-Dick test pack should be placed horizontally at the bottom front of the sterilizer near the door, in an otherwise empty chamber for 3.5 minutes.
4. The time-temperature charting devices and temperature-pressure gauges should be calibrated after any repair affecting sterilizer performance and at least every 6 months or at the interval recommended by the sterilizer manufacture.
5. A maintenance record should be kept for each sterilizer and should include at least:
   a. Date of Service.
   b. Model number of sterilizer.
   c. Serial number of sterilizer.

d. Location of equipment.
e. Description of service performed.
f. Description and quantity of parts replaced.
g. Results of biological indicator and/or Bowie-Dick test following sterilizer repair.
h. Name of person performing service.
i. Name of authorizing individual from health care institution requesting service.
j. Signature and title of person acknowledging completed work.

Rationale
1. Daily cleaning includes washing and rinsing all surfaces of the sterilizer to prevent accumulation of grease residue from materials being sterilized. The strainers located in the opening of the chamber discharge line should be removed daily and cleaned to insure that pores are free from lint and sediment.[42]
2. Periodic cleaning of the discharge system will prevent build up of grease residues and clogging substances that may retard air and condensate discharge from the chamber.[43]
3. The Bowie-Dick test evaluates the ability of prevacuum sterilizers to reduce air residuals effectively from the chamber space. If air has not been sufficiently removed, steam will drive air back into the load, air pockets will develop, and sterilizing conditions will not occur. The Bowie-Dick test pack consists of 100% cotton, freshly laundered huckaback towels (surgical towels). The towels are folded no smaller than 9 inches (24 cm) by 12 inches (30 cm) and stacked one on top of another until the stack measures 10 to 11 inches (25 to 27 cm). The Bowie-Dick type test sheet is placed in the center of this pack. A single wrapper is then loosely applied.[44] Disposable Bowie-Dick test packs are available.

Recommended Practice XIII
A high-level disinfectant should be used if an item is to be disinfected rather than sterilized.

Interpretive Statements:
1. Products selected for disinfection should be registered with the EPA. The manufacturer's written instructions should be followed for use.
2. Items to be disinfected should be thoroughly cleaned, rinsed and as dry as possible to avoid interference with the disinfecting process or dilution of the disinfectant.
3. All surfaces, including lumens and channels, of the item(s) should be in contact with the disinfectant solution for the recommended exposure time.
4. The disinfection process should occur:
a. prior to storage, and
b. immediately prior to use.
5. Prior to use, items should be aseptically removed from the disinfectant, rinsed thoroughly with sterile water and dried in a manner which minimizes the risk of contamination.
6. An expiration date, determined according to manufacturer's written recommendations, should be marked on the container of the disinfectant solution currently in use.
7. High-level disinfectant contact with skin, mucous membrane and eyes should be avoided.
8. High-level disinfectant solutions should be kept covered and used in a well ventilated area.

Rationale
1. In general, chemical disinfection differs from sterilization by its power to kill spores.[45]
2. Disinfection is divided into 3 levels: high, intermediate and low. A high-level disinfectant can be sporicidal as well as bacteriocidal and virucidal if contact time is sufficient. An intermediate-level disinfectant is not sporicidal but will kill the more resistant bacteria and viruses. A low-level disinfectant is not sporicidal and will kill only less resistant bacteria and viruses.[46]
3. The time required to achieve high-level disinfection varies depending on factors including the nature of the contaminating microorganisms, length of exposure to the agent, bioburden, and temperature.[47]
4. All disinfectants will cease to remain effective after repeated use due to dilution, inactivation, and/or instability.[48]
5. Some high-level disinfectant solutions have been reported to be irritating to the skin and the eyes.[49]

Recommended Practice XIV
Policies and precedures for sterilization and disinfection should be written, reviewed at least annu-

ally, and be readily available within the practice setting.

Interpretive Statements:
1. The policies should establish authority, responsibility, and accountability for sterilization and disinfection processes within the practice setting.
2. Procedures for sterilization and disinfection processes should include, but are not limited to:
   a. Preparation of items for processing.
   b. Processing of limited use items.
   c. Loading of the sterilizers.
   d. Use of chemical and biological indicators.
   e. Type of process and length of time for sterilization and disinfection of individual items.
   f. Use of each type of sterilizer and disinfectant within the practice setting.
   g. Specific aeration requirements for each type of material EO sterilized.
   h. Maintenance of sterilizers and aerators and records of same.
   i. Safety precautions associated with use of sterilizers, aerators, and disinfectants.
   j. Handling and storage of sterilized instruments and supplies.
   k. Designation of shelf life.
   l. Recall and/or disposal or reprocessing of outdated sterile supplies.
3. This information should be included in the orientation and ongoing education of all appropriate personnel in the practice setting.

Rationale
Documentation aids in communication, provides a mechanism for evaluation of nursing care, and service as evidence of care in legal matters.[50]

Guidelines
1. The following are some considerations when selecting the method of sterilization or disinfectant of surgical instruments, drapes, and other items:
   a. Availability/efficiency of sterilant/disinfectant.
   b. Physical properties of the item
   c. Urgency of need
   d. Standards of practice
   e. Hazard of toxic residue
   f. Infection control
   g. Manufacturer's recommendations
   h. Decontamination requirements
   i. Packaging requirements
   j. Ease of transport and storage
   k. Environmental/disposal requirements
   l. Cost containment
2. Reprocessing and/or reuse of single use items is a controversial subject. Research regarding this issue is minimal and inconclusive. Factors to be considered in the decision to reprocess and/or reuse include but are not limited to:
   a. Item function and safety following reprocessing
   b. Legal and ethical issues associated with the item
   c. Economics

   It is suggested that each single use item to be reprocessed or reused be considered on an individual basis after careful validation of the safety and efficacy of the device following reprocessing. Single use items that cannot be cleaned, sterilized, or disinfected without damage to the integrity and/or function should not be reprocessed. If a single use disposable item is reused, the liability for that device reverts to the user.[51]
3. These guidelines provide information on sterilizing and processing issues not frequently used in a health care facility.
   a. Dry Heat Sterilization

   Dry heat sterilization requires a dry-heat sterilizer and may be used for sterilization of anhydrous oils, powders, and greases. Sterilization by dry heat requires higher temperatures and longer sterilization times than moist heat sterilization. Death of microorganisms is achieved primarily by moist heat sterilization. Death of microorganisms is achieved primarily by oxidation rather than coagulation of protein.[52]

   One time-temperature ratio for dry heat sterilization is difficult and impractical to establish. The article to be sterilized, method of preparation, packaging and loading of sterilizer are all factors that influence this ratio.[53]
   b. Solution Sterilization

   Preparation and sterilization of liquids in the health care facility is discouraged as:
   1) Health care facilities are not equipped to monitor each sterilizer load to assure

sterility and non-pyrogencity and;
2) There is a great potential for burns from hot liquids if bottles burst.

If an emergency situation does arise where it is necessary to sterilize liquids, the sterilizer manufacturer's exposure period and cycle setting should be followed.

Precautions:
1) Sterilize separately from any other items.
2) Do not use prevacuum cycle.
3) Process in flasks, bottles or closures specifically designed for liquid sterilization.
4) Do not use screw caps or rubber stoppers with crimped seal.[54]

Glossary

1. *Ambient Air*—surrounding room air.

2. *Bioburden or bioload*—the microbial population of a specified item.

3. *Biological indicators*—a commercially prepared device with known population of highly resistant microorganisms to test the method of sterilization being monitored. The indicator is used to demonstrate that conditions necessary for sterilization were met during the cycle being monitored.

4. *Bowie-Dick type test*—a method of monitoring the adequacy of air removal from the chamber and porous load during the prevacuum stage in a high vacuum steam sterilizer. The Bowie-Dick test is not a test for sterilization.

5. *Chemical indicator*—a commercially prepared device to monitor all or part of the physical conditions of the sterilization cycle. There are 3 types of chemical indicators; the melting pellet type, the wicking type, and the thermochromic (color-change) ink type.

6. *Decontamination*—a process whereby the number of microorganisms on an item is eliminated or reduced.

7. *Exposure time*—the minimum length of time required for sterilization at a designated temperature.

8. *Heat-up time*—the time required for the entire load to reach the selected sterilizing temperature.

9. *Pack density*—size of pack expressed in cubic inches, divided by 1728, equals cubic feet of pack; weight of pack in pounds, divided by cubic feet of pack, equals density in pounds per cubic foot.

10. *Reuse*—cleaning and sterilization or disinfection of an item labeled single use disposable.

11. *Saturated steam sterilization*—the process that utilizes moist heat, at a temperature related to a water saturated steam pressure, for sufficient time to remove or destroy all viable forms of microorganisms. The process is a measure of a probability function.

12. *Superheating*—raising the temperature of a confined vapor above that normally corresponding to the saturation temperature at a given pressure. Saturated steam (containing as much water in the vapor state as physically possible and no liquid water) can only have one temperature at any given pressure. At sea level 15 pounds of pressure above atmospheric pressure will always produce a temperature 121°C. (250°F.) in saturated steam. If the steam loses water vapor, it can achieve a higher temperature at that pressure and thus become superheated.

Notes

1. "Good Hospital Practice: Steam Sterilization and Sterility Assurance", (Arlington, VA: Association for the Advancement of Medical Instrumentation, 1980) 3; Bertha Litsky, "Microbiology of sterilization," *AORN Journal* 26 (August 1977) 339-342; Seymour S Block, *Disinfection, Sterilization and Preservation,* (Philadelphia: Lea and Febiger, 1983) 11-14; Robert F Smith, "Reader clarifies item in "Q and A" column," *AORN Journal* 36 (September 1982) 350.

2. "Good hospital practice: Steam," 1-3.

3. John J Perkins, *Principles and Methods of Sterilization in Health Sciences,* (Springfield, IL: Charles C Thomas, 1982) 258.

4. "Good hospital practice: Steam," 3; "Questions," *Journal of Hospital Supply, Processing and Distribution,* 3 (March-April 1985) 71.

5. Perkins, *Principles and Methods of Sterilization in Health Sciences,* 260.

6. Ibid, 213-215; "Good hospital practice: Steam," 2-3; Peter Jancke, "Superheated Steam in porous load sterilizers," *Hospitals* (January-February 1983) 61-63; Block, *Disinfection, Sterilization and Preservation,* 23-24.

7. Perkins, *Principles and Methods of Sterilization in Health Sciences,* 193-194.

8. Ibid, 230-231

9. "Recommended Practices for Inhospital Packaging Materials," *AORN Standards and Recommended Practices for Perioperative Nursing,* (Denver: Association of Operating Room Nurses, Inc., 1983) Part III, Section 7, 1-3.

10. David Birnbaum and Robert Smith, "The emperor has no clothes: Sterilization quality assurance revisited," *Journal of Hospital Supply, Processing and Distribution* 2 (March-April 1984) 38-39; "Cleaning disinfection and sterilization of hospital equipment, *Guidelines for Hospital Environment Control,* (Atlanta: Centers for Disease Control, 1985) 11.

11. Thomas A. Augurt, "Sterilization and sterility assurance," *Journal of the Operating Room Research Institute* 20 (June 1982) 57; "Chemical Indicator Location," *Journal of Hospital Supply, Processing and Distribution* 2 (March-April 1984) 42.

12. Cherl-Ho Lee, Thomas Montville, Anthony Sinskey, "Comparison of the efficacy of steam sterilization indicators," *Applied and Environmental Microbiology* 37 (June 1979) 1113-1117.

13. Daniel E Mayworm, "Dan's Desk: The 12 x 12 x 20 Syndrome," *Tower Topics* 2 (1978) 2; Augurt, "Sterilization and sterility assurance," 20.

14. "Cleaning, disinfection and sterilization of hospital equipment," 12; "Good hospital practice: Steam," 8.

15. "Cleaning, disinfection and sterilization," 13, *Accreditation Manual for Hospitals, 1985* (Chicago: Joint Commission on Accreditation of Hospitals, 1984) 57.

16. "Cleaning, disinfection and sterilization of hospital equipment," 11.

17. "Good hospital practice: Steam," 8.

18. "Good hospital practice: Performance evaluation of ethylene oxide sterilizers—ethylene oxide test packs," (Arlington, VA: Association for the Advancement of Medical Instrumentation, 1985) 6, 8.

19. Ibid, 2-3.

20. Ibid, 5.

21. "Cleaning, disinfection and sterilization of hospital equipment," 12.

22. Perkins, Principles and Methods of Sterilization in Health Sciences, 493. American Society for Hospital Central Service Personnel of the American Hospital Association (ASHCSP/AHA), "Ethylene Oxide Use, 1982, 72.

23. "Good hospital practice: Steam," 9; "Good hospital practice: Performance evaluation of ethylene oxide sterilizers," 7; *Accreditation Manual for Hospitals, 1985,* 56; "Cleaning, Disinfection and Sterilization of hospital equipment," 4, 6.

24. "Good hospital practice: Performance evaluation of ethylene oxide sterilizers," 7.

25. "Are biological indicators the 'ultimate' sterilizer test?", *Hospital Infection Control* (September 1981) 115.

26. Perkins, *Principles and Methods of Sterilization in Health Sciences,* 239.

27. Ibid, 193

28. Litsky, "Microbiology of sterilization," *AORN Journal* 26 (August 1977) 339-342.

29. Perkins, *Principles and Methods of Sterilization in Health Sciences,* 514; "Good hospital practice: Performance evaluation of ethylene oxide sterilizers;" ASHCSP/AHA *Ethylene Oxide Use,* 44-45.

30. ASHCSP/AHA, *Ethylene Oxide Use,* 65-66.

31. Ibid, 83-85; "Good hospital practice: Ethylene oxide gas ventilation recommendations and safe use," (Arlington, VA: Association for the Advancement of Medical Instrumentation, March 1981), 8.

32. ASHCSP/AHA, *Ethylene Oxide Use,* 32-34.

33. Ibid, 83.

34. U S Department of Labor, Occupational Safety and Health Administration, *Federal Register,* "Occupational exposure to ethylene oxide," Vol. 49, No. 122 (June 22, 1984) 25734.

35. Ibid.

36. "Good Hospital Practices: Steam," 6.

37. Perkins, *Principles and Methods of Sterilization in Health Sciences,* 219.

38. Paul G Standard, Don C Mackel, G F Mallison, "Microbial penetration of muslin and paper-wrapped sterile packs stored on open shelves and in closed cabinets," *Applied Microbiology* 22 (September 1971) 435-436; Linda K Groah, *Operating Room Nursing: The Perioperative Role* (Reston, VA: Reston Publishing Co, Inc., 1983) 195; Dan Mayworm, "Sterile shelf life and expiration dating," *Journal of Hospital Supply, Processing and Distribution* 2 (November-December, 1984) 32-35.

39. *Accreditation Manual for Hospitals, 1985,* 56.

40. "Good hospital practice: Steam sterilization

using the unwrapped method (Flash sterilization)" (Arlington, VA: Association for the Advancement of Medical Instrumentation, June 1986) sec. 4.4.1.2,5.

41. Association for the Advancement of Medical Instrumentation, *In Hospital Sterility Assurance— Current Perspectives,* "Flash Sterilization," (Arlington, VA: Association for the Advancement of Medical Instrumentation, 1982) 63-64; Perkins, *Principles and Methods of Sterilization in Health Sciences,* 157; "Flash sterilization—A special report," *Journal of Hospital Supply, Processing and Distribution,* 3 (May-June 1985) 57-69.

42. Perkins, *Principles and Methods of Sterilization in Health Sciences,* 188.

43. Ibid.

44. "Good hospital practice: Steam," 9.

45. Earle Spaulding, "Chemical disinfection and antisepsis in the hospital," *Journal of Hospital Research* 9 (February 1978) 13.

46. Ibid, 13-15.

47. Ibid, p. 8.

48. Lucy Jo Atkinson and Mary Louise Kohn, *Berry and Kohn's Introduction to Operating Room Technique,* 5th ed. (New York: McGraw-Hill, Inc., 1978) 103-104.

49. Block, *Disinfection, Sterilization and Preservation,* 79-80.

50. "Recommended practices for documentation of perioperative nursing care," *AORN Standards and Recommended Practices for Perioperative Nursing* (Denver: Association of Operating Room Nurses, Inc., 1987) Part III, Section 3, 1-3.

51. Association for the Advancement of Medical Instrumentation (AAMI), "Reuse of disposables," (Arlington, VA: AAMI, 1983); CDC, *Guidelines for Handwashing and Environmental Control* (1985) 11-12; "Reusing disposables, examining the risks and benefits," *Hospital Infection Control* (September 1983) 114-132; "Reuse of disposable medical devices in the 1980s," (Washington DC: Institute for Health Policy Analysis, Georgetown University Medical Center, 1984) 6.

52. Block, *Disinfection, Sterilization, and Preservation,* 27-30, Perkins, *Principles of Sterilization,* 63.

53. Perkins, *Principles of Sterilization,* 289.

54. "Good hospital practice: Steam," 4.

Originally published August 1980, *AORN Journal.*
Format revision July, 1982.
Revision February 1987, *AORN Journal.*

Protocols for Sterilization of Office Surgical Units

Any discussion of cleanup methods must be based on the concept that every surgical procedure deserves the same care as every other—that is, every patient merits the same degree of safety and precaution. Additionally, personnel working in surgery must be protected. Therefore every case should be treated as potentially contaminated. Cleanup techniques must be set up to contain and confine organisms to prevent contaminating the entire operating suite.

Considerations

1. Blood and tissue fluids from any patient may contain organisms that are pathogenic to other persons.
2. Operating room practices have been developed that provide complete isolation for each patient.
3. Isolation procedures should be put into effect for the patient who, in addition to a surgical wound, has a known communicable disease.

Purpose

The purpose of cleaning the operating room is to prevent an infectious organism from being transmitted from one part of the body to another on the same patient and from one patient to another.

Procedure
General

1. Excess furniture and equipment need not be removed from the room. Place as far from contamination as possible.
2. The only contaminated articles in the room are the furniture and equipment in direct contact with the operative field.
3. Use as much disposable linen as possible.
4. All personnel wear shoe covers and change before leaving the room.
5. The scrub nurse should have sufficient water in her basin to submerge the open instruments.

Preoperative Preparations

1. All personnel entering even an empty operating room must be properly dressed and wearing a cap and mask.
2. Using an alcohol-soaked cloth, wipe down all flat

surfaces of tables, equipment, and overhead lights at least 1 hour before scheduled surgery.
3. At the same time, the tops and rims of autoclaves and counter tops in substerile rooms should be damp dusted with an alcohol-soaked cloth.
4. Place a plastic bag inside the trash container for disposables.

Operative Period

1. Areas contaminated by organic debris (blood and sputum) during the operation should be sprayed with a germicide and wiped up immediately.
2. Sponges should be discarded into plastic-lined kick buckets.
3. Use a glove or sponge stick to count sponges. Place counted sponges directly into a plastic bag and tie it. Do not place sponges on any item on the floor.
4. Once the patient is in the room and surgery has started, supplies and equipment should not be removed from the room.
5. Traffic in and out of room must be kept at a minimum to curtail dust turbulence.
6. The circulating nurse should anticipate needs to avoid having to leave and return frequently.
7. The circulating nurse keeps the floor and room neat and clear of debris.

Interim Cleaning

As soon as surgery is completed and the patient is taken from the room, cleanup is initiated to ready the room for the next patient.

1. Be sure the surgeon removes his gown first and then his gloves.
2. All personnel should change bloody shoe covers as they leave the operating room.
3. The scrub nurse places all linen and disposable drapes in appropriate hampers, then clears the back table of all disposable items and places them in a garbage bag. The needle book is disposed of in its designated box. All sponges in or out of plastic bags are placed in appropriate containers by the scrub nurse.
4. The scrub nurse assembles unused instruments and places them in a tray.

Patient_____ _____ Age_____ Chart No._____

Procedure_____ _____ Date of procedure_____

Site of infection_____ _____ Date of diagnosis_____

Specimen source_____ _____

Medications patient taking_____ _____
before infection
                                                 _____

Medications prescribed today_____ _____

                                                           Nurse: _____

Culture report: Organisms   Sensitive to   Resistant to

Date_____

                                                           Nurse: _____

Physician review: Significant previous   History of prior
                            medical history   infections

Clinical follow-up:
  (Date)

Recommendations:

                                                    Physician:_____

Example of an infection control report.

5. The scrub nurse removes her gown but leaves her gloves on.
6. The scrub nurse takes the tray of instruments and basin of dirty instruments to the sink area for cleaning. After cleaning, the instruments are flashed for the next case or the tray is covered with a plastic bag and carried to the instrument processing area.
7. The circulating or scrub nurse removes the back table cover by folding it toward the center to prevent spreading of airborne contaminants.

Interim Housekeeping

1. Horizontal surfaces of tables and equipment involved in the surgical procedure should be cleaned with detergent germicide.
2. Wet-mop floors using a fresh mop and bucket of detergent germicide.
3. Saline solution from the back table may be disposed of in the sink.
4. The room is prepared for the next case.

It is important to provide a mechanism for retrospective analysis to assure that, in fact, procedures can be performed safely and effectively. As mentioned previously, there is a difference of opinion as to the type of ventilatory systems needed within an office surgical environment. Because of this, it is imperative that the physician closely monitor infection rates. If the infection rate rises to an unacceptable level, the physician must review his sterilization, cleaning, and sanitizing protocols for the office surgical area and reevaluate both the surgical environment and his surgical technique. If, on the other hand, the infection rate remains acceptable or at a level below the community norms, this is further justification that surgery can be performed safely in this office surgical unit.

BIBLIOGRAPHY

Accreditation Association for Ambulatory Health Care, Inc.: Accreditation Handbook, Skokie, Ill.

Aglietti, P., et al.: Effect of a surgical horizontal unit of directional filtered air flow unit on wound bacterial contamination and wound healing, Clinical Orthopedics 101:99–104, 1974.

Alexakis, P.G., et al.: Airborne bacterial contamination of operative wounds, Western Journal of Medicine 124:361–369, 1976.

American Academy of Facial Plastic and Reconstructive Surgery: Establishing a facial plastic surgery practice—development of an office surgery center (monograph), 1985.

American College of Surgeons, Clinical Congress Reports: From design to evaluation of OR suite, A.O.R.N. Journal 23:101, 1976.

American College of Surgeons, Committee on Operating Room Environment: Definition of surgical microbiologic clean air, Bulletin, American College of Surgeons 61:19, 1976.

American College of Surgeons, Committee on Operating Room Environment, Air Quality Sub-Committee: Recommendations for reports of various air environments, Bulletin, American College of Surgeons, 62:12, 1977.

Amstutz, H.C.: Clean air symposium: prevention of operative infections, Cleveland Clinic Quarterly 40:125–131, 1973.

Analyzing air pollution in the OR, Medical World News, Apr. 13, 1973.

AORN recommended practices for traffic patterns in the surgical suite, A.O.R.N. Journal 35:750, 1982.

Ayre, P.: Music in hospitals, Anesthesiology 35:233–234, 1980.

Beck, W.C.: Color problems in hospitals, Guthrie Bulletin 46:39–48, 1976.

Beck, W.C.: Choosing surgical illumination, American Journal of Surgery 140:327–331, 1980.

Birren, F.: Human response to color and light, Hospitals 53:93–96, 1979.

Brock, L.: The importance of environmental conditions especially temperature in the operating room and intensive care ward, British Journal of Surgery 62:253–258, 1975.

Brodsky, J.B.: Exposure to anesthetic gases: a controversy, A.O.R.N. Journal 38:132, 1983.

Buchberg, H., et al.: Evaluation and optimum use of directed horizontal filtered air flow for surgeries, Clinical Orthopedics 111:151–155, 1975.

Campbell, D., et al.: Comparison of personal pollution monitoring techniques for use in the operating room, British Journal of Anaesthesia 52:885–892, 1980.

Cleaner air symposium: Clean air in operating room, Cleveland Clinic Quarterly 40:99–114, 1973.

Clean air for the OR, Modern Health Care 2:82–83, 1974.

Clarke, B.H.: Guidelines for design of surgical suite, Hospital TOP 57:45–46, 1979.

Cricke, C.: Patients wait for surgery in "twilight zone," A.O.R.N. Journal 22:980, 1975.

Current status of special air handling systems in operating rooms, Journal of the Association of Advanced Medical Instrument 7:7–15, 1973.

Design points way to infection control, Modern Health Care 1:44–47, 1974.

Drake, T.C., et al.: Environmental air and airborne infections, Annals of Surgery 185:219–223, 1977.

Fitzgerald, R.H., Jr.: Microbiologic environment of the conventional operating room, Archives of Surgery 114:772–775, 1979.

Gunderman, K.O.: Spread of microorganisms by air conditioning systems—especially in hospitals, Annals of the New York Academy of Science 353:209–217, 1980.

Harvey, C.K., et al.: Recommendations for proper temperature in OR suite, A.O.R.N. Journal 83:392, 1983.

Herndon, C.H.: Clean air operating room at university hospitals of Cleveland, Cleveland Clinical Quarterly 40:183–190, 1973.

Howorth, F.H.: Air flow patterns in the operating theater, Eng. Med. 9:87–92, 1980.

Keep, P.J.: Stimulus deprivation in windowless rooms, Anesthesiology 32:598–602, 1977.

Keesee, M.A.: Central sterile work core adds space, reduces contamination, Hospital 50:119, 1976.

Kerr, D.R., et al.: Electrical design and safety in the operating room and intensive care unit, International Anesthesiology Clinics 19:27–48, 1981.

Kethley, T.W., and Crown, W.B.: What is the quality of the air in your operating room? Guthrie Bulletin 46:25, 1976.

Klebanoff, G.: Operating room design, American College of Surgeons Bulletin 64:6–10, 1979.

Kubota, Y.: Windows in operating theaters, Anesthesiology 35:922, 1980.

Laurence, M.: Ultraclean air, Journal of Bone and Joint Surgery 65:375–377, 1983.

Lewis, R.G., et al.: Operating rooms: subtle plate assessment of airborne infections, Dimensions of Health Service 51:13, 1974.

Lighting the surgical suite, Contemporary Surgery 12:9, 1978.

LoCicero, J. III, and Nichols, R.E.: Environmental health hazards in the operating room, Bulletin of the American College of Surgeons May 1982.

Lomando, K., et al.: A worktable plan for OR quality assurance, A.O.R.N. Journal 35:1291–1295, 1982.

MacClelland, D.C.: Music in operating rooms, A.O.R.N. Journal 29:252–260, 1979.

Mallison, G.F.: Housekeeping in operating suites, A.O.R.N. Journal 21:2, 1975.

Mayo, C.G.: Theater ventilation: a comparison of design and observed values, British Journal of Anesthesia 50:157–163, 1978.

Marsh, R.C., et al.: Comparing surgical clean room filters, Contemporary Surgery 7:33–34, 1975.

Modern architectural design in the operating room, Hospital TOP 52:41–42, 1974.

Olson, R.: Continuous power to the OR and other critical care areas, Dimensions of Health Serv. 52:29–30, 1975.

Pastorek, N.J.: Psychological and aesthetic considerations in outpatient facial plastic surgery, Otolaryngology Head and Neck Surgery 92 (6):611, 1984.

Perin, J.G., et al.: The office based elective surgery center, Annals of Plastic Surgery 4:94–99, 1980.

Ritter, M.A.: Laminer flow, is it still justified? Contemporary Orthopedics 5:23–26, 1980.

Schonholtz, G.J., et al.: Maintenance of aseptic barriers in the conventional operating room, Journal of Bone and Joint Surgery 58-A:439–445, 1976.

Schultz, J., et al.: Cleaning of ceiling-mounted surgical lighting tracks, A.O.R.N. Journal 29:898, 1979.

Sebben, J.E.: Avoiding infection in office surgery, Journal of Dermatologic Surgery and Oncology 8:455–458, 1982.

Sell, J.: Mechanical needs in the operating and delivery suites, Hospitals 48:79, 1974.

Shaparo, S.L., et al.: Office and hospital post-surgical infection: a survey, Journal of Foot Surgery 19:32–33, 1980.

Society for Office Based Surgery: Annual meeting, Los Angeles, Calif., Jan, 1983.

Suggested bacterial standards for air and ultraclean operating rooms, Journal of Hospital Infection 4:133–139, 1983.

Symposium on office surgery, Clinics in Plastic Surgery, 10(2):, 1983.

Symposium on the operating room environment, Archives of Surgery 114:771, 1979.

The importance of airborne bacterial contamination of wounds, Journal of Hospital Infection 3:123–135, 1980.

Thomas, D.V.: Noise in the modern operating room, Anesthesiology 54:523, 1981.

Toronello, J.D.: When I build my OR "dream and reality," A.O.R.N. Journal 30:44–48, 1979.

Unbacked drywall construction: a problem in the operating room, Bulletin of American College of Surgeons, 67:6–7, 1980.

Wall material in operating rooms, A.O.R.N. Journal 29:1222, 1979.

Wiley, A.M., et al.: The prevention of surgical sepsis: clean surgeons and clean air, Clinics of Orthopedics 96:168–175, 1973.

Appendix 15: Recommended Practices for Surgical Tissue Banking

The following recommended practices were developed by the AORN Recommended Practices Coordinating Committee and have been approved by the AORN Board of Directors. They were published as proposed recommended practices in the August 1990 *AORN Journal* for comment by members and others.

These recommended practices are intended as achievable recommendations representing what is believed to be an optimal level of practice. Policies and procedures will reflect variations in practice settings and/or clinical situations that determine the degree to which the recommended practices can be fulfilled.

AORN recognizes the numerous different settings in which perioperative nurses practice. The recommended practices are intended as guidelines adaptable to various practice settings. These practice settings include traditional operating rooms, ambulatory surgery units, physicians' offices, cardiac catheterization laboratories, endoscopy rooms, radiology departments, and all other areas where surgery may be performed.

Purpose
These recommended practices reflect current medical and technical methodology for processing, preserving, and storing selected human tissue. Human tissue selected for banking can include, but is not limited to, skin, bone, cartilage ossicles. These recommended practices provide guidance for developing institutional procedures that are specific and compatible with the practice setting's facility, patient needs, and personnel capabilities or expertise.

A tissue bank should be established only where a need exists. Before the decision is made to establish a tissue bank, consideration should be given to personnel, equipment, and practical operational requirements for providing safe, reliable, and biologically useful tissue grafts.

Recommended Practice I
Tissue for transplantation should be procured from suitable donors.

Interpretive Statement 1:
The donor or donor's responsible party should sign an informed consent. Nonliving donors whose deaths have resulted from trauma or unknown circumstances should be released according to local, state, or federal regulations where applicable.

Rationale:
All states within the United States have legislation protecting the rights of potential donors.[1]

Interpretive Statement 2:
A history and assessment of the donor should be obtained to identify contraindications before implantation of tissue. The donor should be free of
- transmissible infection,
- malignancy,
- autoimmune disease (eg, systemic lupus erythematosus),
- neurologic disease of unknown etiology, and
- human derived growth hormone,
- other disease of known or unknown etiology.

Rationale:
The potential donor is screened to avoid transmission of infection or disease.[2]

Recommended Practice II
Tissue should be collected under aseptic conditions.

Interpretive Statement 1:
A sterile field should be established and maintained in accordance with AORN's "Recommended practices for basic aseptic technique."

Rationale:
Aseptic technique is used to prevent contamination of the tissue.[3]

Interpretive Statement 2:
The donor site and/or operative site should be prepared in accordance with AORN's "Recommended practices for preoperative skin preparation of patients."

Rationale:
Adequate skin preparation may reduce microbial count of the tissue.[4]

Interpretive Statement 3:
Cultures including, but not limited to, aerobic and

Reprinted with permission from *AORN Standards and Recommended Practices for Perioperative Nursing*, 1991. Copyright © AORN Inc, 10170 East Mississippi Avenue, Denver, CO 80231.

anaerobic bacteria, and serologic testing (eg, for HIV, hepatitis B virus, hepatitis C virus, cytomegalovirus), should be done when procuring allografts and may be done for autografts.

Rationale:
The screening evaluation is designed to prevent transfer of infection to the recipient.[5]

Discussion:
Standards set by the American Association of Tissue Banks (AATB) should be referenced for further information on developing quality control measures. A major concern in tissue banking is HIV. As of March 1990, the AATB recommends an initial HIV test of living bone donors immediately after donation and recommends quarantining of the bone for 90 days.[6] Only after a negative HIV test result can the bone be released for clinical use.[7] Because there are many unknown factors concerning the length of time for HIV seroconversion, practice settings must have policies and procedures that are current with the ever changing standards of practice.

Recommended Practice III
Tissue should be stored in a controlled, safe environment.

Interpretive Statement 1:
Tissue that will not be sterilized should be transferred to the sterile storage container under aseptic technique.

Rationale:
Aseptic technique is used to prevent contamination of tissue.[8]

Interpretive Statement 2:
The storage container should be labeled indicating contents including solution composition.

Rationale:
Certain solutions may require copious rinsing of the tissue to prevent recipient reaction.[9]

Interpretive Statement 3:
Refrigeration and freezer units used for storing tissue should be monitored for temperature deviation. Records should be maintained.

Rationale:
Temperature fluctuations outside recommended temperature range, may render tissue unusable. Documentation of temperature readings provides evidence of monitoring.[10]

Recommended Practice IV
Each practice setting should develop donor, graft, and recipient records to ensure that pertinent data are retrievable.

Interpretive Statement 1:
Records should be maintained according to the practice setting's policy and procedures and should contain the following information:
- donor name,
- identification number,
- pertinent medical information,
- donor history,
- pathology reports,
- culture and serology reports,
- type and anatomical site of tissue,
- date and time of collection,
- method of collection,
- preservation solution and composition,
- recipient of graft,
- identification number,
- date and time of transplantation,
- anatomical site of transplantation, and
- informed consents.

Rationale:
Documentation aids in clinical evaluation and in protecting a potential recipient if an adverse reaction is identified.[11]

Interpretive Statement 2:
A form attached to the graft container should include the following donor information:
- name (may be coded),
- identification number,
- pertinent medical information,
- pathology reports,
- type and anatomical site of tissue being preserved,
- date and time of collection,
- method of collection,
- preservation used, if applicable, and
- final culture and serology report.

Rationale:
Documentation facilitates communication from one member of the health care team to another.[12]

Recommended Practice V
Tissue for transplantation should be transplanted immediately or processed and stored in a controlled, safe environment.

Interpretive Statement 1:
Skin should be maintained for future grafting in low temperature storage.

Rationale:
Viability declines in direct proportion to storage time. Controlled cooling reduces metabolic activity of the cells.[13]

Discussion:
One acceptable method of short-term storage is to place skin in an isotonic solution (eg, normal saline or balanced salt solution) or tissue medium and refrigerate at 1°C (33.8°F) to 10°C (50°F) for up to 14 days.[14]

For long-term storage, skin should be maintained in a cryoprotectant under controlled cooling and freezing conditions. Freeze by cooling skin to at least −70°C (−94°F) at a rate of decline between 1°C (1.8°F) to 5°C (9°F) per minute. The skin can then be stored in a liquid nitrogen freezer.[15]

Data is inconclusive on the addition of antimicrobial solutions.

Increased tissue viability and longer effective storage time are achieved by exposing skin to tissue nutrient media.[16]

Freezing too rapidly causes osmotic dehydration and intracellular ice. Cooling too slowly causes extensive osmotic dehydration, concentration of electrolyte solutions, and mechanical distortion of the cell.[17]

Interpretive Statement 2:
Immediately before use, skin should be warmed rapidly at a rate of 50°C (90°F) to 70°C (126°F) per minute, attained by immersion in 42°C (107.6°F) sterile water baths (warming time 3.2-4.5 minutes).

Rationale:
A warming temperature of 42°C (107.6°F) provides the maximal warming rate compatible with cellular viability.[18]

Interpretive Statement 3:
Bone and cartilage should remain frozen then rapidly thawed immediately before grafting.

Rationale:
Bone retains favorable biomechanical properties when stored for long periods of time. If bone thaws, enzymes such as collagenases and proteases, may become active and degrade the tissue.[19]

Discussion:
One acceptable method for storage is to culture the bone, cut it to desired shape and size, and place it into a sterile, moisture-proof container. A cryoprotectant may be used. For short-term storage (less than six months), bone should be maintained at −15°C (5°F).[20] Long-term storage (indefinite) has been reported at −20°C (−4°F), −70°C (−94°F), and −170°C (−274°F) with clinical success.[21]

Interpretive Statement 5:
Ethylene oxide gas or radiation should be used when sterilizing bone.

Discussion:
For processing bone by ethylene oxide gas or radiation, refer to the *Technical Manual for Surgical Bone Banking*[22]. Shape, size, density of bone, and prior processing will determine the ethylene oxide exposure and necessary aeration time. The literature does not comment on the efficacy of steam sterilization, and no sterilization parameters are defined.[23]

Recommended Practice VI
Policies and procedures on storing, preserving, and maintaining tissue should be established.

Discussion:
Policies should establish authority, responsibility, and accountability for tissue handling and appropriate donor testing within the practice setting. Procedures for tissue handling should include but are not limited to
- obtaining informed consent from the donor,
- providing information and obtaining informed

consent from recipient,
- monitoring temperature during storage,
- handling of frozen tissue if there is a freezer malfunction/power outage,
- preserving tissue,
- warming/reconstituting preserved tissue,
- rinsing solutions from tissue,
- documenting implanted tissue in an easily retrievable format, and
- notifying the recipient if and adverse reaction is identified.

These recommended practices should be used as guidelines for developing policies and procedures for tissue banking within the practice setting. Policies and procedures establish authority, responsibility, and accountability and serve as operational guidelines. An introduction and review of tissue banking policies and procedures should be included in the orientation and ongoing education of personnel to assist in the development of knowledge, skills, and attitudes that affect patient care.

Glossary

Allografts: Grafts taken from a living or nonliving donor for transplantation to an unrelated recipient.

Autographs: A graft of tissue derived from another site in or on the body of the organism receiving it.

Nonviable: Tissue that is nonliving.

Viable: Tissue capable of living.

Notes:

1. A M Sadler, Jr, B L Sadler, E B Stason, "The uniform anatomical gift act: A model for reform," *Journal of the American Medical Association* 11 (Dec 9, 1968) 2505-2506.

2. G E Friedlaender, "Bone banking: In support of reconstructive surgery of the hip," *Clinical Orthopaedics and Related Research* 225 (December 1987) 17-21.

3. W W Tomford et al, "1983 bone bank procedures," *Clinical Orthopaedics and Related Research* 174 (April 1983) 15-21.

4. "Recommended practices for the preoperative skin preparation of patients" in *Standards and Recommended Practices for Perioperative Nursing* (Denver: Association of Operating Room Nurses, Inc, 1990) III:10-1.

5. Friedlaender, "Bone banking: In support of reconstructive surgery of the hip," 18.

6. *Standards for Tissue Banking* (Arlington, Va: American Association of Tissue Banks, 1987); "Canada recommends 6-month quarantine to screen living donors for HIV," *American Association of Tissue Banks Newsletter,* 13 no 2 (1990) 1-8.

7. K R Buckham, "Surgical bone banking: Recommendations for setting up a program," *AORN Journal* 50 (October 1989) 765-783.

8. Friedlaender, "Bone banking: In support of reconstructive surgery of the hip," 18.

9. S Friedler, L C Guidice, E J Lamb, "Cryopreservation of embryos and ova," *Fertility and Sterility* 49 (May 1988) 743-764; S R May, F A DeClement, "Skin banking methodology: An evaluation of package format, cooling and warming rates, and storage efficiency," *Cryobiology* 17 (February 1980) 33-45.

10. Standards for Tissue Banking, 9.

11. *Ibid,* 8.

12. *Ibid,* 16.

13. S J Aggerwal, C R Baxter, K R Diller, "Cryopreservation of skin: An assessment of current clinical applicability," *Journal of Burn Care Rehabilitation* 6 (November/December 1985) 469-475.

14. S R May, J F Wainwright, "Integrated study of the structural and metabolic degeneration of skin during 4°C storage in nutrient medium," *Cryobiology* 22 (February 1985) 18-34.

15. Aggarwal, Baxter, Diller, Cryopreservation of skin: An assessment of current clinical applicability," 472.

16. M D Rosenquist, A E Cram, G P Kealey, "Short-term skin preservation at 4°C: Skin storage configuration and tissue-to-volume medium ratio," *Journal of Burn Care Rehabilitation* 9 (January/February 1988) 52-54.

17. Aggarwal, Baxter, Diller, "Cryopreservation of skin: An assessment of current clinical applicability," 470.

18. *Ibid,* 475.

19. W W Tomford et al, "Methods of banking bone and cartilage for allograft transplantation," *Orthopedic Clinics of North America* 18 (April 1987) 241-247.

20. *Technical Manual for Surgical Bone Banking,* (McLean, VA: American Association of Tissue Banks, 1987) 10.

21. Tomford, et al, "1983 bone bank procedures," 17.

22. *Technical Manual for Surgical Bone Banking,* 10.

23. Tomford, et al, "1983 bone bank procedures," 17.

Suggested Reading

Hart, M M; Campbell, E D; Kartub, M G. "Bone banking: A cost effective method for establishing a community hospital bone bank" *Clinical Orthopaedics and Related Research* 206 (May 1986) 295-300.

Originally published September, 1984, *AORN Journal.*
Revised April, 1991.

Index

Accreditation, 3–4
  anesthesia and surgical services, 12–13
  standards, 6–13
    facilities and environment, 10–12
    medical records, 9–10
    quality assurance, 8–9
    quality of care, 7
Accreditation Association for Ambulatory Health Care, 58, 60, 62, 76, 77
Administrative forms. *See* Forms
Adverse reactions, to anesthesia, 55–56
Advertising. *See* Marketing
Aesthetic Plastic Surgery: A Medical Corporation, 139–140
Air conditioning, of office, 63, 117–118
Alarms, of office, 119
Ambulatory surgery. *See* Surgery, ambulatory
American Society of Anesthesiologists' risk categories, 55
American Society of Outpatient Surgeons, 58
Anesthesia
  accreditation standards, 12–13
  avoiding problems, 55–56
  forms, 149–159
  miscellaneous, 56–57
  outpatient surgery and, 51–57
  preoperative medications, 52–55
    bupivacaine, 55
    diazepam, 52–53
    dimenhydrinate, 53
    dyclonine hydrochloride, 55
    hydromorphone hydrochloride, 53
    hydroxyzine, 53
    innovar, 54
    ketamine hydrochloride, 54
    lidocaine hydrochloride, 55
    local, 54–55
    lorazepam, 53
    mepivacaine hydrochloride, 55
    physostigmine salicylate, 53
    procaine hydrochloride, 55
    scopolamine, 53
    tetracaine hydrochloride, 55
    twilight, 52
  surgical care protocol, 147–148
Associated Facial Plastic and Cosmetic Surgery, 141–143

Banks, 99, 100
Beeson Facial Surgery Post-Op Recovery Record, 157
Beeson Facial Surgery Pre-Operative Record, 155–156
Blepharoplasty, 220, 228–229
Building construction, of office, 117–119
Bupivacaine, 55
Business office, design of, 121

Calcium antagonists, 57
Cardiac problems, 52, 57
Certification, 3–4
Cocaine, 52, 54–55
Computerization
  analyzing needs, 109
  future of, 114
  managing data processing, 112–114
  purchasing mechanisms, 112
  safeguarding data, 112–114
  selecting hardware, 111–112
  selecting software, 110–111
Confidentiality
  of office finances and affairs, 182
  patient, 182
Consulting room, design of, 123
Consultations
  forms for, 236–237
  and medical questionnaire, 207–208
Crash cart, 64
  check sheet, 233
Credit, 108

Dantroline sodium, 56
Data
  employee records, 180–181
  management of, 112–114
  safeguarding, 112–114
Dermabrasion, 219
Diazepam, 52–53
Dimenhydrinate, 53
Direct mail, marketing by, 73–74
Disinfection, practices for, 255–265
Droperidol, 51
Dyclonine hydrochloride, 55

Electrocardiogram, 52
Employees
  code of ethics, 16–17
  disciplinary action, 18–19
  evaluation of, 18
  forms
    application, 198–201
    confidentiality, 182
    corrective action notification, 202
    data records, 180–181
    job performance appraisal
      office/clerical personnel, 183–185
      personnel action form, 189
      technical/professional personnel, 186–188
    physical exam and medical profile, 178–179
  job description, 15, *16*
  leaves and holidays, 17–18
  lounge, 124

274 *(Numbers for Tables and Figures are in italic)*

orientation of, 20–21
policies and procedures, 16–19, 190–197
professional development, 18
records of, 19
rights, 17
salary and fringe benefits, 17
termination of, *19*
training
    daily duties, 160
    nurse's check lists, 161–162
    weekly duties, 160
Environment
    accreditation, 10–12
    for operating room, 245–250
Epinephrine, 56
Equipment
    bathrooms, 67
    cleaning, 67
    crash cart, 64–65
    emergency power, 60–61
        sample calculations for, 61
    lease or buy, *121*
    maintenance and repair, 66
    medical gases and suction, 65
    monitors, 64
    music, 64
    operating room tables, 65
    recovery, 66–67
    repair of, form for, 231
    sterilization, 65–66
    storage, 67
Examination room, 123

Facial Plastic and Cosmetic Surgical Center, 135–136
    forms of, 149–154, 226–229
Facial surgery, 221, 227
Facilities
    accreditation standards, 10–12
    color, 59
    electrical circuitry, 60
    layout, 61–61
    lighting, 59–60
        emergency, 60
    size, 58–59
    suite design, 58
    ventilation, 62–64
    See also Equipment
Fee agreement, 204
Fentanyl citrate, 51
Financing a practice, 99–108
    credit criteria, 108
    lending institution, choice of
        commercial banks, 99
        life insurance policies, 100
        other institutions, 100
        savings and loans, 100
        small business administration, 100
        small loan companies, 100
    loan package
        breakdown of loan proceeds, 104
        business financial status, 104
        cash flow projections, 104, *106*
        perform a balance sheet, 104
        personal financial status, 101–104
            cost-of-living budget, *105*
        personal statement, *102–103*

        practice plan, 104
            business plan, *107*
        projected earnings, 104
            income statement, *106*
        resume, 101
    loan restrictions, 108
    loan review, 104, 108
    money needed, 99
    types of loans
        intermediate term, 101
        long term, 101
        short term, 100–101
Fire alarms, for office, 118
Forms
    administrative, 230–237
        consults for the week, 236–237
        crash cart check sheet, 233
        equipment repair, 231
        in-service record, 235
        inventory sheet, 234
        patient telephone log, 230
        purchase authorization, 232
    anesthesia, 149–159
    of Beeson facial surgery, 155–159, 206–211, 215–225, 230–237
    building comparisons, *122, 129*
    employee, 178–189, 198–202
    of Facial Plastic and Cosmetic Surgery Center, 149–154, 226–229
    fee agreement, 204
    history and physical exam, 209–211
    in-service record, 235
    inventory, 234
    medical record worksheet, 168
    nurse's check lists, 161–162
    patient care, 203–205
    patient information, 213–214
    patient instructions, 215–229
    patient questionnaire, 207–208
    patient registration, 78–81
    quality assurance, 165–167
    for repair of equipment, 231
    risk management, 170–171
    treatment record, 206
    work sheets, *87–88*, 168

Gilmore, Jim, 141–143

Hair transplants, 217
Halothane, 51
Health Care Committee of the Illuminating Engineering Society, 59–60
Heating, of office, 117–118
Hiring, of staff
    attracting quality staff, 23–24
    performance factors, 25
    personal disposition factors, 26–27
    six steps for success, 27–42
    useful questions, 43–46
Holidays, 17–18
Hospitals
    access to, 116
    instruction sheets, 222–223
Hydromorphone hydrochloride, 53
Hydroxyzine, 53

Illness prevention, 90
Infection control report, 170

Infectious medical waste, facilities and environment, 172–176
Injury prevention, 90
Innovar, 54
In-service record, form for, 235
Instruction sheets, 215–225
Insurance, 100, 131
Inventory sheet, 234
Isoflurane, 51

Joint Commission of Accreditation of Hospitals, 77

Ketamine hydrochloride, 54

Laboratory, 124
  tests, 51
Laser, safe use of, 240–244
Lease
  agreement, 124–133
    commencement date, 125
    construction of improvements, 125, 127
    defaults and remedies, 132
    insurance, 131
    lessee
      indemnification of lessor, 131–132
      obligations of, 129–130
    lessor
      obligations of, 129
      rights reserved to, 130
    miscellaneous, 132–133
    operating expenses, 127–129
    premises, 124–125
      samples, *125, 126–127*
    rent, 127
      calculation of, *128*
    rights in event of eminent domain or casualty, 131
    security deposit, 131
    signature page, 122
    space measurement, *128*
    term, 125
  building cost comparison, *129*
  of equipment, *121*
  negotiating, 124
Legal considerations, 91–98
  business contracts, 92–93
    adhesion, 93
    employment, 93
    goods and services, 93
  employee policies, 93–95
  malpractice
    avoidance of, *94–95*
    court behavior, *97*
    informed consent, 97
    locality rule, 96–97
    pretrial discovery, 98
    screening panels, 98
    standard of care, 96
    trial, 98
    types of suits, 96
  patient records, 91–92
    complete, 91–92
    confidential, 91
    consent form, *92*
  peer review, 95–96
  preemployment guide, 47–50
Leave of absence, 17–18
Lidocaine hydrochloride, 52, 55

Lighting, 59–60
  emergency, 60
Loans, 99–108
Lorazepam, 53

Magazines, advertising in, 72
Malignant hyperthermia, 56
Malpractice, 96–98
Mangat, Devinder S., M.D., 144–145
Marketing
  direct mail, 73–74
  magazines, 72
  medical ethics and, 68–71
  newspaper, 72–73
  outdoor advertising, 73
  radio, 72
  television, 71–72
  yellow pages, 71
Medical ethics
  code of, 16–17
  marketing and, 68–71
Medical records, accreditation standards and, 9–10
Medications
  cocaine, 52, 54, 55
  crash cart, 64–65
  preoperative
    bupivacaine, 55
    diazepam, 52–53
    dimenhydrinate, 53
    dyclonine hydrochloride, 55
    hydromorphone hydrochloride, 53
    hydroxyzine, 53
    innovar, 54
    ketamine hydrochloride, 54
    lidocaine hydrochloride, 55
    lorazepam, 53
    mepivacaine hydrochloride, 55
    physostigmine salicylate, 52, 53, 55
    procaine hydrochloride, 55
    scopolamine, 53
    tetracaine hydrochloride, 55
    twilight anesthetic, 52
Mepivacaine hydrochloride, 55
Monitors, 64
Music, in office, 64

National Fire Protection Association, 58, 59, 60
Newspapers, advertising in, 72–73
Nitrous oxide, 51

Office of Architecture and Engineering Health Care Facilities Service, 58
Office facility, 134–145
  of Gilmore, Jim, M.D., 141–143
  of Mangat, Devinder S., M.D., 144–145
  of Patseavouras, Louie L., M.D., F.A.C.S., 137–138
  of Strahan, Ronald W., M.D., 139–140
  of Tobin, Howard, M.D., 135–136
Office space
  building comparisons, 122
  building construction factors, 117–119
    air conditioning, 117–118
    alarms, 119
    building shell, 117
    ceiling heights, 118
    central control, 119
    core area, 117

elevators, 118, 119
emergency power, 118
emergency stairs, 119
exterior skin, 117
fire alarms, 118
fire control panel, 119
floor load, 118
heating, 117–118
interior improvements, 117
life safety, 118–119
plumbing, 118
security systems, 118–119
smoke detectors, 119
sprinkler systems, 118–119
standards, *119*
tenant improvements, 117
ventilation of, 117–118
design factors, 119–124
business office, 121
consultation room, 123
employee lounge, 124
examination rooms, 123
comfort factors, 123
efficiency factors, 123
size and number, 123
laboratory, 124
layout efficiency, 119–120
private office, 124
reception, 120–121
storage, 123
toilets, 123
utility space, 124
waiting room
arrangement, 120–121
decor, 121
size, 120
development of, 115, *116*
negotiating, 124
equipment, *121*
ergonomics, *120*
maintenance, 66
site selection factors, 115–117
ancillary facilities, access to, 116
"curb appeal," 117
expansion potential, 117
growth area, 115
hospital, access to, 116
parking availability, 117
physician mix, 116
prestigious area, 115
restaurants, availability of, 116
shopping, availability of, 116
transportation to office, ease of, 116
travel time to, 116
visibility, 116
tenants, tips for, *120*
Office surgical center
chain of command, 15
hiring process
attracting quality staff, 23–24
performance factors, 25
personal disposition factors, 26–27
six steps for success, 27–42
useful questions, 43–46
job description, 15, 16
legal pre-employment guide, 47–50
organizational decisions, 15
orientation, 20–21
personnel, 14–15
policies and procedures manual, 16–19
code of ethics, 16–17
disciplinary action, 18–19
employee rights, 17
evaluations, 18
leaves and holidays, 17–18
nepotism, 19
office goals and philosophy, 16
personnel records, 19
professional development, 18
salary and fringe benefits, 17
recruiting and interviewing, 19–20
Office surgery, *See* Surgery, ambulatory
Operating room
environmental sanitation, 245–250
size of, 58–59
tables, 65
Outdoor advertising, 73
Outpatient surgery, 51–57, 215
Outpatient Surgical Center, 137–138

Packaging material, selection and use of, 251–254
Patient care
forms, 203, 205, 211–212
Beeson facial surgery treatment record, 206
Beeson patient questionnaire, 207–208
Beeson pre-operative history and physical exam, 209–211
consultation and medical questionnaire, 213–214
surgical fee agreement, 204
perioperative, quality, 238–239
Patient instruction sheets
for blepharoplasty, 220
for dermabrasion, post-operative, 219
for facial surgery, 221
for hair transplant post-operative care, 217
for hospital patients, preoperative, 222–223
for outpatient surgery, 215
for rhinoplasty, 216
after surgery, 224–225
for wound care, postoperative, 218
for quality assurance, 84–86
Tobin instruction sheets
for blepharoplasty, post-operative, 228–229
for facial cosmetic surgery, pre-operative, 227
for surgery, 226
Patient records, 91–93
work sheet, 168
Patient risk classification, 55
Patient telephone log, 230
Patseavouras, Louie L., M.D., F.A.C.S., 137–138
Peer review, 95–96
Physical examination, 52
Physician's orders, 86–89
Physostigmine salicylate, 52, 53, 55
Policies and procedures, for employees, 190–197
for quality assurance, 77–78
Procaine hydrochloride, 55
Public relations, *See* Marketing
Purchase authorization, 232

Quality assurance
accreditation standards and, 8–9
forms
AAAHC medical record work sheet, 168
evaluation form, 165
tracking sheet, 166–167

Quality assurance (*continued*)
  plan, 163–164
  studies, 76–89
    consultation notes, 81, *82*
    credentialing, 76
    fee quotation, 84, *85*
    follow-up letter, 81, *83*, 84
    operative permit, 86
    operative report, 89
    patient instructions, 84, 86
    patient registration form, 78, *79–80*, 81
    physician's orders, 86–89
    policy and procedures, 77–78
Quality of care, 3
  accreditation standards and, 7
  perioperative, 238–239

Radio, advertising on, 72
Recovery room, 66–67
Rhinoplasty, 216
Risk management, 89
  classification for, 55
  forms
    incident report, 170
    infection control report, 171
  program, 169

Scopolamine, 53
Security systems, for office, 118–119
Seizures, 56
Smoke detectors, for office, 119
Staff, *See* Employees; Office surgical center
Sterilization, 65–66
    practices for, 255–265
    protocols for office surgical units, 265–268
Storage, space for, 67, 123
Strahan, Ronald W., M.D., 139–140
Succinylcholine, 56
Suite design, 58, 134–145
Surgery
  ambulatory
    accreditation, 3–4
      standards, 6–13
    certification, 3–4
      and quality of care, 5
      reasons for, 4
      types of, 4
    history of, 1–2
    legal considerations, 91–98
    liability, 4–5
    office setting for, 2
    quality of care, 5
    requirements of, 2–3
  care protocol, 147–148
  fee agreement, 204
  instruction sheets, 224–225, 226
  outpatient, 51–57, 215
  preoperative considerations, 51–52
  preoperative medications, 52–55
  work sheet, *87–88*

Television, advertising on, 71–72
Tenants, tips for, *120*
Tetracaine hydrochloride, 55
The Facial Plastic and Cosmetic Surgery Center, 144–145
Tissue banking, practices for, 269–273
Tobin, Howard, M.D., 135–136
  forms of, 149–154
  instruction sheets
    for blepharoplasty, 228–229
    for facial cosmetic surgery, 227
    for surgery, 226
  surgery work sheet, *87–88*
Toilets, 123
Training, of employees, 160–162
Twilight anesthesia, 52

Utility space, 124

Ventilation, of office, 62–64

Waiting room, 120–121
Waste disposal protocol, 177
Wound care, 218

Yellow pages, advertising in, 71